MARIJUANA

EFFECTS ON HUMAN BEHAVIOR

CONTRIBUTORS

Howard Cappell
Charles F. Darley
Fonya Lord DeLong
Rhea L. Dornbush
William G. Drew
Robert B. Forney
Erich Goode
James A. Halikas
Glen F. Kiplinger
Harry Klonoff
Bernard I. Levy
Morton D. Low
Barbara R. Manno
Joseph E. Manno
Loren L. Miller
Patricia Pliner
Jared R. Tinklenberg
Abraham Wikler

MARIJUANA
EFFECTS ON HUMAN BEHAVIOR

Edited by
LOREN L. MILLER

Laboratories of Behavioral Neurophysiology
Department of Psychiatry
University of Kentucky
Albert B. Chandler Medical Center
Lexington, Kentucky

ACADEMIC PRESS

New York San Francisco London 1974

A Subsidiary of Harcourt Brace Jovanovich, Publishers

COPYRIGHT © 1974, BY ACADEMIC PRESS, INC.
ALL RIGHTS RESERVED.
NO PART OF THIS PUBLICATION MAY BE REPRODUCED OR
TRANSMITTED IN ANY FORM OR BY ANY MEANS, ELECTRONIC
OR MECHANICAL, INCLUDING PHOTOCOPY, RECORDING, OR ANY
INFORMATION STORAGE AND RETRIEVAL SYSTEM, WITHOUT
PERMISSION IN WRITING FROM THE PUBLISHER.

ACADEMIC PRESS, INC.
111 Fifth Avenue, New York, New York 10003

United Kingdom Edition published by
ACADEMIC PRESS, INC. (LONDON) LTD.
24/28 Oval Road, London NW1

Library of Congress Cataloging in Publication Data

Miller, Loren L
    Marijuana; effects on human behavior.

    Includes bibliographies.
    1. Marihuana–Psychological aspects. 2. Marihuana
–Physiological effect. I. Title. [DNLM: 1. Behavior–Drug effects. 2. Cannabis–Pharmacodynamics.
3. Psychopharmacology. QV109 M648m]
BF209.M3M55   615'.782   74-10216
ISBN 0–12–497050–8

PRINTED IN THE UNITED STATES OF AMERICA

CONTENTS

List of Contributors xi
Preface xiii

Chapter 1
THE LOGISTICS OF MARIJUANA RESEARCH: METHODOLOGICAL, LEGAL, AND SOCIETAL
Harry Klonoff

    I. Introduction 1
    II. Clinical Research Planning 3
    III. Clinical Study at the University of British Columbia 10
    IV. Driving Research Planning 19
    V. Summary 22
    References 23

Chapter 2
THE MARIJUANA CONTROVERSY
Abraham Wikler

    I. Introduction 25
    II. Biological Issues 26
    III. Aesthetic Issues 39
    IV. Social Issues 40
    References 42

Chapter 3

MOTOR AND MENTAL PERFORMANCE WITH MARIJUANA: RELATIONSHIP TO ADMINISTERED DOSE OF Δ^9-TETRAHYDROCANNABINOL AND ITS INTERACTION WITH ALCOHOL

Joseph E. Manno, Barbara R. Manno,
Glen F. Kiplinger, and Robert B. Forney

I. Introduction	46
II. Preparation and Calibration of Marijuana Cigarettes for Administration of Uniform Dosage	47
III. Establishment of Experimental Procedures	49
IV. Marijuana Dosage Form	55
V. Motor Performance	56
VI. Mental Performance and Ataxia	59
VII. Physiological Reactions to THC and Alcohol	59
VIII. Subjective Reactions	64
IX. Significance and Conclusion	69
References	71

Chapter 4

MARIJUANA AND MEMORY

Charles F. Darley and Jared R. Tinklenberg

I. Introduction	73
II. Purposes of Marijuana–Memory Research	74
III. A Working Memory Model	76
IV. Experimental Tasks and Specific Experiments with Marijuana	78
V. Locus of the Storage Deficit	88
VI. Evidence of State-Dependent Retrieval	92
VII. Alternative Interpretations of Experimental Results	94
VIII. New Directions and Promising Research	96
IX. Outlook for Marijuana–Memory Research	99
References	100

Chapter 5

A MODEL OF ATTENTION DESCRIBING THE COGNITIVE EFFECTS OF MARIJUANA
Fonya Lord DeLong and Bernard I. Levy

I. Introduction	103
II. A Model of Attention	104
III. Summary	117
References	117

Chapter 6

PSYCHOLOGICAL AND NEUROPHYSIOLOGICAL EFFECTS OF MARIJUANA IN MAN: AN INTERACTION MODEL
Harry Klonoff and Morton D. Low

I. Introduction	121
II. Methods	130
III. Results	135
IV. Discussion	145
References	153

Chapter 7

CANNABIS: NEURAL MECHANISMS AND BEHAVIOR
Loren L. Miller and William G. Drew

I. Introduction	158
II. Cognitive Effects of Cannabis in Man	158
III. Hippocampus and Memory	160
IV. Hippocampus and Internal Inhibition	163
V. Cholinergic System, Memory, and Inhibition	164
VI. Comparison of Cannabinoids, Anticholinergics, and Hippocampectomy	165
VII. Evidence That Cannabinoids Exert Actions within the Limbic System	171
VIII. Evidence That Cannabinoids Exert Actions on Cholinergic Mechanisms	173

IX. Data Inconsistent with the Cholinergic Hypothesis	175
X. Effects of THC on Neuroendocrine Systems	177
XI. Comparison of THC, the Extraadrenal Actions of ACTH, and Hippocampectomy	178
XII. Summary	181
References	182

Chapter 8

MARIJUANA AND BEHAVIOR: HUMAN AND INFRAHUMAN COMPARISONS
Loren L. Miller

I. Introduction	189
II. Memory and Acquisition	191
III. Timing Behavior	202
IV. State-Dependent Learning	206
V. Attention and Habituation	212
VI. Summary and Discussion	216
References	217

Chapter 9

THE LONG-TERM EFFECTS OF CANNABIS USE
Rhea L. Dornbush

I. Introduction	221
II. Studies of Chronic Use in Created Populations	222
III. Studies in Animals	226
IV. Studies of Chronic Use in Existing Populations	228
V. Summary	230
References	231

Chapter 10

CANNABIS INTOXICATION: THE ROLE OF PHARMACOLOGICAL AND PSYCHOLOGICAL VARIABLES
Howard Cappell and Patricia Pliner

I. Introduction	233

II.	Recent Evidence	235
III.	The Experimental Program	242
IV.	Conclusions	261
	References	263

Chapter 11

MARIJUANA USE AND PSYCHIATRIC ILLNESS
James A. Halikas

I.	Statement of the Problem	265
II.	Pitfalls in Marijuana Research	267
III.	Psychiatric Syndromes Described in Association with Marijuana Use	277
IV.	Correlations of Marijuana Use with Psychiatric Illness	289
V.	Conclusion	297
	References	299

Chapter 12

MARIJUANA USE AND THE PROGRESSION TO DANGEROUS DRUGS
Erich Goode

I.	Introduction	303
II.	Logical Issues—Descriptive Studies	305
III.	Methodological Issues—Descriptive Studies	313
IV.	Logical Issues—Causal Mechanisms	320
V.	Methodological Issues—Causal Mechanisms	327
	References	336

Chapter 13

MARIJUANA AND HUMAN AGGRESSION
Jared R. Tinklenberg

I.	Introduction	339
II.	Basic Considerations	340
III.	Sources and Limitations	344
IV.	Laboratory Data	345
V.	Field Studies of Marijuana and Human Aggression	347
	References	354

Chapter 14
EFFECTS OF MARIJUANA ON DRIVING IN A RESTRICTED AREA AND ON CITY STREETS: DRIVING PERFORMANCE AND PHYSIOLOGICAL CHANGES
Harry Klonoff

I.	Introduction	359
II.	Methods	362
III.	Results	372
IV.	Discussion	388
V.	Conclusion	394
	References	396

Subject Index   399

LIST OF CONTRIBUTORS

Numbers in parentheses indicate the pages on which the authors' contributions begin.

Howard Cappell (233), Addiction Research Foundation, Toronto, Ontario, Canada

Charles F. Darley (73), Department of Psychiatry, Stanford University School of Medicine, Stanford, California, and Veterans Administration Hospital, Palo Alto, California

Fonya Lord DeLong (103),* Department of Psychology, George Washington University, Washington, D.C.

Rhea L. Dornbush (221), Department of Psychiatry, New York Medical College, New York, New York

William G. Drew (157), Department of Psychiatry, University of Kentucky, Lexington, Kentucky

Robert B. Forney (45), Department of Toxicology, Indiana University Medical Center, Indianapolis, Indiana

Erich Goode (303), Department of Sociology, State University of New York, Stony Brook, New York

James A. Halikas (265), Department of Psychiatry, Washington University School of Medicine, St. Louis, Missouri

Glen F. Kiplinger (45), The Lilly Research Laboratories, Eli Lilly and Company, Indianapolis, Indiana

Harry Klonoff (1,121,359), Division of Psychology, Department of Psy-

---

* Present address: 4840 Glenbrook Rd., N.W., Washington, D.C.

chiatry, University of British Columbia, Vancouver, British Columbia, Canada

Bernard I. Levy (103), Department of Psychology, George Washington University, Washington, D.C.

Morton D. Low (121), Department of Neurology, University of British Columbia, Vancouver, British Columbia, Canada

Barbara R. Manno (45), Veterans Administration Hospital, Shreveport, Louisiana

Joseph E. Manno (45), Department of Pharmacology and Therapeutics, Louisiana State University School of Medicine, Shreveport, Louisiana

Loren L. Miller (157,189), Laboratories of Behavioral Neurophysiology, Department of Psychiatry, University of Kentucky, Albert B. Chandler Medical Center, Lexington, Kentucky

Patricia Pliner (233), Department of Psychology, Erindale College, University of Toronto, Clarkson, Ontario, Canada

Jared R. Tinklenberg (73,339), Department of Psychiatry, Stanford University School of Medicine, Stanford, California, and Veterans Administration Hospital, Palo Alto, California

Abraham Wikler (25), Department of Psychiatry, University of Kentucky Medical Center, Lexington, Kentucky

PREFACE

The use of marijuana in the United States during the past decade has burgeoned. Yet, until recently, a paucity of objective evidence existed pertaining to the behavioral and physiological actions of the drug. Although efforts have been made recently to research the marijuana problem, the use of the drug has increased at such an alarming rate that it is doubtful that such efforts will keep pace with the discovery of new social consequences concerning its continued use. In addition, much research to date has been hampered by political and social issues surrounding the use of marijuana on a widespread basis. Whether or not marijuana ingestion has long range detrimental effects on the mental and physical health of members of our society is certainly a polemic question with no final answers but only more questions. Unfortunately, debating the relative merits of using or not using marijuana has in numerous instances clouded an important issue: that of scientifically determining in a systematic and objective manner the effects of this agent on human behavior. Eschewing the use of marijuana without an unbiased evaluation of the drug's actions and at the same time offering moralistic arguments makes no more sense than promoting the use of the drug on the basis of subjective evaluations such as "it makes me feel more creative" and "insightful" or "more well-rounded." Numerous types of arguments for or against its consumption can be contrived, but most suffer from speciosity and from what Harry Stack Sullivan has termed paritaxical reasoning.

Although a plethora of research on marijuana has been conducted in the past three to four years, the majority of it has been devoted to defining and characterizing such variables as the pharmacological and chemical properties of cannabis and its basic physiological effects. Surprisingly, systematic research concerning the effects of marijuana on human behavior is minimal compared with some of the above-mentioned research areas when in fact this area is of vital importance from a scientific as well as social point of view.

This book attempts to synthesize much of the existing experimentation concerning the acute and chronic effects of marijuana and its derivatives on human behavior.

Loren L. Miller

MARIJUANA

EFFECTS ON HUMAN BEHAVIOR

Chapter 1

THE LOGISTICS OF MARIJUANA RESEARCH: METHODOLOGICAL, LEGAL, AND SOCIETAL

HARRY KLONOFF

I. Introduction	1
II. Clinical Research Planning	3
A. Strategy and Tactics for Clinical Research on Marijuana	3
B. A Model for Marijuana Clinical Research	6
C. A Model for Self-Reporting of Marijuana Experiences	9
III. Clinical Study at the University of British Columbia	10
A. Criteria for Volunteers and Screening Procedure	10
B. Background Characteristics of Subjects	11
C. Experimental Design and Examination Procedure	11
D. Marijuana and Placebo	12
IV. Driving Research Planning	19
A. Strategy and Tactics for Research on Marijuana and Driving	19
B. A Model for Driving and Marijuana	20
V. Summary	22
References	23

I. INTRODUCTION

The progress of science is the work of creative minds. Every creative mind that contributes to scientific advance works, however, within two limitations. It is limited, first, by ignorance, for one discovery waits upon that other which opens the way to it. Discovery and its acceptance are, however, limited also by the habits of thought that pertain to the culture of any region and period, that is to say, by the *Zeitgeist:* an idea too strange or preposterous to be thought in one period of western civilization may be readily accepted as true later. Slow change is the rule—at least for the basic ideas. On the other hand, the more superficial fashions as to what is important, what is worth doing and talking about, change much more rapidly, depending partly on discovery and partly on the social interaction of the wise men most concerned with the particular matter in hand—the cross-stimulation of leaders and their followers, of protagonists and their antagonists (Boring, 1950).

This chapter is directed to those scientists and researchers who are willing to persevere in their search for explanation, understanding, and prediction, in spite of *Zeitgeist* protagonists and antagonists of marijuana usage.

Is the drug problem of today really as unique and mysterious as many would have us believe? From a historical perspective, the use of mind-altering agents may be as timeless as man, the motivation in all probability deriving from the need to make life more pleasurable or from the desire to diminish the stress of human existence. The Sumerians, 7000 years ago, described on clay tablets the cultivation and preparation of opium (Neligan, 1927). Alcohol, with all its distressing consequences, is described in the Old Testament. The Chinese, 4000 years ago, used cannabis as a remedy (Nahas, 1973). In turning from the historical to the contemporary, a National Commission on Marijuana and Drug Abuse survey estimated that the total number of persons who have used marijuana in the United States may exceed 24 million (National Institute of Mental Health, 1972). Fejer *et al.* (1971), in surveying students in grades 7, 9, 11, 12, and 13, found that marijuana use increased 173% in Toronto between 1968 and 1970, and 162% in Halifax between 1969 and 1970. It should also be noted that in addition to nonprescribed mind-altering agents ingested in North American society there has been an explosion of prescribed psychotropic drugs (major tranquilizers, minor tranquilizers, antidepressants, stimulants, sedatives, and hypnotics). Between 1958 and 1967, there was a 65% increase in new psychotropic drug prescriptions filled in the United States; in 1967, psychotropic drugs accounted for 17% or 178 million prescriptions; mixture of psychotropic and nonpsychotropic drug prescriptions was 275 million or 25% of all prescriptions written; extent of use was 133.1 new and refill prescriptions for every 100 of adult population; one-quarter of all adults took a psychotropic agent in the 12 months preceding the survey; prescribing occurs in the over 20 age group, principally ages 40 to 59; and females account for 67% of all psychotropic drug usage (Balter and Levine, 1969).

Le Dain (1973) lists the following causes which interact to predispose and encourage the individual to engage in nonmedical drug use: personality of the user; his close personal relations—family, school, and peer group; social and economic conditions; and the general attitude of society toward drug use as reflected by advertising media and the practices of the adult population.

Some of the hysteria surrounding marijuana use is abating and the climate for research on marijuana is improving. But those concerned with social action and legislative change are still searching for credible information, and it would seem that there are four streams of relevant investigation that might help to bridge the information gap. The first area of investigation is that of the acute effects of marijuana. Researchers have been active in this area and the acute effects of marijuana have been documented in Canadian studies (Le Dain Commission, 1972, 1973; Klonoff, 1973a,b; Klonoff et al., 1973; Low et al., 1973; Marcus et al., 1974), as well as numerous studies in the United States (National Institute of Mental Health, 1972). The second area is that of the effects of marijuana on driving in a real life situation, and only two studies have been reported in this area (Le Dain Commission, 1972; Klonoff, Chapter 14). The third area is that of the chronic use of marijuana, particularly heavy chronic use, and in a relevant culture. There is no reported study in this area that can withstand critical scrutiny. The fourth area would involve a consideration of the effects on society if two mind-altering agents (marijuana and alcohol, rather than only alcohol) were available on demand, possibly using the ecosystems approach of Fisher and Strantz (1972).

Regarding the fourth area of investigation, Milner (1973) outlines some of the relevant variables that would be worthy of investigation before moving into the legalization of marijuana, and these are as follows: adverse effects, driving hazards, multiple drug use, incorrect evaluation, consumer culture, alcohol and marijuana, example to children, rights of the less-privileged, prejudiced assessments, community testing, legal control difficulties, social group alienation problems, regard for the law, and social goals.

II. CLINICAL RESEARCH PLANNING

A. Strategy and Tactics for Clinical Research on Marijuana

Weil et al. (1968) pointed out that research on marijuana is fraught with a large number of legal and attitudinal hurdles and obstacles. The situation they described still obtains today. Accordingly it might be helpful to provide first-hand information and data regarding the nature of such obstacles and, even more important, the ways and means of meeting the necessary demands in order to embark on marijuana research. Figure 1 outlines the channels—university, medicolegal, funding, Food and Drug, and law enforcement—that one must go through before beginning a systematic inquiry on marijuana.

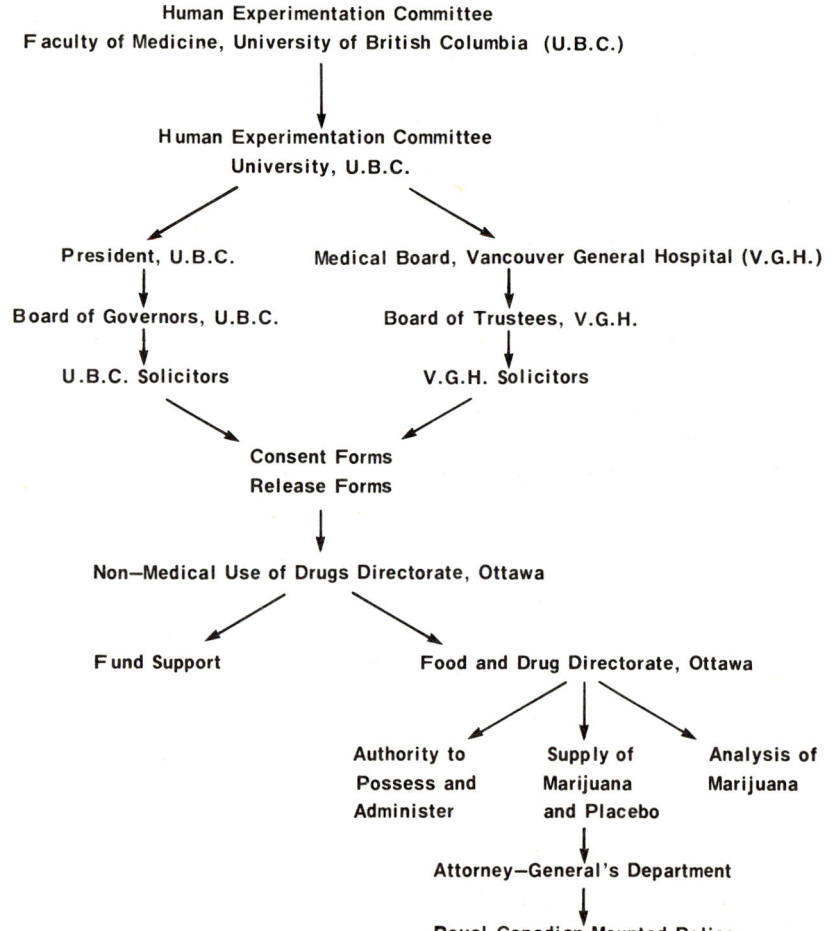

Fig. 1. Channels for initiating research on marijuana.

The process of endorsement begins with the university human experimentation committee. The human experimentation committee at the University of British Columbia passes on the proposed research and certifies that the procedures planned are acceptable on ethical grounds and, in particular, that: (a) the safety, welfare, and rights of the subject(s) are adequately protected; (b) the amount and kind of information communicated to the subject(s) is appropriate in order to secure informed consent* within the best definition of that term; (c) suitable precautions are taken to minimize risks; and (d) the subject is made aware that he has the right to withdraw from the research at any time. In addition, the matter of confidentiality regarding the identity and data of the volunteers must be made explicit, and such confidentiality must be maintained by agreement with the various levels of law enforcement. It should be stressed that human experimentation committees are concerned with the ethical and legal aspects and implications of the proposed research and not with the scientific credibility of the research. The researchers on marijuana at the University of British Columbia obtained approval from a Faculty of Medicine human experimentation committee, and subsequently from a more general university human experimentation committee.

As the research project was to be carried out in the University hospital (Health Sciences Centre), University of British Columbia, as well as the Vancouver General Hospital, it was necessary to obtain the approval from the University administration, specifically, the President of the University and the Board of Governors of the University, as well as from the Vancouver General Hospital administration, specifically, the Medical Board and the Board of Trustees of the Vancouver General Hospital. University and hospital administrations, before endorsing the project, requested their respective solicitors to review the proposals as submitted and to draw up a release and consent form as well as an acknowledgment and certificate form.

The release and consent form made explicit the following: that information had been provided regarding the proposed experiment; the nature, expected duration, and means of administration of the marijuana; potential risks; the nature of supervision during the experiment; freedom to withdraw; assurance that an offence was not being committed against the laws of Canada; and release of the University and the Vancouver General Hospital and their respective staffs from liability. The release and consent form was signed by the volunteer before participating in the project and was witnessed and then endorsed by a physician on the project.

The acknowledgment and certificate form was signed by the volunteer

---

* Informed consent is defined within the terms of reference of the Declaration of Helsinki—Recommendations Guiding Doctors in Clinical Research (1964).

after each experimental procedure, regardless of whether marijuana or placebo had been used, in order to maintain the double blind procedure. The acknowledgment and certificate form was signed by the volunteer after the effects of the marijuana had worn off and was witnessed and endorsed by a physician on the project. The acknowledgment and certificate form made explicit that the subject felt no ill effects from having participated in the research, that he considered himself capable, and was able to proceed from the hospital without further supervision.

The research proposal was then submitted to the next level, the Non-Medical Use of Drugs Directorate, Ottawa. This Directorate is concerned with funding of projects. When the application for funding was endorsed, the project moved to the next level, the Food and Drug Directorate, Ottawa. The Food and Drug Directorate provides accredited investigators (those investigators who have satisfied the criteria of all the levels noted above) with: "authorization to possess cannabis in amounts only for the purposes of and subject to the conditions contained in the study" (for nonphysicians); "authorization to possess and administer cannabis in amounts only for the purposes of and subject to the conditions contained in the study" (for physicians). The Food and Drug Directorate also provided the supplies of standardized *Cannabis sativa* as well as a placebo prepared in their laboratories. Finally, the Food and Drug Directorate laboratories provided analyses of the agents. Records, inspection, and security precautions with respect to marijuana must conform to the requirements of Section 48 of the Narcotic Control Regulations.

The final level involved liaison with the provincial Attorney General's Department and related law enforcement agencies.

B. A Model for Marijuana Clinical Research

In addition to legal and logistical problems, there are many inherent methodological problems that must be faced in research on marijuana. In spite of the almost frenetic reporting on the symbols of social conflict—psychoactive drugs and, more particularly, marijuana—during recent years, a good deal of literature in the field is still replete with fear, mythology, and overgeneralization, rather than systematic inquiry.

Generalizations regarding the effects of marijuana, in order to be scientifically valid for man, should be based on human research rather than, or in addition to, preclinical research on animals. While animal behavior is based on anthropomorphic assumptions and may be valid for biochemical and neurophysiological processes, it does not follow that animal behavior and human behavior are similarly affected by psychoactive drugs (Newmark, 1971). Second, clinical-experimental observation should counterbalance anecdotal-descriptive reports, for the latter are often confounded by retrospective falsification of the examinee and biases of the examiner. Third, findings must relate to the sociocultural matrix. Fourth, findings should be reproducible.

A model is accordingly proposed which would enable the planning of more meaningful clinical research on the effects of marijuana and, equally important, would provide benchmarks for critical evaluation of reports and literature on marijuana. The components of such a model and the associated methodological problems are as follows.

1. PHARMACOLOGY

Unresolved problems include: source and composition; chemical structure; biological actions; toxic effects; routes of administration; absorption; physiological fate; distribution and excretion; duration of action; tolerance, reverse tolerance, and cross-tolerance; therapeutic potential; and dose response with standardized amounts of Δ^9-THC as well as response to amounts usually smoked by subjects (subjective high). Comparative assessment of research is well-nigh impossible unless there is a specification of pharmacological variables, particularly those variables which relate to potency of Δ^9-THC.

2. NATURE OF EFFECT

Most clinical studies to date have dealt with short-term effects. Statements regarding long-term effects invariably derive from anecdotal reports that may not be related to the sociocultural matrix, or from retrospective clinical studies where the design and inferences are highly suspect.

3. SET

The expectancies, attitudes, and motivation of subjects, as well as learned skills for modifying the drug experience, should be taken into account. The expectancies and attitudes of examiners may also influence results.

4. SETTING

Anecdotal statements about the effects of marijuana in social settings, using an illicit agent, may be misleading. Rigid systematic clinical enquiry in a sterile laboratory environment may also result in artifact. In the design of research into the effects of marijuana, one should accordingly strive to create a setting that is socially and clinically relevant.

5. SUBJECTS

Interpretation of drug effects should take into account the following: physical health; personality characteristics; possible sex differences; and drug history including light, moderate, or heavy usage of prescribed and nonprescribed drugs.

6. CONTROLS

Serious studies on drug effects should include controls, specifically, one placebo group or condition.

7. DEPENDENT VARIABLES

The most obvious basic requirements for drug evaluation are stable and reproducible baselines against which to assess drug-correlated changes. Objective dependent variables are urgently needed to assess changes due to psychoactive drug effects. These would include: cognitive-perceptual measures, personality measures, rating scales and behavioral inventories, and electrophysiological measures. Subjective drug effects questionnaires are useful adjunctive measures. In all instances of drug evaluation, there should be a clear-cut specification as to whether the effects being measured are short term or long term.

Even when all criteria but the last are satisfied, the study may be methodologically sound but psychologically naive. The current state of psychometric sophistication and psychological theory has been reflected minimally in published studies on marijuana. The inclusion of psychological tests in marijuana studies should be predicated on the following: information is processed by a number of modalities (visual, auditory, and tactile); perceptual-sensory measures should be counterbalanced by motor variables; mental abilities include complex skills such as concept formation, multimodality memory, and sequential learning, in addition to simple motor skills; tests should be sufficiently extensive to ensure reliability; tests must have norms, if one is to engage in meaningful generalizations; there should be a specification as to whether differences between drug and control (placebo) conditions are within or beyond established psychological test norms; the tests included should enable differentiation between immediate drug effect and effect on subsequent learning; and the tests included in a battery should relate to theoretical models of explanation.

C. A Model for Self-Reporting of Marijuana Experiences

A good deal of the current literature on marijuana derives from subjective statements of users, and published studies on self-reporting inventories run the gamut from the anecdotal to the chain letter (mailing of questionnaires to a restricted number of users and imploring those who are willing to cooperate to distribute the questionnaires to their friends who are also users) to the captive audience (students and military personnel) to the epidemiologic approach with predetermined sampling procedures to clinical research where a questionnaire is an integral part of the methodology. Unfortunately, there has been no concerted effort to devise a self-reporting inventory that would reflect the antecedent factors, drug use patterns, attitudes toward marijuana, and effects of marijuana. Researchers accordingly fall back on devising situational inventories that lack reliability and validity.

In the construction of a self-reporting inventory: content validity or theoretical underpinnings should be the basis for assembling, selecting, and grouping items; a decision should be made regarding the relative merit of forced choice compared with open-ended questions; social desirability or group conformity may be a contributory factor that detracts from reliability; faking and retrospective falsification may be particularly relevant with a soft drug group in that proselytizing is not unusual, particularly in light of the confusion about soft drug terminology even in the minds of experts; and the guarantee of confidentiality and anonymity is extremely important in that this may well determine the degree of sincerity and seriousness with which the respondent completes the questionnaire. In the experience of the author, a self-reporting inventory format which is built into the design of the overall clinical investigation on marijuana ensures greater reliability and permits cross-validation of statements with other data. Other safeguards to increase reliability and the total return of data include standardization of instructions and the setting, guarantees of confidentiality, and interview after completion of the questionnaire to ensure that all items have been completed.

The remainder of this chapter will deal with the logistics of marijuana research. The first frame of reference presented is generic and applicable to any study in which marijuana is administered to human subjects and where the focus is the determination of psychological and physiological effects. An example of a study that has incorporated many of the strategies outlined will be cited and this will then serve as a prelude to Chapter 6 of this volume. The second frame of reference presented is specific and applicable only to studies determining the effects of marijuana on driving. This will then serve as a prelude to Chapter 14 of this volume.

III. CLINICAL STUDY AT THE UNIVERSITY OF BRITISH COLUMBIA

A. Criteria for Volunteers and Screening Procedure

The procedures about to be described are exemplary of the more methodologically precise human studies that have been reported. All subjects in the study at the University of British Columbia were volunteers who met the following criteria: (1) age between 19 and 31; (2) light and restricted use of psychoactive drugs (24 subjects—15 men and 9 women—had experimented with psychoactive drugs other than marijuana or hashish at some time, but not during the past year); (3) not on any form of prescribed drug regimen; (4) good physical health; and (5) no signs of serious personality disorder. There was no advertising for volunteers, and interested individuals became aware of the project through the grapevine.

Prospective subjects were initially interviewed by the project coordinator, informed about the general nature of the experiment, given an opportunity to ask relevant questions regarding the project, and were then given the opportunity to volunteer or not volunteer for the study. Enough volunteers of each sex were chosen to yield a male:female ratio of approximately 1:1. Those volunteers who satisfied all the above criteria were then interviewed by a psychiatrist. The purposes of the interview were (1) to determine general health; (2) to screen out volunteers with evidence of serious personality disorder; and (3) to obtain the psychiatric status and drug history (prescribed and nonprescribed) of a group of marijuana users in a standardized manner. The psychiatrist also assumed responsibility for obtaining the signature of the volunteers on the release and consent form.

Volunteers who met all the above-noted criteria were then given the Wechsler Adult Intelligence Scale and the Minnesota Multiphasic Personality Inventory. In addition, a questionnaire was completed. Volunteers were asked to refrain from using psychoactive drugs one week prior to the experimental session or during the course of the experiment.

B. Background Characteristics of Subjects

The project population consisted of 81 volunteers, 38 men and 43 women. Men and women were selected on an approximately 1:1 basis as women are purportedly becoming involved in almost as much experimentation with soft drugs as men (DeFleur and Garrett, 1970, men: women, 1:1; Goode, 1971, men:women, 3:2). Mean age was 22.51 years (SD 2.81, range 19–31 years). Age range was included as a criterion because it is consistent with the ages of individuals in our society who are the primary users of soft drugs, and to enable comparison with other published studies that have also used this age range. The lower limits of our age range were so specified because of statutes regarding legal responsibility. Educational level of the population was as follows: highschool, 7%; 1 year of university, 19%; 2 to 4 years of university, 46%; bachelor's degree, 17%; master's degree, 4%; and doctorate or medical degree, 7%. This is a highly educated group, the large majority being university trained and 28% having university degrees. Occupation was classified into the following five categories: postsecondary students, 60%; professional, 10%; semiprofessional, 4%; service, technical, and clerical, 11%; and skilled and semiskilled, 15%. The study sample was heavily skewed toward the university educated and higher occupational status, and these characteristics are also consistent with the subjects included in current reports on marijuana. Of the group, 74% were single, 18% married, and 8% divorced or separated or living common law.

C. Experimental Design and Examination Procedure

For the neuropsychological examination and reexamination, subjects were assigned to one of the following four counterbalanced experimental conditions for the high-dose level of drug: marijuana/marijuana, marijuana/placebo, placebo/marijuana, and placebo/placebo. For the low-dose level, subjects were assigned to one of the following three counterbalanced experimental conditions: marijuana/marijuana, marijuana/placebo, and placebo/marijuana. The placebo/placebo group was used for high- then low-dose level analyses. This counterbalanced design enabled each subject to serve as his or her own control, allowed for assessment of placebo effects, controlled for practice effects between the two sessions, and permitted an evaluation of the action of marijuana on learning. For the electrophysiological examination, subjects were assigned to one of three experimental conditions: marijuana low- or high-dose levels or placebo.

The subjects had been informed during the screening that they would receive either marijuana or placebo, but were unaware of the experimental sequence or the dose. The research assistants may or may not have been aware of the dose level. The examinations were conducted in a comfortable clinical environment.

The examination began directly after the smoking of the marijuana or placebo. After completion of the examination and an appropriate interval of time, the volunteer was seen by a physician and the acknowledgment and certificate form was completed. The volunteer agreed not to drive a vehicle until the following morning and was driven home by taxi. The volunteer phoned in the day following the examination to report on his or her condition. The interval between sessions was approximately one week.

During the initial session and the subsequent session one week later, the same battery of neuropsychological tests as well as a projective personality test were administered. After each marijuana or placebo session volunteers dictated their reactions to the sessions into a tape recorder. During the third session, baseline electrophysiological data were obtained, followed by electrophysiological monitoring during the marijuana or placebo experience.

D. Marijuana and Placebo

1. SOURCE, DOSE, SMOKING PROCEDURE

The marijuana and placebo used in this project were supplied by the Food and Drug Directorate, Ottawa. Low dose was defined as standardized *Cannabis sativa* labeled as containing 0.69% Δ^9-THC, and high dose as containing 1.3% Δ^9-THC. The batch label regarding percentage of Δ^9-THC was confirmed by Food and Drug laboratory analysis. The batches of standardized cannabis with higher percentages of Δ^9-THC were mixed with placebo in order to ensure that a constant (in terms of grams of cigarette) and standard (in terms of milligrams of THC) quantity of marijuana was administered to all subjects. Reanalysis by Food and Drug laboratories confirmed the percentage of Δ^9-THC in low- and high-dose batches used in the research.

The placebo was also provided by the Food and Drug Directorate. The physical characteristics of the placebo were identical to those of the *Cannabis sativa* plant material. Food and Drug laboratory testing of the placebo showed that 1 gm extracted in the normal manner gave a

1. The Logistics of Marijuana Research

negative result on chemical testing for the cannabinols. The placebo, when smoked, smelled and tasted like the marijuana cigarettes made from the unextracted plant material.

Marijuana and placebo were administered in the form of cigarettes of standard size and weight made with a hand-operated rolling machine. This route of administration was used because marijuana is most frequently smoked in a social context. For the neuropsychological examination, the low- and high-doses of marijuana were one cigarette of 0.7 gm followed by half a cigarette of 0.35 gm 1 hour later. Approximately 4.8 mg Δ^9-THC was contained in the initial cigarette smoked by the low-dose group and 9.1 mg Δ^9-THC by the high-dose group. The second cigarette smoked 1 hour later contained 2.4 mg Δ^9-THC for the low-dose group and 4.5 mg Δ^9-THC for the high-dose group. Weil et al. (1968) reported that the effects of marijuana diminished after 30 to 60 minutes. Truitt (1971) subsequently found that THC has a half-life of roughly 30 minutes in man. A reinforcing dose of marijuana was accordingly included at the end of the first hour in order to maintain a more consistent level of "high" throughout the examination. For the electrophysiological examination, the low dose of marijuana was 0.7 gm (4.8 mg Δ^9-THC) and the high dose 0.7 gm (9.1 mg Δ^9-THC). The amount of marijuana administered to the high-dose group was arrived at empirically during the pilot phase of the project. In experimenting with varying dosage levels of marijuana, it was found that 0.7 gm (9.1 mg Δ^9-THC) of marijuana smoked in a standardized procedure was the optimal level of intoxication readily tolerated by volunteers, and furthermore that 0.35 gm (4.5 mg Δ^9-THC) of marijuana again smoked in a standardized procedure was required 1 hour later to maintain this optimal level of intoxication. Placebo was administered in an identical manner, i.e., a 0.7 gm cigarette initially, followed by a 0.35 gm cigarette 1 hour later (reinforcing dose included only for the neuropsychological examination).

In order to deal with the problem of quantification in delivery of smoked marijuana, the smoking was standardized. As has been pointed out by Manno et al. (1970), approximately 50% of the total THC content of the cigarette is delivered to the subject, provided the butt is fully smoked. The smoking of marijuana and placebo was standardized and timed with a stopwatch as follows: subject inhaled smoke (forced) for 3 seconds, inhaled air for 1 second (to clear mouth of smoke), held breath for 15 seconds, exhaled and rested for 15 seconds; this procedure was followed until the cigarette was completely smoked. It took approximately 10 minutes to smoke a 0.7 gm cigarette, including the "roach" (butt of cigarette).

Comparison of findings in studies assessing psychological effects is possible only if the potency of the marijuana and the smoking procedure are specified. Reporting to date has been variable, and potency of marijuana is seldom confirmed by independent analysis. Even when investigators have been more precise in reporting dosage levels, the percentage of Δ^9-THC has been variable, regardless of the route of administration. Studies reporting on Δ^9-THC delivered by smoking have included Weil et al. (1968), 4.5 and 18 mg Δ^9-THC; Caldwell et al. (1969), 3.9 and 6.3 mg Δ^9-THC; Manno et al. (1970), 2.5 and 5.0 mg Δ^9-THC; Kiplinger and Manno (1971), 5 mg Δ^9-THC; and Dornbush and Freedman (1972), 7.5 and 22.5 mg Δ^9-THC. Le Dain (1972), after reviewing the literature, reported that in North America most users smoke less than 10 mg Δ^9-THC to get "stoned." In the four studies conducted by Le Dain and subsequently included in the Commission Report (1972), doses ranged from 0.7 to 6.8 mg Δ^9-THC. Studies reporting on oral doses of marijuana have included Hollister and Gillespie (1970), 32 mg Δ^9-THC; Melges and Tinklenberg (1970), 20, 40, and 60 mg Δ^9-THC; Waskow et al. (1970), 20 mg Δ^9-THC; and Rafaelsen et al. (1971), 8 to 16 mg Δ^9-THC. The dose levels in the neuropsychological portion of the present study of 4.8 and 9.1 mg Δ^9-THC administered initially, followed by 2.4 and 4.5 mg Δ^9-THC administered 1 hour later, are modest in comparison with some of the studies but high in comparison with others.

2. SUBJECTIVE EVALUATION OF MARIJUANA AND PLACEBO

At the conclusion of each experimental session, marijuana or placebo, the subject was asked to rate the "high" state experienced compared with previous "high" states, on a scale of 0 to 10, 0 indicating no effect and 10 indicating maximal effect (Table I). In comparing the subjective impressions of volunteers who smoked low doses of marijuana with those who smoked high doses, the following conclusions emerge (based on average ratings and distribution among no effect, minimally high, moderately high, and very high categories): (1) there was generally a positive relationship between dose level and subjective rating of extent of "high"; (2) subjective ratings were related to low- and high-dose levels when marijuana was administered initially or when marijuana was smoked in both sessions; and (3) the volunteers did not discriminate between low- and high-doses when marijuana administered in the second session was preceded by placebo in the initial session. In comparing the subjective impressions of low- and high-dose marijuana conditions with placebo conditions, the following conclusions emerge (based on average ratings and distribution among no effect, minimally high, moderately high, and very high categories): (1) Placebo during the second session, preceded by placebo during the initial session, was misidentified (mod-

TABLE I
Subjective Evaluation of Effects of Marijuana and Placebo[a]

Subjective rating	Low dose						High dose					
	Marijuana 1st session $n = 18$	Marijuana 2nd session (marijuana 1st) $n = 9$	Marijuana 2nd session (placebo 1st) $n = 8$	Placebo 1st session $n = 21$	Placebo 2nd session (marijuana 1st) $n = 9$		Marijuana 1st session $n = 28$	Marijuana 2nd session (marijuana 1st) $n = 13$	Marijuana 2nd session (placebo 1st) $n = 14$	Placebo 1st session $n = 27$	Placebo 2nd session (marijuana 1st) $n = 15$	Placebo 2nd session (placebo 1st) $n = 13$
No effect (0)	0	0	0	3 (14)	7 (78)		0	1 (8)	1 (7)	7 (26)	7 (47)	3 (23)
Minimally high (1–2)	1 (6)	0	0	9 (43)	1 (11)		0	0	1 (7)	9 (33)	6 (40)	3 (23)
Moderately high (3–6)	6 (33)	3 (33)	3 (37)	7 (33)	1 (11)		6 (21)	2 (15)	2 (14)	8 (30)	2 (13)	6 (46)
Very high (7–10)	11 (61)	6 (67)	5 (63)	2 (10)	0		22 (79)	10 (77)	10 (72)	3 (11)	0	1 (8)
Average rating	6.5	6.7	7.2	2.8	0.7		7.8	7.3	7.0	2.5	1.2	2.8

[a] Percentage in parentheses.

erately high and very high rating) by 54% of the volunteers assigned to this condition; (2) placebo administered initially was not identified as such by either low- (43%) or high- (41%) dose groups; and (3) misidentification by low- (11%) and high- (13%) dose groups was, however, infrequent when placebo was administered during the second session and preceded by marijuana in the initial session.

These findings reflect the importance of learned expectancies, set and attitude, as well as prior experience with the drug. For example, the highest incidence of misjudgment in the placebo condition might have been a result of an expectancy by the volunteers that they would receive one drug and one placebo experience. Differences in discrimination in the other two experimental conditions might have been the result of the presence or absence of a prior laboratory experience with marijuana. The findings of this study are consistent with those of Manno et al. (1970) and Meyer et al. (1971) who also found that subjects were unable to differentiate placebo from marijuana. Jones (1971) in administering marijuana followed by placebo found that many subjects rated their subjective level of intoxication after smoking placebo as identical to that after smoking marijuana.

No distinctive trend was noted in comparing the subjective ratings of men as compared with women. Reanalysis of the data, excluding subjects who had used other psychoactive agents in addition to marijuana or hashish, produced approximately the same results. From the results of the present study, we concluded that the placebo prepared by the Food and Drug Directorate met specifications for a control group agent in marijuana research.

3. SUBJECTIVE EVALUATION OF EFFECTS AFTER A DRUG EXPERIENCE

As a first step in the evaluation of drug effects, definition of terms would be in order. From a pharmacological frame of reference, there is a differentiation between the main (desired) drug effect and side (unpleasant) effects. From the point of view of the marijuana user, the main drug effect is to become "high" and side effects would include the unpleasant, negative, unexpected, or adverse reaction during the drug experience (bad trip) or shortly thereafter (hangover) or subsequent to the experience (flashback). Unpleasant effects, however, as threshold of effect can be related to personal attitudes and expectancies, social norms regarding drug experiences, and cultural attitudes regarding the desirability or undesirability of experiencing altered states of consciousness.

The subjects in the study being reported spent approximately 5 minutes at the conclusion of each session dictating an account of their reactions to the marijuana or placebo experience. Subjective effects reported by a subsample of 17 volunteers who were administered low doses of marijuana and 24 volunteers who were administered high doses* during the initial session were analyzed. In order to place the effects reported directly after a marijuana experience in a controlled clinical setting into a broader context, the findings on the subsample were compared with two sets of questionnaire data: the first derives from the sample of 81 subjects included in this study (which subsumes the subsample), the questionnaires having been completed prior to the experimental procedures; the second derives from an independent study of 213 heavier drug users. Both questionnaires dealt with antecedent factors regarding marijuana use, reported use of marijuana, attitudes toward marijuana, and drug effects. The effects reported on the questionnaires by these marijuana users may accordingly be viewed as expectancies, and such expectancies should be included as one of the factors that influence the nature of the drug experience. At the same time, there is no reason to presume that there would be a one-to-one relationship between expectancies and the actual drug experiences.

The initial portion of the data analyzed on the subsample of 41 volunteers dealt with the feeling state that resulted from the drug experience. Statements by these volunteers regarding feeling state were categorized as positive (1—happy, content, relaxed; 2—increased sensory awareness with a pleasant connotation; and 3—fatigued but content) for 71% of the low- as well as the high-dose group, and as negative (1—anxious, suspicious; 2—confused thinking, difficulty in concentration and verbalization; and 3—fatigued but not content) for 29% of both groups. A comparison of the findings that derive from a marijuana experience in a controlled clinical setting on the subsample of 41 volunteers (71% of effects were positive and 29% negative) with the expectancies that derive from a questionnaire of the group of 81 (75% of effects were positive and 25% negative) revealed a very close fit. In comparing the subsample of 41 volunteers who were lighter marijuana users with the expectancies that derive from a questionnaire of the group of 213 heavier marijuana users, there is also a high degree of concordance in the ratio of positive (64%) to negative (36%) effects reported by the heavier marijuana users. The expectancy of positive effects, by lighter as well as heavier marijuana users, may accordingly be one of the reinforcing factors in their continued usage of marijuana.

The second area of analysis on the subsample of 41 volunteers dealt with unusual experiences that resulted from the drug experience. State-

---

* Data were not obtained on one volunteer of the low-dose group and four volunteers of the high-dose group.

ments regarding unusual experiences were categorized in terms of regression, suspiciousness and projection, somatic references, somatic delusions, and delusions. The incidence of unpleasant experiences was high for both the low- (47%) and high- (46%) dose groups; the more striking experiences during the acute intoxication stage reflect abnormal mental content. The abnormal mental content was transient and subsided shortly after the termination of the session. The relative isolation of the volunteer (only one examiner was present during the examination procedure) and the dose of marijuana administered may have contributed to the high incidence of unpleasant experiences, including the frank abnormal content noted.

The presence of adverse effects including hallucinations, impaired mental processes, and high anxiety during marijuana intoxication have been documented by others (Keeler, 1967; Halikas et al., 1971). The unresolved question is the relative incidence of usual as compared with adverse effects during marijuana intoxication. The present study suggests that unusual or adverse effects are quite frequently encountered, particularly in laboratory settings. Le Dain (1972) confirms that researchers have reported acute reactions under laboratory conditions using doses exceeding 10 mg Δ^9-THC.

Whereas there was consistency regarding feeling state reported by the subsample and the two comparison groups, divergence characterized the reporting of unusual experiences. Specifically, 46% of the subsample of 41 volunteers reported unpleasant experiences which often shaded over into abnormal mental content, but only 14% of the comparison group of 81 and 20% of the comparison group of 213 reported such experiences. Minimization, denial, retrospective falsification, tolerance of the unpleasant as the price of a "high," or flirting with states of unreality may be possible explanations for the divergence of reported unusual experiences for those subjects who were reflecting on their previous experiencs compared with those subjects who had a marijuana experience.

The third area of analysis on the subsample of 41 volunteers dealt with wishes that followed on the heels of the drug experience. Rank order of statements regarding what the subsample of 41 volunteers would have liked to have done subsequent to the drug experience was as follows: do something passive, eat, do something active, do something artistic or musical, and unusual.

4. SUBJECTIVE EVALUATION OF EFFECTS THE FOLLOWING DAY

Analysis of the verbal statements (taken over the phone the morning after the initial marijuana session) of 18 volunteers in the low-dose group and 28 in the high-dose group revealed the following: 82% of the low-dose group and 75% of the high-dose group felt fine and had returned to *status quo ante;* 6% (one volunteer) and 14% (four volunteers), respectively, of the low- and high-dose groups mentioned feeling fatigued; 6% and 4%, respectively, of the low- and high-dose groups reported headaches; and 6% and 7% (two volunteers), respectively, of the low- and high-dose groups felt "slightly high." These data suggest that residual effects the next morning are not infrequent, such effects having been noted by 22% of the sample (17% of the low-dose group and 25% of the high-dose group).

IV. DRIVING RESEARCH PLANNING

A. Strategy and Tactics for Research on Marijuana and Driving

With one exception to date, namely, the pilot study conducted by the Le Dain Commission (1972) using an airport runway, all research dealing with the effects of marijuana on driving have used laboratory simulator paradigms. The use of driving simulators in a laboratory environment to determine the effects of marijuana would necessite the same strategy as described above. In order to proceed from laboratory clinical research and simulator paradigms to driving in a real life situation, a list of additional administrative problems must be solved. In the planning of our experimental study to determine the effects of marijuana on driving, initially in a restricted area free of traffic, and subsequently on city streets, a series of complicated legal and logistical problems had to be resolved.

The endorsement by the University Human Experimentation Committee and university administrative channels was similar to that noted under clinical research. Appropriate release and consent as well as acknowledgment and certificate forms were drawn up by university solicitors. Since the project was done in two phases, the first in a restricted driving area, the major hurdle to resolve was automobile liability insurance. An international insurance carrier agreed to provide the insurance policy for this project with third party liability coverage in the amount of $500,000. In order to insure that the policy issued was legally valid, permission was obtained from the Superintendent of Insurance, British Columbia, to remove from the statutory conditions of the policy those sections prohibiting the driving of a vehicle while under the influence of a drug. The policy was issued with the undertaking that the following precautions would be taken: volunteers would be selected in terms of stated criteria; a dual control vehicle (double brakes and double ignition) would be used; a driving observer would be present in the vehicle with the subject; and appropriate supervision and monitoring of the volunteers would be provided before, during, and after the driving experience. The restricted driving area initially selected and used for the pilot portion of the study was a very large parking lot within the confines of the university. The area used for the experimental portion of the study included the runways on a military base which was in the process of being turned over from the Department of National Defence to the Parks Board of the City of Vancouver.

In order to move into the second phase of the driving project, namely, onto city streets and through downtown Vancouver, it was necessary to obtain permission in writing from the various levels of law enforcement within the province of British Columbia, namely, the Attorney General of British Columbia, the Assistant Commissioner, Royal Canadian Mounted Police, and the Chief Constable of the City of Vancouver. Such permission was granted with commitment on the part of the investigators that the criteria noted above would obtain and with the proviso that the dual controls on the vehicle would include double steering. The final caveat was that the insurance carrier would extend the liability coverage to take effect while the vehicle was being driven on city streets. A revised release and consent form was drawn up by the university solicitors before approaching the insurance company. After negotiation, the insurance carrier modified the coverage to include third party liability while the vehicle was being driven on city streets. It was then necessary to renegotiate through the university administrative channels.

B. A Model for Driving and Marijuana

The methodological problems confronting the researcher interested in evaluating the effects of marijuana on driving are even more frustrating than for the clinical researcher on marijuana, primarily because of the underdevelopment of driving research in general. The timidity of investigators has relegated them to the laboratory with the result that the marijuana and driving literature to date has focused on laboratory psychomotor skills and driving simulator paradigms. The predictive validity of both of these approaches with respect to actual driving has yet to be demonstrated, and generalizations from simulator paradigms to actual driving should accordingly be viewed with caution if not skepticism. The urgency of moving from the laboratory to the "street" in driving studies becomes obvious when confronted with data that driving under the influence of marijuana is a frequent occurrence (Benjamin, 1972; Klonoff, Chap. 14, this volume). A model is accordingly proposed which would assist in the planning of research into the effects of marijuana on driving. Such a model should encompass the components noted under clinical research on the effects of marijuana as well as the following which are directly related to driving.

1. DRIVER CHARACTERISTICS

Selection of subjects should take into account the following: age, sex, driving experience, previous accident record, safety attitudes, range of speed normally driven, risk taking threshold, and personality characteristics.

2. DRIVING CONDITIONS

Environmental factors—external and internal—include: visibility, traffic pattern (downtown compared with residential side streets), traffic events (right compared with left turns), external environmental distractions (billboards and pedestrians), and internal environmental distractions (passengers and radio).

3. SITUATIONAL DETRIMENTAL FACTORS

The more relevant variables are fatigue and drugs.

4. DRIVER BEHAVIORAL MEASURES

Driving behavior can be inferred from psychomotor measures such as reaction time or from a task that requires motor coordination and attention, but the question of validity remains unanswered. Quantifiable procedures have recently been developed for simulator research, and these show promise for investigating the effects of marijuana on driving. The first is signal detection procedure (Wilde and Curry, 1970; Moskowitz et al., 1973). The second breaks down the components of driving into a search and scan task, a perceptual judgment task, a decision-making/ cognitive-response task, and the execution of physical response task (Ellingstad et al., 1973). Other quantifiable procedures have been used for real life driving situations, and these include the following.

a. Component Movements. Accelerator movements, steering action, and use of brakes.

b. Driving Skills. General driving habits (starting-stopping, carelessness with driving regulations, turning, lane changing, and regard for traffic signals), speed, care while driving, judgment, concentration, confidence, tension, aggression, and risk taking.

c. Spare Capacity. Capacity for intake and processing of information is greater than normally required by the driving conditions and this may be used to compensate for emergent events or factors such as fatigue or drugs; e.g., the comparison of error rates on subsidiary tasks while driving in an easy residential area and a difficult heavy-traffic shopping area (Wilde and Curry, 1970).

5. DRIVER PHYSIOLOGICAL MEASURES

Measures such as heart rate, galvanic skin response, electroencephalogram, and respiratory rate provide independent indices of arousal which can be related to driving behavior.

Even with a methodology that can withstand critical scrutiny, there remains the problem of an appropriate statistical design. The statistical analysis should extend beyond effects (statistically significant differences) between experimental conditions and include a measure of subject performance with respect to cutoff points; i.e., proviso should be made in the design for subject improvement in performance as well as no change in performance and deterioration in performance.

V. SUMMARY

Before undertaking clinical research on marijuana or research on the effects of marijuana on driving, certain demands must be met in the following areas: educational and health facilities, the legal position, funding, and Food and Drug Directorate regulations and law enforcement. Methodological problems in clinical research include those concerned with pharmacology, nature of effect, set, setting, subjects, controls, and dependent variables. The second portion of this chapter described the methodology and findings of a clinical study of 81 volunteers, selected according to specified criteria, screened psychiatrically and psychologically, then assigned to one of seven experimental groups. Dosage and smoking procedure were standardized for both marijuana and placebo. The experience was evaluated subjectively by the volunteers at the end of each experimental session and again on the following morning. The third portion of this chapter reviewed the methodological problems in planning driving research on marijuana that should be considered, namely, driver characteristics, driving conditions, situational detrimental factors, driver behavioral measures, and driver physiological measures.

ACKNOWLEDGMENTS

This research was supported by Grant 610-25-1, National Health Grants, Ottawa, Canada, and by a grant from the British Columbia Alcohol and Drug Commission. The author wishes to express his appreciation to A. M. Marcus, M.D., Associate Professor and Head, Division of Forensic Psychiatry, Department of Psychiatry, University of British Columbia; M. Low, Ph.D., M.D., Associate Professor (Neurology), Department of Medicine, University of British Columbia, and Head, EEG Department, Vancouver General Hospital; H. Sanders, Ph.D., Associate Professor, Department of Pharmacology, University of British Columbia; C. Fibiger, Ph.D., Post-Doctoral Fellow, Department of Psychiatry, University of British Columbia; B. Simpson, R.N., and H. Hoodless, B.Sc., research assistants, Division of Psychology, Department of Psychiatry, University of British Columbia; the Health Sciences Centre Hospital, University of British Columbia and the Vancouver General Hospital, for their cooperation and for providing the necessary research facilities.

REFERENCES

Balter, M. B., and Levine, J. (1969). *Psychopharmacol. Bull.* **5**, 3–13.
Benjamin, F. B. (1972). In "Current Research in Marijuana" (M. F. Lewis, ed.), pp. 205–219. Academic Press, New York.
Boring, E. G. (1950). "A History of Experimental Psychology," p. 3. Appleton, New York.
Caldwell, D. F., Myers, S. A., Domino, E. F., and Merriam, P. E. (1969). *Percept. Mot. Skills* **29**, 755–759.
Declaration of Helsinki. (1964). "Recommendations Guiding Doctors in Clinical Research."
DeFleur, L. B., and Garrett, G. R. (1970). *J. Couns. Psychol.* **17**, 468–476.
Dornbush, R. L., and Freedman, A. M. (1972). *Psychopharmacol. Bull.* **8**, 19–20.
Ellingstad, V. S., McFarling, L. H., and Struckman, D. L. (1973). Contract No. DOT-HS-191-2-301. University of South Dakota, Vermillion.
Fejer, D., Smart, R. G., Whitehead, P. C., and LaForest, L. (1971). *Pub. Opin. Quart.* **35**, 235–241.
Fisher, G., and Strantz, I. (1972). *Amer. J. Pub. Health* **62**, 1407–1414.
Goode, E. (1971). *Nature (London)* **234**, 225–227.
Halikas, J. A., Goodwin, D. W., and Guze, S. B. (1971). *J. Amer. Med. Ass.* **217**, 692–694.
Hollister, L., and Gillespie, H. (1970). *Arch. Gen. Psychiat.* **23**, 199–203.
Jones, R. T. (1971). *Pharmacol. Rev.* **23**, 359–369.
Keeler, M. H. (1967). *Amer. J. Psychiat.* **124**, 674–677.

Kiplinger, G. F., and Manno, J. E. (1971). *Pharmacol. Rev.* **23**, 339–347.
Klonoff, H. (1973a). *Can. Med. Ass. J.* **108**, 145–150.
Klonoff, H. (1973b). *Can. J. Pub. Health* **65**, 552–561.
Klonoff, H., Low, M., and Marcus, A. (1973). *Can. Med. Ass. J.* **108**, 150–157.
Le Dain Commission. (1972). "A Report of the Commission of Inquiry into the Non-Medical Use of Drugs." Information Canada, Ottawa.
Le Dain Commission. (1973). "Final Report of the Commission of Inquiry into the Non-Medical Use of Drugs." Information Canada, Ottawa.
Low, M., Klonoff, H., and Marcus, A. (1973). *Can. Med. Ass. J.* **108**, 157–164.
Manno, J. E., Kiplinger, G. F., Haine, S. C., Bennett, I., and Forney, R. (1970). *Clin. Pharmacol. Ther.* **11**, 808–815.
Marcus, A., Klonoff, H., and Low, M. (1974). *Can. Psychiat. Ass. J.* **19**, 31–39.
Melges, F. T., and Tinklenberg, J. R. (1970). *Arch. Gen. Psychiat.* **22**, 204–210.
Meyer, R. E., Pillard, R. C., Shapiro, L. M., and Mirin, S. M. (1971). *Amer. J. Psychiat.* **128**, 198–204.
Milner, G. (1973). *Med. J. Aust.* **2**, 285–290.
Moskowitz, H., McGlothlin, W., and Hulbert, S. (1973). Contract No. DOT-HS-150-2-236. University of California, Los Angeles.
Nahas, G. G. (1973). "Marihuana—Deceptive Weed." Raven Press, New York.
National Institute of Mental Health. (1972). "Report on Marihuana and Health." US Govt. Printing Office, Washington, D.C.
Neligan, A. R. (1927). *In* "The Opium Problem" (C. E. Terry and M. Pellens, eds.), p. 53. The Haddon Craftsman, Camden.
Newmark, C. S. (1971). *Psychol. Rep.* **28**, 715–723.
Rafaelsen, L., Bech, P., Christrup, H., and Rafaelsen, O. J. (1971). Rigshospitalet Psychochemistry Institute, Copenhagen (unpublished manuscript).
Truitt, E. B. (1971). *Pharmacol. Rev.* **23**, 273–278.
Waskow, I. E., Olsson, J. E., Salzman, C., and Katz, M. (1970). *Arch. Gen. Psychiat.* **22**, 97–107.
Weil, A., Zinberg, N., and Nelsen, J. (1968). *Science* **162**, 1234–1242.
Wilde, G. J. S., and Curry, G. A. (1970). "Psychological Aspects of Road Research: A Study of the Literature, 1959–1968." Kingston, Ontario.

Chapter 2

THE MARIJUANA CONTROVERSY *

ABRAHAM WIKLER

    I. Introduction 25
   II. Biological Issues 26
       A. Dose-Response Relationships (Δ^9-THC) 26
       B. Impairment of Immediate Memory 27
       C. Alteration of Time Sense 30
       D. "Adverse" Reactions 32
       E. Tolerance and Dependence 36
 III. Aesthetic Issues 39
 IV. Social Issues 40
      References 42

I. INTRODUCTION

The purpose of this chapter is to separate and discuss the issues that have beclouded the question of legalization of marijuana in the United States. Though they overlap, these issues may be classified, for purposes of discussion, as biological, aesthetic, and social. The biological issues are concerned with quantitative data on dose-response relationships, and tolerance to and dependence on cannabis products (including marijuana) in man, or, more specifically, to their Δ^9-tetrahydrocannabinol (Δ^9-THC) content. Among the aesthetic issues are the use of terms such as "high,"

---

* Preparation of this article was supported, in part, by Research Grant No. DA 00044 from the National Institute of Drug Abuse with funds made available by the Special Action Office for Drug Abuse Prevention.

"turning on," "psychedelic," and "transcendental" experiences in referring to the qualitative effects of cannabis products or other agents. The social issues include the justice and efficacy of "criminalization" of marijuana users, the proclivity of heavy marijuana users to use other drugs, and the incongruity of the legal status and practically unrestricted use of alcoholic beverages. Judgments on legalization of marijuana may vary, depending on the importance one attaches to the biological, aesthetic, or social aspects of the problem, but it is hoped that separation of these issues will, at least, clarify the basis of positions taken in the current marijuana controversy.

II. BIOLOGICAL ISSUES

A. Dose-Response Relationships (Δ^9-THC)

The full range of possible biological effects of cannabis products was investigated by Isbell et al. (1967), Isbell and Jasinski (1969), and Hollister et al. (1968). In placebo-controlled studies on former opioid addicts, Isbell and his co-workers (1967) demonstrated that at dose levels of 120 and 480 µg/kg orally, or 50 and 200 µg/kg by smoking, Δ^9-THC produced dose-related changes in mood (usually euphoric), alterations in subjective time sense and visual and auditory perceptions (subjectively "keener") at the lower dose levels, and marked distortion of visual and auditory perceptions, visual and auditory hallucinations, depersonalization, and derealization at the higher dose levels in most subjects. Cardiac rate also increased as a function of dose, and chemosis and ptosis were observed at the higher dose levels. Isbell and Jasinski (1969) compared the effects of 75 and 225 µg/kg of Δ^9-THC by smoking with those of 0.5 and 1.5 µg/kg of LSD-25 by intramuscular injection in former opioid addicts, using the vehicles (ethanol or saline) by the oral and intramuscular route as control substances. Though LSD-25 was 160 times as potent as Δ^9-THC (on a milligram per body weight basis), the effects of the two drugs on a "psychotomimetic" scale (63 items) were dose-related and parallel. On "drug specific" scales (scales that differentiate the effects of a given drug from those of all other drugs), Δ^9-THC but not LSD-25 produced dose-related effects on a "marijuana" scale; on an "LSD" scale, Δ^9-THC was less effective than LSD in producing dose-related responses. In contrast to Δ^9-THC, LSD-25 also produced pupillary dilation, increased body temperature, increased blood pressure, decreased knee jerk threshold, and only a moderate increase in pulse rate.

Hollister et al. (1968) compared the effects of oral doses of Δ^9-THC (341–946 µg/kg; median, 581 µg/kg) with those of synhexyl (633–2666 μg/kg; median, 1370 μg/kg) in volunteer subjects who were not former opioid addicts. On a milligram per body weight basis, Δ^9-THC was 3 times as potent as synhexyl, and the effects of the latter were slower in onset. Nevertheless, both drugs produced dose-related effects that, in general, were similar to those obtained by Isbell and co-workers. These included increased acuity of hearing, visual distortions, visual hallucinations, alteration of time sense, euphoria, bursts of uncontrolled laughter, difficulty in concentration, sedation, and dreaminess. Physiological changes included tachycardia, chemosis, and muscular weakness as measured by a finger ergograph.

From these studies, it may be concluded that Δ^9-THC, like LSD-25, is a psychotomimetic drug. However, their effects are apparently mediated by different mechanisms, inasmuch as Isbell and Jasinski (1969) also demonstrated no cross-tolerance to Δ^9-THC in LSD-25 tolerant subjects; the reverse test of cross-tolerance (the effects of LSD-25 in Δ^9-THC tolerant subjects) has not yet been done in man. In rats, however, Silva and Carlini (1968) reported an absence of cross-tolerance between Δ^9-THC, on the one hand, and LSD-25 or mescaline, on the other. After development of tolerance to the performance-impairing effects of Δ^9-THC, a challenging dose of LSD-25 or mescaline produced impairment, and after development of tolerance to LSD-25 or mescaline, a challenging dose of Δ^9-THC produced impairment.

B. Impairment of Immediate Memory

Perhaps the most obvious feature of acute marijuana intoxication (so-called "high") is the difficulty the (nonintoxicated) observer has in understanding what the subject is saying. In 1934, Bromberg described this vividly:

> Speech is rapid, flighty, the subject has the impression that his conversation is witty, brilliant, ideas flow quickly. . . . When the user wishes to explain what he has thought, there is only confusion. . . . The flighty ideas are not deep enough to form an engram that can be recollected—hence the confusion that appears on trying to remember what was thought.

Similarly, Ames (1958) described the effects of a cannabis extract on memory as follows:

> Some degree of thought disorder was invariably present. In many cases, this consisted primarily of an inability to recall what had just happened, so that the subject was often totally unable to sustain a conversation unless prompted about a recent remark by the observer. In some subjects, the whole process of thinking seemed broken off abruptly, or they complained

of "fragmentation" of thought and described thinking as having no beginning and no end and such a tenuous reality that it was continually being shattered by other disconnected pieces of thoughts.

Of course, there is no way of judging the dose of Δ^9-THC which produced the effects on memory described above. However, more recent studies indicate that such effects can very well be produced by doses of Δ^9-THC that are in the range of those found in marijuana cigarettes.

Thus, Weil and Zinberg (1969) published an analysis of 5-minute speech samples obtained in an earlier study (Weil et al., 1968) in which they had found that habitual marijuana users showed no impairment in performance on the Digit Symbol Substitution Test and on the Pursuit Rotor Test ("naive" subjects showed impairment on both tests). The published analysis of the speech samples were obtained from habitual marijuana users who smoked a "high" dose (2 gm marijuana, 0.9% Δ^9-THC), although it is said that "naive" subjects showed similar but lesser effects. The speech samples were obtained in response to a request to relate an "interesting or dramatic experience" in their lives. Both presmoking and postsmoking speech samples were rated by "blind" judges on a 7-point bipolar scale (narrative quality, coherence, unity, awareness of a listener, thought completion, time orientation, free associative quality, degree of intimacy, and nature of imagery). The results indicated marked impairment, and the authors commented,

> . . . We think the problem is this: A "high" individual appears to have to expend more effort than when not intoxicated to remember from moment to moment the logical thread of what he is saying. . . . This speech difficulty has two principal manifestations: simple forgetting of what one is going to say next and a strong tendency to go off on irrelevant tangents because the line of thought is lost. . . .

and they conclude that marijuana may interfere with retrieval of information from immediate storage in the brain.

Likewise, illustrative of the impairment of immediate memory by marijuana, is the study of Drew et al. (1972). These investigators read the Babcock Story (which can be scored quantitatively) to 24 subjects (occasional users of marijuana) 30 minutes after smoking either marijuana cigarettes that were calibrated to deliver a dose of 25 μg/kg of Δ^9-THC (corresponding for a 70 kg man, to about 3.5 mg of Δ^9-THC in the cigarette—a "low" dose!) in 12 subjects, or cannabinoid-exhausted marijuana cigarettes (placebo) in the other 12 subjects. Half of the subjects in each group had also received a total of 40 mg of propranolol orally 24 hours before smoking, while the other half received an oral placebo. A few seconds after finishing the reading of the Babcock Story to the subjects, they were asked to repeat the story in as much detail as they could. Propranolol was found to exert no effects on recall, either alone or in interaction with Δ^9-THC. However, recall of the Babcock Story was impaired after smoking marijuana containing Δ^9-THC. In particular, "out of place memories" were increased significantly. The total number of "distortions" also tended to be moderately elevated, and the number of correct memory units tended to be decreased. The bizarre nature of distortions and out of place memories is revealed in samples of the material "recalled."

In an attempt to define more precisely the nature of the memory disturbance produced by marijuana, Melges et al. (1970a,b) studied the effects of an extract of marijuana on a task termed "goal directed serial alternation" (GDSA task). This "required that the subject simultaneously hold in mind and coordinate information as well as mental operations relevant to pursuing a goal. After giving the subject a number between 106 and 114, we asked him to subtract 7, then add 1, 2, or 3, and repeat such alternate subtraction and addition until he reached an exact goal between 46 and 54 that we specified for each trial. We asked the subject to recite his mental operations out loud and to work as rapidly and accurately as possible, without his using written props." Scores were based on time taken to perform the task and on the number of mistakes made (the higher the score, the greater the "temporal disintegration"). Subjects were 8 male graduate students and the doses of the extract contained 20, 40, and 60 mg of Δ^9-THC, given *orally*. Inasmuch as Δ^9-THC is approximately 2.6–3.0 times as potent when smoked than when ingested (Isbell et al., 1967), the highest dose of Δ^9-THC given orally would correspond to the Δ^9-THC content of "potent" marijuana cigarettes. The study was performed in a placebo-controlled double-blind manner. The results showed a dose-related impairment of GDSA performance, with the poorest performance taking place 1½ hours after ingestion of Δ^9-THC, and the impairment lasting longer with increased dosage. To a lesser but still significant extent, conventional digit span recall was impaired but no impairment was found on regular serial subtraction of sevens. Melges et al. (1970a) conclude: "This temporal incoordination of recent memories with intentions may account, in fact, for the disorganization of speech patterns that occurs under marijuana intoxication." In another study with the same extract and the same dose ranges, Melges et al. (1970b) employed the GDSA test together with a Temporal Integration Inventory and a Depersonalization Inventory. Changes in all these scores were positively and significantly correlated, confirming the hypothesis that as the subjects became more temporally disorganized, they simultaneously became depersonalized.

C. Alteration of Time Sense

Subjects intoxicated with marijuana frequently state that time seems to pass slowly. An early attempt to define this change objectively was made by Williams et al. (1946). Subjects were former opioid addicts who volunteered to smoke "good weed" (Δ^9-THC content unknown). Time estimation was tested by requiring 6 subjects to report when they thought 20 seconds had elapsed after a prearranged signal. Control estimates ranged from 10.4 to 17.7 seconds. After smoking marijuana, the range was 7.5 to 13.0 seconds. These results suggest that marijuana "speeds up the internal clock," but the mean pre- and postsmoking differences were not significant because of between-subject variability.

More definitive results were obtained by Clark et al. (1970), who administered a fixed dose of marijuana extract (Δ^9-THC content 0.3 mg/lb, or 46.2 mg/70 kg body weight) *orally* to 18 subjects, none of whom admitted marijuana use. The subjects were asked to guess the time required to complete digit-symbol matching tests which were designed to take approximately 15, 90, and 180 seconds. Both overestimates and underestimates were scored as "errors," which increased with the task duration under both control and drug conditions, but far more so under drug. Overestimation errors (total) were 89, 437, and 618 seconds for the 15, 90, and 180 second task durations, respectively, under control conditions, and 144, 620, and 1,309, respectively, for the drug condition. Underestimation errors were 26, 213, and 285 under control and 23, 35 and, 0 for the drug condition. There was no significant difference in the actual time subjects took to complete the tasks under control and drug conditions. It should be noted that the instructions to the subjects in the studies of Clark et al. (1970) required them to estimate open-ended durations of time, whereas in the studies of Williams et al. (1946) they were required to estimate when a fixed duration of time (20 seconds) had elapsed. The results of both studies indicate speeding up of the internal clock, though at first glance the data seem to be in opposite directions. Thus, if one can imagine the subjects looking at their internal clocks, which had been speeded up by marijuana, by actual time they would underestimate the time required for 20 seconds to elapse and overestimate the time required to complete a task for which no time specification was given.

The same interpretation applies to the data of Hollister and Gillespie (1970), who administered 27-39 mg (median dose 32 mg) of Δ^9-THC contained in a marijuana extract *orally* to 12 young subjects, most of whom had used marijuana occasionally, in a comparative study of the effects of marijuana, dextroamphetamine, 13–18 mg (median dose 15 mg), and alcohol, 50–68 gm (median dose 57 gm), as well as placebo. "Subjects were instructed to pay close attention to the duration of a tone, try to conceive a period of time exactly one-half the duration of the tone, and then after a lapse of 4 seconds to match that interval by depressing a telegraph key the appropriate length of time." The actual duration of the tones were 2, 7, and 12 seconds (relatively short, as compared with the tasks required by Clark et al., 1970). None of the drugs produced any significant changes except marijuana (for the 7-second tone) which, relative to placebo, prolonged the time estimate, again illustrating speeding up of the internal clock by marijuana.

In a comparison of the effects of "social" doses of alcohol (0.7 mg/kg of 95% alcohol), marijuana extract (Δ^9-THC content 0.35 mg/kg or 24.5 mg/70 kg body weight), and placebo given orally to young men who had used alcohol and marijuana (the latter no more often than once or twice a week), Tinklenberg et al. (1972) found that only marijuana had significant effects on the subjects' estimation of when 30, 60, and 120 seconds had elapsed (a task similar to that employed by Williams et al., 1946). In this study, time was "underproduced" by the subjects, suggesting speeding up of the internal clock. The investigators note that marijuana also increases the amplitude of the "expectancy wave" or Contingent Negative Variation (CNV) (Kopell et al., 1972), and that both speeding up of the internal clock and increased CNV amplitude had been reported for the psychotomimetic drug, LSD-25. In the study of Tinklenberg et al. (1972), neither marijuana nor alcohol produced significant changes in GDSA performance. The mean scores showed a consistent trend toward poorest performance under marijuana, the dose of which was roughly equivalent to the lowest of the three doses used in the earlier studies (Melges et al., 1970a,b), which showed dose-related impairment of performance on the GDSA.

Speeding up of the internal clock by marijuana is also suggested by the findings of Cappell et al. (1972), who studied differential reinforcement of low rate responding (pressing a key at intervals of at least 20 seconds, with "holds" of 0.5–4.0 seconds) for monetary reinforcement after subjects smoked two cigarettes, each containing placebo or marijuana (2, 4, and 8 mg Δ^9-THC), or drank a fluid containing a commercial orange drink or a cocktail of the orange drink with 0.48, 0.72, and 0.96 gm/kg or ethanol in the same fluid volume (producing blood ethanol levels of 48, 65, and 108 mg% at 20 minutes after completion of drinking). Marijuana produced a dose-related increase in the ratio of premature to premature plus late responding, as well as a dose-related increase in pulse rate and in self-rating of "marijuana high," whereas ethanol had no consistent measurable effect on performance. It should be noted that in this study "external" control (subjects received immediate feedback indicating whether each response was premature, correct, or late) was strong, yet marijuana impaired performance in the direction of premature responding.

In a comparison of the effects of cannabis resin given orally in the form of cakes (containing 8, 12, or 16 mg of Δ^9-THC) with those of alcohol (peak blood alcohol levels 67–129 mg%) on simulated automobile-driving ability, Bech et al. (1973) found that, unlike alcohol, cannabis produced a significant dose-related overestimation of time elapsed and of distance traversed. Though both effects were significantly dose-related, "subjective" time and distance estimation (How long and how far do you really *feel* you have been driving?) was more markedly affected than "objective" estimation. (How long and how far do you really *think* you have been driving?) The only significant effect of alcohol was overestimation of time elapsed when driving at 70 km/hour; no effect was observed when driving at 40 km/hour. After cannabis, the subjects reported spontaneously that time seemed to pass very slowly.

The impairment of "immediate" or "recent" memory and speeding up of the internal clock may be related effects of marijuana and other psychotomimetic agents. As formulated by L. L. Miller (personal communication), under marijuana,

> . . . an event that occurred recently in objective time is perceived as having occurred remotely in subjective time. This may result in an inability to sequentially integrate associations in long term store along a temporal dimension of recency. This, in effect, would increase the search time necessary to choose an association in long term storage for the purpose of matching it with information in the short term store. This would result in information in short term stores undergoing decay because relevant associations are not found quickly enough to block normal decay processes.

D. *"Adverse" Reactions*

From the biological point of view, the impairment of short-term memory and speeding up of the internal clock produced by marijuana are certainly "adverse," regardless of the evaluation by the subject of his own state, usually reported as a high. Popularly, however, adverse has been used to refer to bad trips, by which is meant extreme anxiety reactions or grossly psychotomimetic reactions that *alarm the user or his confrères*. As the studies of Isbell and co-workers (1967, 1968) and of Hollister et al. (1968) have shown, the possibility of the occurrence of paranoid reactions, hallucinations, and depersonalization (all adverse effects whether or not they alarm the user or his observers) increases with the dose of Δ^9-THC, given the same subjects, subject-expectancies, and experimental setting. In most of the cases of bad trips reported in the literature, the doses of Δ^9-THC smoked or ingested are unknown. However, Bromberg (1934) described 11 patients who, after smoking marijuana, exhibited visual and auditory hallucinations, manic states, depression, paranoid reactions, or catatonic excitement. The New York Mayor's Committee report (1944) contains descriptions of 9 individuals (among 72 subjects) who displayed "psychotic reactions" after administration of marijuana or cannabis extract. Keeler (1967) reported 11 cases of adverse reactions described retrospectively by marijuana smokers. Talbott and Teague (1969) described 12 psychotic reactions lasting 1–11 days after smoking marijuana cigarettes during a 1-year period among United States soldiers in Viet Nam. Wikler (1970) reported on two experimental subjects who became acutely paranoid after smoking a few marijuana cigarettes. Very recently, Chopra and Smith (1974) reported that 22 of 200 patients who were seen at the Drug Addiction Clinic in Calcutta, India, exhibited transient psychoses of variable duration after use of marijuana, bhang, ganja, or charas. Undoubtedly, many adverse (in the sense of bad trips) reactions to marijuana are not reported in the literature. Some indication of their frequency may be gained from the study of Ungerleider *et al.* (1968) who reported on a survey conducted in Los Angeles over an 18-month period to which 1584 of 2700 selected physicians and psychologists responded. These stated that they had seen 2389 cases of adverse reactions to LSD and 1887 to marijuana, but only 19–145 such cases as responses to other (probably far less frequently used) drugs.

The effects of heavy, long-term use of marijuana are difficult to assess because of cultural and socioeconomic differences in parts of the world where marijuana use is common, and the restrictions placed on experimental chronic intoxication with marijuana or Δ^9-THC in the United States. In 1946, Williams *et al.* reported on behavioral changes in 6 former opioid addicts who were allowed to smoke "good weed" (Δ^9-THC content unknown) *ad libitum* for 39 consecutive days. The "euphoric" effects of marijuana disappeared after a few days, following which subjects showed decreased activity, indolence and nonproductivity, and neglect of personal hygiene. During this period, chemosis, mydriasis, increased pulse rate, and increased appetite (especially for sweets) were noted initially, but declined later. Intellectual functioning (Stanford-Binet test) was slightly impaired. On the MacQuarrie Test for Mechanical Ability, performance was improved when speed alone was the relevant factor, but impaired when coordination and manual skills were necessary. No consistent changes were noted in the electroencephalogram. On abrupt cessation of smoking marijuana, all subjects complained of "jitteriness" during the first day or two, but no objective signs of a withdrawal syndrome were found. Thereafter, the subjects' behavior returned rapidly to their presmoking pattern, which was characterized by attention to their occupations and prison-research ward "rules," as well as maintenance of good personal hygiene.

The behavior of these subjects during chronic marijuana intoxication is reminiscent of the "amotivational syndrome," described by West (1970) for many chronic marijuana users in the "national scene":

> . . . the experienced clinician observes . . . personality changes that may grow subtly over long periods of time: diminished drive, lessened ambition, decreased motivation, apathy, shortened attention span, distractibility, poor judgment, impaired communication skills, loss of effectiveness, introversion, magical thinking, derealization and depersonalization, diminished capacity to carry out complex plans or prepare realistically for the future, a peculiar fragmentation of thought, habit deteriorations and progressive loss of insight. There is a clinical impression of organicity to this syndrome that I simply cannot shake off or explain away.

Similar findings have been reported by Kolansky and Moore for 38 adolescents and young adults (1971), who smoked marijuana two or more times weekly, and for 13 adults, who smoked marijuana 3–10 times per week for 16 months to 6 years (1972). The authors, psychoanalytical psychiatrists, found no evidence of pre-marijuana psychopathology in these patients and noted that in most cases the behavioral and mental changes (which included 8 cases of psychosis among the 38 adolescent and young adults) disappeared or improved after cessation of marijuana smoking. Other drug use (LSD-25, amphetamines) was minimal or absent, and the authors concluded that the etiological factor was marijuana alone, producing "organic" changes in the brain. In the latter connection, Campbell et al. (1971) have reported air-encephalographic studies on 10 "chronic cannabis smokers" (who also used LSD-25, amphetamines, and, occasionally, other drugs) which revealed dilation of the cerebral ventricles, possibly due to damage to the caudate nuclei, basal ganglia, and the structures adjacent to the third ventricle, in comparison with ventricular measurements made on "normal" air-encephalograms that had been obtained for diagnostic reasons on 13 controls who displayed no neurological signs or increased protein in the cerebrospinal fluid. Though the subjects of this study were not "pure" marijuana users, the findings are of great interest and may conceivably be checked by appropriate animal research.

On the other hand, Bowman and Pihl (1973) found no significant differences whatever in performance on a battery of tests between a total of 24 nonusers of marijuana and 30 chronic heavy users (tested not less than 4 hours after smoking) recruited from "the lower social classes" in Jamaica. The tests were designed to assess physiological, sensory and perceptual-motor functioning, concept formation, abstracting ability and cognitive style, as well as memory (some tests with a delay condition). The marijuana smoked by the users was very potent, the Δ^9-THC content of two-thirds of the samples being in excess of 4–5%. The authors mention that they often observed users smoking large quantities of marijuana, showing only minimal behavioral effects, and conclude that this points to the development of behavioral adaptation or tolerance. Contrasting their findings with those reviewed above, these investigators suggest that the latter may represent "cultural artifacts rather than drug effects," or that the adverse behavioral changes reported in the literature were observed in populations that did not use marijuana sufficiently heavily for tolerance to have been developed. It should be noted, however, that the battery of tests administered by Bowman and Pihl (1973) are unlikely to be sensitive to such changes as the development of more passive, inward turning, relaxed and careless drifting, apathy, loss of effectiveness and diminished willingness to carry out long-term plans, endure frustration, successfully master new material, impairment of verbal facility in speaking or writing, and preoccupation with childlike magical thinking, which characterize the "amotivational syndrome" described "anecdotally" by McGlothlin and West (1968) and which can have serious consequences for middle-class persons in a competitive, industrialized society. Far from being a cultural artifact, the requirements for long-range planning, goal-directedness, verbal facility, and sophisticated thinking in such a society constitute an important set of variables for "higher" nervous system functioning, on which chronic heavy use of marijuana might exert deleterious effects. Bowman and Pihl (1973) also state that their study gave no indications of organic brain damage among the marijuana users because the latter scored normally on tests (concept formation and memory) that reveal impairment in chronic heavy alcohol use. This, of course, does not rule out the possibility of mild degrees of cerebral atrophy reported by Campbell *et al.* (1971), discussed above.

Adverse effects of chronic heavy use of hashish (Δ^9-THC content higher than that in American marijuana) among soldiers stationed in West Germany has been reported by Tennant and Groesbeck (1972). In 392 "moderate" users (smoking up to 10 or 12 gm of hashish per month) no ill effects were observed other than "hash throat" (rhinopharyngitis). However, in 110 "heavy" users (50–600 gm of hashish per month for 3–18 months) all showed apathy, dullness, lethargy, mild to severe impairment of judgment, concentration and memory, poor hygiene, and slowed speech. Such changes disappeared after cessation of hashish smoking in 16 of 32 subjects, but persisted for longer periods in the other 16, after detoxification. Persistent schizophrenic reactions were observed in 112 soldiers who had smoked 250–500 gm of hashish per month and who had used hallucinogens and/or amphetamines as well as alcohol. With hashish alone, 5 first-time users developed "panic" reactions and 13 developed acute toxic psychoses. Over a period of 3 years, 85 cases of such psychoses were noted in soldiers who used hashish, hallucinogens, amphetamines, alcohol, or "downers" (tranquilizers, sedatives, and analgesics). "Flashback" phenomenon could not be documented in any soldier who used only hashish, but 15 soldiers experienced the hallucinations of a previous LSD-25 trip while under the influence of hashish.

E. Tolerance and Dependence

It has been documented in animals (pigeons, rats, dogs, and monkeys) that tolerance develops on repeated administration of marijuana or Δ^9-THC (Carlini, 1968; McMillan et al., 1971; Harris, 1971; Deneau and Kaymakcalan, 1971). Deneau and Kaymakcalan also described an abstinence syndrome in monkeys which appeared 12 hours and lasted 5 days after abrupt withdrawal of Δ^9-THC, consisting of anorexia, yawning, piloerection, irritability, biting fingers, hair-pulling, tremors, twitches, photophobia, and apparent hallucinations. At the start of the study, none of the 6 monkeys initiated self-injections of Δ^9-THC, and the drug was then given by automatic injection; during the appearance of the abstinence syndrome, 2 of the monkeys initiated self-injection and maintained themselves on Δ^9-THC.

In man, however, experimental investigations on chronic marijuana smoking (or administration of Δ^9-THC) have been very few. The fact that habitual heavy marijuana users can smoke large quantities of high potency marijuana without *grossly* obvious harm (see review by Nahas, 1973) is certainly indicative of tolerance. Yet, it has been claimed that habitual marijuana smokers display "reverse tolerance," i.e., they will report a high after smoking a Δ^9-THC standardized cigarette which, in naive subjects, does not produce a high (Weil et al., 1968). However, careful study of the paper by Weil et al. (1968) reveals that although the naive subjects did not report a high they did report that "things seemed to go slower," "a sense of the past disappearing," "fits of silliness," "I would keep forgetting what I was doing"—changes that, had they been properly "educated," would have been interpreted as a high. In contrast to their impaired performance on the Digit Symbol Substitution and Pursuit Rotor tests, improvement rather than impairment was observed in the habitual marijuana smokers who reported a high. The failure of marijuana to impair performance in the habitual smoker is indicative of tolerance in the classical sense; their report of a high may, perhaps, be explained as a placebo effect, inasmuch as Jones (1971) found in a double-blind study on 25 infrequent and 25 frequent users of marijuana that whereas the infrequent users did distinguish placebo and marijuana cigarettes on a global subjective rating scale, the frequent users did not. Jones (1971) concluded that "with the frequent users, the correct smell and taste seem to be an adequate cue to induce an identifiable subjective state not distinguishable from that induced by marijuana. These data do not support the pharmacological interpretation of the phenomenon of 'reverse tolerance' . . ." Quite the contrary, Jones (1971) presents evidence that after smoking marijuana (9 mg of Δ^9-THC), acceleration of the pulse rate, salivary flow decrease, impairment on the Digit Symbol Substitution test, and increase in complex reaction time were significantly less for frequent than for infrequent marijuana users, differences that indicate the greater development of tolerance in the former.

The development of tolerance to the "euphorigenic" effects of smoking marijuana cigarettes has been alluded to above in connection with the early study of Williams et al. (1946). More recently, Volavka et al. (1971) reported similar findings in 4 former opioid addicts who smoked two marijuana cigarettes (6.5 mg Δ^9-THC per cigarette) twice daily for a scheduled 22 days.

> During the initial days, postsmoking euphoria was prevalent. Dysphoria first appeared during the third to sixth days and persisted for the remaining sessions. Paranoid thoughts and depression developed. In subjects 1 and 2, dysphoria was so pronounced that their participation was discontinued on the 17th and 10th days, respectively. The other two subjects were persuaded to complete the entire 22-day schedule. These symptoms completely disappeared within 5 days after the last administration of *Cannabis.*

Biochemical studies also indicate the development of at least "metabolic" tolerance to Δ^9-THC. Lemberger et al. (1971a,b) reported that after intravenous injection of a "nonpharmacological" dose (0.5 mg) of radioactively labeled Δ^9-THC, the disappearance of the drug from plasma occurred in an initial rapid phase, followed by a slower phase. The half-life of the slower phase was 57 hours in the nonusers of marijuana, but only 28 hours in the long-term users. An active metabolite, 11-hydroxy-Δ^9-THC appeared in the plasma of both nonusers and long-term users of marijuana within 10 minutes after intravenous injection of Δ^9-THC. Only the long-term users reported marijuana-like effects and these investigators speculated on the possibilities of increased enzyme induction (which might convert Δ^9-THC more rapidly into 11-hydroxy-Δ^9-THC), cumulative effects on repeated administration, increased receptive sensitivity, or a learned response, to account for this phenomenon.

No physiological abstinence syndrome has been observed in man following withdrawal of marijuana. However, the persistence of marijuana use despite severe social consequences in many societies suggests that the drug can produce what has been called "psychic" dependence. Soueif (1967), discussing hashish use in Egypt, points out that

> ... there is a definite pattern of oscillation of temperamental traits, swinging between two opposite poles, that of social ease, a desire to mix, acquiescence, elation and agreeableness (globally called euphoria) when under immediate drug effect and that of ascendancy, seclusiveness, negativism, depression of the mood and pugnacity (which may be considered as the main components of a psychic withdrawal syndrome) when Ss are deprived of the drug. *This pattern of oscillation of temperament may be considered the behavioral core of a state of psychic dependence.* One of the most salient characteristics of this state is a need to continue taking the drug not only to attain the feeling of well-being, but also to avoid feeling low.

The term, psychic dependence, is extremely vague, sometimes referring to processes of social reinforcement, sometimes to reinforcement through reduction of tensions that existed prior to first drug use, and sometimes to reinforcement through reduction of tensions generated by previous drug use in the absence of demonstrable physiological changes (Wikler, 1971). Etiologically, there would seem to be no justification for designating behavioral changes (including verbal reports) as "psychic," in contradistinction to "physical" (physiological) changes, even though both types of change may be unconditioned or conditioned. If it could be shown that the "oscillation of temperament" was a *consequence* of heavy hashish smoking, and not an antecedent, then this phenomenon (also noted in the few experimental studies reported on chronic marijuana smoking) should be classified as evidence of "physical" dependence (on the properties of Δ^9-THC). Further research on the behavioral changes *following* the marijuana high during chronic marijuana smoking in persons previously free from oscillation of temperament is needed to verify or refute the popular impression that if dependence on marijuana develops at all, it is of the psychic rather than the physical variety.

The data reviewed in this section indicate that, from the biological point of view marijuana, with Δ^9-THC content usually found in American cigarettes of moderate strength produces adverse effects measurable in terms of speeding up the internal clock and impairment of the ability to organize thoughts in a temporal sequence leading to a goal, with consequent impairment of certain kinds of immediate, or short-term memory. Furthermore, these adverse effects are dose related. In addition, smoking marijuana of ordinary strength can induce bad trips (paranoid reactions, anxiety, and panic) unpredictably, and smoking of marijuana with higher Δ^9-THC content can predictably produce hallucinations, depersonalization, and derealization, very similar to those produced by higher doses of LSD-25 (whether or not these are also called bad trips depends on the aesthetic orientation of the subject and/or his observer). Tolerance to Δ^9-THC develops with repeated frequent use, though the rates of development of tolerance to different effects remain to be elucidated. There is also suggestive evidence indicating that conditioning of marijuana effects proceeds with repeated use (cf. the placebo effect) and that repeated, heavy use can lead to dependence (physical, not psychic). Finally, the question of organic brain damage in heavy marijuana users (amotivational syndrome; cerebral ventricular dilatation) needs to be investigated further.

III. AESTHETIC ISSUES

Throughout history, man has used two frames of reference for appraisal of reality. One is a set of terms and concepts based on experiences connected with problems of survival and domination of the physical world; to the extent that such terms and concepts can be tested for predictive utility, they are called "scientific." The other represents an attempt to explain the unknown in terms of the undefined—terms and concepts which cannot be defined publicly and thereby be subjected to the test of predictive utility. These may be called "mystical" and are particularly prominent in the discourses and writings of certain religionists, poets, writers, and social philosophers as well as some scientists. The difference in aesthetic values between the mystical and scientific orientations is apparent in the use of the term high to refer to effects of marijuana that are biologically adverse. After proper indoctrination by his peers, the user reports that marijuana induces clarity of thinking, original, brilliant ideas, heightened perception, and novel insights (all of which are, presumably, subsumed under the term high), whereas the observer can detect only distortions of time-sense and impairment of logical thought as revealed by speech analyses. Furthermore, the marijuana user *learns* to regard such a high as pleasurable (Becker, 1968). Similar considerations apply to the term "psychedelic" ("consciousness" or "mind-expanding") which is sometimes used to refer to the effects of marijuana (Leary, 1968). "Mind-expansion" implies that a scale exists, along which the dimensions of "mind" can be measured. In the nonintoxicated state, illogical thought, distortions of perception, hallucinations, and paranoid reactions would be classed as "errors"; to the psychedelists, however, when produced by marijuana (or LSD-25), they are considered evidence of mind-expansion.

Recently, the term "recreational drug" has come into vogue among the supporters of legalization of marijuana (Becker, 1968). By recreational is meant "pleasure-giving," without the compulsive use to repeat the experience, as in the case of addicting drugs. As already noted, the pleasurable effects of marijuana are a learned derivative of the high which, in turn, is a derivative of mystical interpretations of the effects of marijuana on time-sense, logical thinking, and perception. The same may be said of many drugs (psychotomimetics, sedative hypnotics, and tranquilizers) which differ markedly in terms of their biological effects. Therefore, all that would be necessary to qualify an agent as a recreational drug would be social reinforcement of the concept of pleasurable as applied to the mystically perceived effects of such an agent. The social consequences of acceptance of the concept of recreational drug would be the permeation of our society with adherents of numerous cultists deriving primary reinforcement from varieties of drugs and secondary reinforcement from drug cult ideologies.

IV. SOCIAL ISSUES

Consideration of the social issues necessarily brings in dimensions which are difficult to assess scientifically. Among these is the fact that in all societies the habitual user of particular drugs has inevitably come to reflect certain particular orientations to life, which may or may not represent that of the dominant groups within the society. In the United States, alcohol is by far the most popular drug and reflects, in general, the need for assertiveness and aggressiveness (McClelland, 1973). In contrast, marijuana is the favorite drug of the "hippie" subculture and of many youths who share certain hippie values, such as noncompetitiveness and mystical preoccupation. Acceptance of one drug or the other therefore entails acceptance of sizeable numbers of persons who display such deviant patterns of behavior. Furthermore, the unrestricted use of alcohol has brought with it a very serious situation in which some 5–6 million people are said to have "alcohol problems," ranging from disruption of family life to delirium tremens and postalcoholic organic brain disease (American Medical Association, 1967). Therefore, the failure of Prohibition in the United States must be regarded as a disaster, at least from the standpoint of health. The possible health consequences of legalization of marijuana are more difficult to assess. It may be expected that a great increase in the number of casual users and inevitably of heavy users of marijuana would follow such an action, thereby increasing the problems associated with marijuana dependence. Furthermore, increasing use of marijuana would lead to an increasing use of other drugs, notably LSD-25 and other hallucinogens. Thus Brill et al. (1971), surveying young college students, report that

> Use of other drugs is clearly related to marijuana use. . . . A total of 100% of the daily marijuana users and 84% of the weekly marijuana users have tried drugs, in contrast to 22% of the monthly marijuana users, 18% of the less frequent users, 20% of the ones who tried marijuana but quit, and 0% of the subjects who never tried marijuana. The types of other drugs tried . . . in order of frequency of mention are: hallucinogens, "downers," "uppers," marijuana-type drugs (hashish, tetrahydrocannabinol), and "hard" drugs (heroin, opium and cocaine).

Pillard (1970) states, "In short, no one has failed to find a statistical relation between marijuana and the use of other drugs—legal and illegal." Incidentally, this relationship does not exist for the use of alcohol and the use of LSD-25 (Pillard, 1971). The chi-square analysis presented by Pillard (1971) should also be applied to the relationship between marijuana and opioid drug use, ridiculed by Grinspoon (1971), who stated, ". . . doubtless they all drank milk, ate food, read comic books, wore clothes, and rode bicycles before they used either cannabis or heroin, yet, as far as I know, no one has maintained that any of these activities lead to cannabis or heroin use." That, in the United States, the majority of heroin users had smoked marijuana earlier, is well known; they had also used alcohol and, in many cases, amphetamines and other stimulants as well as sedative-hypnotic drugs, but at least with regard to prior use of alcohol there would appear to be no significant statistical relationship to their subsequent use of heroin. In Egypt, Soueif (1971) found a positive relationship between years of hashish consumption and percentage of opium takers among hashish users, and in England, Paton (1968) reported a parallel increase in the number of cannabis offenses and the number of heroin addicts. Such data cannot be ignored!

"Choosing" between alcohol and marijuana (or accepting both) is therefore equivalent to "choosing" between syphilis and gonorrhea. One may ask whether either drug is necessary. One answer to this, Leary's (1968) "second commandment," "Thou shalt not prevent thy fellow man from altering his own consciousness," is presumptuous, since in our culture the use of "mind-altering" drugs is propagated among our youth (who cannot give "informed consent") by their drug-using peers, and this violates the rights and duties of parents in child-rearing. A commentator has the privilege as well as the duty of specifying the kind of society that would be tolerable to him. In the opinion of the writer, a society in which alcoholic inebriation and marijuana intoxication are *contained* would be tolerable. Control of alcohol has failed, due to the all-pervasiveness of alcohol use for many centuries in Western and American societies. If marijuana is legalized, control of its abuse and of more potent Δ^9-THC-containing substances (e.g., hashish) will become increasingly difficult.

On the other hand, methods of containing marijuana use are debatable. Certainly the harsh penalties inflicted on marijuana and other illegal drug users in the United States are unjust in view of the fact that they punish the victim. Furthermore, there is no evidence that the degree of control effected is a function of the severity of the penalty imposed. It would therefore be rational to reduce penalties for possession for personal use of marijuana and all other illegal drugs to fines, weekend work-house sentences, and other substitutes for jail sentences. Difficult as the distinction between possession for personal use and for sale may be, the law should reserve its severe penalties for large-quantity "wholesale" purveyors of illegal drugs. Hopefully, such an approach to drug control will contain the marijuana and other drug problems though it may not eradicate them.

REFERENCES

American Medical Association. (1967). "Alcoholism." Amer. Med. Ass., Chicago, Illinois.
Ames, F. (1958). *J. Ment. Sci.* **104**, 972–999.
Bech, P., Rafaelson, L., and Rafaelson, O. J. (1973). *Psychopharmacologia* **32**, 373–381.
Becker, H. S. (1968). In "The Marihuana Papers" (D. Solomon, ed.), pp. 65–102. Signet Books, New York.
Bowman, M., and Pihl, R. O. (1973). *Psychopharmacologia* **29**, 159–170.
Brill, N. Q., Crumpton, E., and Grayson, H. M. (1971). *Arch. Gen. Psychiat.* **24**, 163–165.
Bromberg, W. (1934). *Amer. J. Psychiat.* **91**, 303–330.

Campbell, A. M. G., Evans, M., Thomson, J. L. G., and Williams, M. J. (1971). *Lancet* **2**, 1219–1225.
Cappell, H. C. D., Webster, B. S., Herring, S., and Ginsberg, R. (1972). *J. Pharmacol. Exper. Ther.* **182**, 195–203.
Carlini, E. A. (1968). *Pharmacology* **1**, 135–142.
Chopra, G. S., and Smith, J. W. (1974). *Arch. Gen. Psychiat.* **30**, 24–27.
Clark, L. A., Hughes, R., and Nakashima, E. N. (1970). *Arch. Gen. Psychiat.* **23**, 193–198.
Deneau, G. A., and Kaymakcalan, S. (1971). *Pharmacologist* **13**, 246.
Drew, W. G., Kiplinger, G. F., Miller, L. L., and Marx, M. (1972). *Clin. Pharmacol. Ther.* **13**, 526–533.
Grinspoon, L. (1971). "Marihuana Reconsidered," p. 246. Harvard Univ. Press, Cambridge, Massachusetts.
Harris, L. S. (1971). *Pharmacol. Rev.* **23**, 285–294.
Hollister, L. E., and Gillespie, H. K. (1970). *Arch. Gen. Psychiat.* **23**, 199–203.
Hollister, L. E., Richards, R. K., and Gillespie, H. K. (1968). *Clin. Pharmacol. Ther.* **9**, 783–791.
Isbell, H., and Jasinski, D. R. (1969). *Psychopharmacologia* **14**, 115–123.
Isbell, H., Gorodetzky, C. W., Jasinski, D., Claussen, U., von Spulak, F., and Korte, F. (1967). *Psychopharmacologia*, **11**, 184–188.
Jones, R. T. (1971). *Ann. N.Y. Acad. Sci.* **191**, 155–165.
Keeler, M. H. (1967). *Amer. J. Psychiat.* **124**, 674–677.
Kolansky, H., and Moore, W. T. (1971). *J. Amer. Med. Ass.* **216**, 486–492.
Kolansky, H., and Moore, W. T. (1972). *J. Amer. Med. Ass.* **222**, 35–41.
Kopell, B. S., Tinklenberg, J. R., and Hollister, L. E. (1972). *Arch. Gen. Psychiat.* **27**, 809–811.
Leary, T. (1968). *In* "The Marihuana Papers" (D. Solomon, ed.), pp. 121–140. Signet Books, New York.
Lemberger, L., Tamarkin, N. R., Axelrod, J., and Kopin, I. J. (1971a). *Science* **173**, 72–74.
Lemberger, L., Axelrod, J., and Kopin, I. J. (1971b). *Ann. N.Y. Acad. Sci.* **191**, 142–154.
McClelland, D. (1973). Paper read at 12th Annu. Meet. Amer. Coll. Neuropsychopharmacol., 1973.
McGlothlin, W. H., and West, L. J. (1968). *Amer. J. Psychiat.* **125**, 370–378.
McMillan, D. E., Dewey, W. I., and Harris, L. S. (1971). *Ann. N.Y. Acad. Sci.* **191**, 83–99.
Melges, F. T., Tinklenberg, J. R., Hollister, L. E., and Gillespie, H. K. (1970a). *Science* **168**, 1118–1120.
Melges, F. T., Tinklenberg, J. R., Hollister, L. E., and Gillespie, H. K. (1970b). *Arch. Gen. Psychiat.* **23**, 204–210.
Nahas, G. G. (1973). "Marihuana—Deceptive Weed," pp. 181–187. Raven Press, New York.
New York Mayor's Committee on Marihuana. (1944). "The Marihuana Problem in the City of New York." Jacques Cattell Press, Lancaster, Pennsylvania.
Paton, W. D. M. (1968). *Advan. Sci.* **25**, 200–212.
Pillard, R. C. (1970). *N. Engl. J. Med.* **283**, 294–303.
Pillard, R. C. (1971). *N. Engl. J. Med.* **285**, 416–417.
Silva, M. T. A., and Carlini, E. A. (1968). *Psychopharmacologia* **13**, 332–340.
Soueif, M. I. (1967). *Bull. Narcotics* **19**, 1–12.
Soueif, M. I. (1971). *Bull. Narcotics* **23**, 17–28.

Talbott, J. A., and Teague, J. W. (1969). *J. Amer. Med. Ass.* **210,** 299–302.
Tennant, F. S., and Groesbeck, C. J. (1972). *Arch. Gen. Psychiat.* **27,** 133–136.
Tinklenberg, J. R., Kopell, B. S., Melges, F. T., and Hollister, L. E. (1972). *Arch. Gen. Psychiat.* **27,** 812–815.
Ungerleider, J. T., Fisher, D. D., Goldsmith, S. R., Fuller, M., and Forgy, E. (1968). *Amer. J. Psychiat.* **125,** 108–113.
Volavka, J., Dornbush, R., Feldstein, S., Clare, G., Zaks, A., Fink, M., and Freedman, A. M. (1971). *Ann. N.Y. Acad. Sci.* **191,** 206–215.
Weil, A. T., and Zinberg, N. E. (1969). *Nature (London)* **22,** 434–437.
Weil, A. T., Zinberg. N. E., and Nelson, J. M. (1968). *Science* **162,** 1234–1242.
West, L. J. (1970). *In* "Psychotomimetic Drugs" (D. H. Efron, ed.), p. 328. Raven Press, New York.
Wikler, A. (1970). *Arch. Gen. Psychiat.* **23,** 320–325.
Wikler, A. (1971). *Psychol. Med.* **1,** 377–380.
Williams, E. G., Himmelsbach, C. K., Wikler, A., Ruble, D. C., and Lloyd, B. J. (1946). *Pub. Health Rep.* **61,** 1059–1083.

Chapter 3

MOTOR AND MENTAL PERFORMANCE WITH MARIJUANA: RELATIONSHIP TO ADMINISTERED DOSE OF Δ^9-TETRAHYDROCANNABINOL AND ITS INTERACTION WITH ALCOHOL*

JOSEPH E. MANNO, BARBARA R. MANNO, GLEN F. KIPLINGER, AND ROBERT B. FORNEY

I. Introduction	46
II. Preparation and Calibration of Marijuana Cigarettes for Administration of Uniform Dosage	47
III. Establishment of Experimental Procedures	49
A. Motor Function Performance	49
B. Delayed Auditory Feedback	51
C. Static Equilibrium	52
D. Subjective Tests	53
E. Setting	53
F. Experimental Protocol	54
IV. Marijuana Dosage Form	55
V. Motor Performance	56
VI. Mental Performance and Ataxia	59
VII. Physiological Reactions to THC and Alcohol	59
VIII. Subjective Reactions	64
IX. Significance and Conclusion	69
References	71

* Supported in part by USPHS Grants MH15864, GM1089, and DA00136.

I. INTRODUCTION

Cannabis has been used for many thousands of years because of its ability to produce euphoria in man. Undoubtedly, many people have noted that smoking too much or too powerful a cigarette made from cannabis (marijuana) can produce intoxication. Although these actions are not as pronounced as the staggering appearance that commonly accompanies alcohol intoxication, nonetheless the subtle changes in memory retention, the inability to perform fine tasks, or coordination changes would certainly be observed. It has not been until recently, however, that the chemistry of the constituents of marijuana, the cannabinols, has been completely understood. It is now felt with reasonable certainty that most of the actions produced by smoking a marijuana cigarette are due to the content of Δ^9-tetrahydrocannabinol (THC) in the marijuana (Mechoulam, 1973).

Before we had the ability to characterize marijuana by its content of THC, several comprehensive investigations into the sociological, medical, psychological, and pharmacological aspects of marijuana were conducted in this country. Perhaps the most comprehensive of these was the investigation commissioned by Mayor LaGuardia (Mayor's Committee on Marijuana, 1944) of New York City in the early 1940's in an attempt to assess marijuana problems in that city. Although their investigation was broad in scope, our discussion will be limited to the psychomotor function effects which they found. Their tests included determinations of static equilibrium, hand steadiness, tapping speed, grip strength, simple and complex reaction times, auditory acuity, as well as perception of time and distance. The simpler psychomotor functions such as speed of tapping and simple reaction time were affected slightly by large doses and negligibly or not at all by small doses of THC extracts administered orally. The more complex functions such as static equilibrium, hand steadiness, and complex reaction time were substantially and adversely affected by both doses of marijuana and marijuana extract. The effects of the large dose were consistently, but not proportionately, greater than the effects of the small dose. Subjects in the La Guardia study were persons who had used marijuana and persons that were naive to the drug. This report indicated that the effects of marijuana were more pronounced in naive subjects than in experienced marijuana users. The first double-blind investigation into the clinical psychological effects of smoking marijuana was reported by Weil *et al.* (1968). These investigators assayed the

3. Motor and Mental Performance with Marijuana

marijuana samples for the content of THC and administered two doses of marijuana in the form of two different size samples as marijuana cigarettes. They also instructed their subjects to smoke in a uniform manner in order to standardize the dose administration. They found that smoking the marijuana cigarette did not produce any effect on some continuous performance tests. However, a decrement in performance was observed in the digit symbol substitution test when it was administered after smoking either the high or the low dose of marijuana. This decrement occurred only in the subjects who had never smoked marijuana previously. They also found a decrement in performance with the pursuit rotor in the same subjects after smoking marijuana.

II. PREPARATION AND CALIBRATION OF MARIJUANA CIGARETTES FOR ADMINISTRATION OF UNIFORM DOSAGE

Although a cigarette is an unusual dosage form for the administration of a drug, it does represent the primary manner by which marijuana is used in this country. As such, it would seem that the act of smoking might have some effect on subjective performance by individuals undergoing clinical testing. In order to lessen the liability of a cigarette as a dosage form, a rigorous procedure of calibration of the marijuana and a highly standardized smoking procedure were used in our investigations so that a uniform dosage could be presented to all subjects utilized in the testing procedure. In order to accomplish this end, as many variables as possible were eliminated. The dry flowering tops from Thailand marijuana were carefully separated from the stems and seeds and passed through a 10–20 mesh sieve. A more smooth burning of the marijuana was assured by this isolation into uniform particle size. This marijuana was then extracted and analyzed by gas chromatography and the exact concentration of THC as well as other cannabinoids was determined. Because our investigations were conducted in a double-blind fashion, it was also necessary to prepare a suitable placebo. This was done by exhaustively extracting the marijuana in a Soxhlet extractor with three different chemical solvents, i.e., petroleum ether, chloroform, and alcohol. After extraction in this manner the marijuana was removed, dried completely, hydrated by soaking in water, and dried at 85°C for 3 hours. Only in this way was it possible to produce a placebo which exactly resembled the natural marijuana in odor, appearance, and burning characteristics. The solvents which we used to extract the marijuana were further analyzed to determine the exact concentration of THC in the marijuana samples.

From our preliminary investigations and the data of other investigators, it was determined that approximately 5 to 10 mg of THC administered as a marijuana cigarette could produce some of the characteristic effects of smoking marijuana (Hollister et al., 1968, 1970; Isbell and Jasinski, 1969; Weil et al., 1968). It was also reasoned that variations in an individual's manner of smoking, for example, the time of inhalation, the amount of time that the smoke is to be held in the lungs, and the amount of the marijuana "joint" that is to be smoked could affect the amount of THC delivered to a person acting as an experimental subject. By observation of experienced marijuana smokers and the manner by which they usually use marijuana, certain standards for smoking a joint in the laboratory were set forth. It was noted that it usually takes from 2 to 4 seconds to inhale a puff of smoke from a marijuana cigarette. Each inhaled puff was held in the lungs for 30–60 seconds before expiration. In order to simulate this process and to determine the approximate amount of cannabinols delivered in the smoke, an artificial smoking machine was devised by attaching a cigarette to a sintered glass tube placed in a side-arm flask filled with chloroform. A Harvard respirator pump was then attached to the side arm of the filter flask and air drawn through the system to "smoke" the marijuana cigarette. Any cannabinols delivered in the smoke were trapped in the chloroform and could be analyzed by gas chromatography.

Perhaps the most difficult variable to control was the amount of smoke inspired by the experimental subject during the smoking process. For example, an average puff inspiration lasts for 2 to 4 seconds; however, certain individuals may inspire for 1 second while some may take up to 5 or 6 seconds. In order to test the effect of this difference in inspiration time, the pump on the artificial smoking machine was set so that inspiration lasted for varied periods of time. Several cigarettes were even smoked so that air was continuously drawn through each marijuana cigarette for the entire period of time required for its complete combustion. For all conditions, the amount of THC delivered in the smoke was approximately 50% ± 10%, indicating that the size of the puff did not seem to be a determining factor in the amount of smoke delivered.

An additional variable requiring elimination was the amount of time that the smoke was held in the lungs of the smoker. The amount of THC expired in the breath of the smoker after holding the smoke for approximately 30–40 seconds was measured by having them blow through a sintered glass tube into chloroform so that any exhaled THC could be quantitated. Less than 1% of inhaled THC was lost in the expired air. The final condition to be controlled was the amount of the marijuana cigarette which was actually consumed. By marking at measured points along the cigarette and smoking through predetermined lengths, we analyzed for the amount of cannabinol delivered in the smoke. Marking and smoking to any point on the cigarette was not an accurate method of delivering a uniform dose of smoke, and variability in THC delivered between cigarettes smoked to the same length was upward of ±20%. To eliminate this variability, we required that our subjects consume the entire cigarette. This was accomplished by attaching mosquito forceps to the end of the cigarette and utilizing the forceps as a means of support. In this manner only a few milligrams of unburned marijuana were left after the subjects had completed the smoking session. All the "roaches" were individually analyzed and the maximum amount of THC remaining in any roach was 0.5 mg.

Since the marijuana which we used contained a relatively high concentration of THC (approximately 3.8%), it was necessary to dilute the marijuana with placebo in order to obtain a marijuana joint with the desired concentration of THC. Placebo material was prepared from marijuana which had had the cannabinols removed by solvent extraction. Solvents were removed by drying and rehydration of the plant material as described for preparation of the marijuana cigarettes. In investigations where THC was administered on a microgram per kilogram basis, varying amounts of placebo were diluted with the amount of drug marijuana necessary to achieve the dosage for each individual subject. The marijuana cigarettes were rolled in a hand cigarette rolling machine, placed in small vials, and sealed under nitrogen. Cigarettes were coded and then stored at 0° under nitrogen until the time of use. This manner of storage prevented any decomposition of the THC in the cigarettes.

III. ESTABLISHMENT OF EXPERIMENTAL PROCEDURES

A. Motor Function Performance

The pursuit meter is designed to provide a visual pattern of known character and adjustable complexity on the screen of a dual-beam oscilloscope. The test subject is provided with a control mechanism (steering wheel) which is operated in response to a preprogrammed pattern. The response pattern and an error signal from the pursuit meter are displayed graphically for evaluation. A block diagram of the pursuit meter is shown in Fig. 1. The signal from one or two low-frequency function generators is applied to the Y axis of the A beam of a dual-beam oscilloscope and

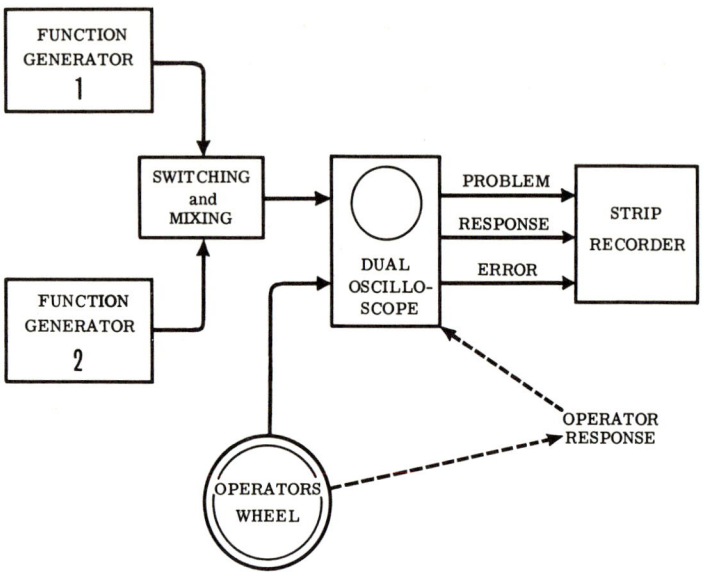

Fig. 1. Block diagram of pursuit meter.

appears as a moving dot of light on the oscilloscope screen. Generators can produce sine-, triangular-, or square-wave functions at varying frequencies. By mixing the signal from two of the generators operating at different frequencies and/or patterns, a more complex task can be presented to the test subject. The operator attempts to superimpose a movable dot of light which he controls upon that which is produced by the function generator by using the steering wheel attached to a variable potentiometer and the Y axis of the B beam of the oscilloscope. The output of this potentiometer is matched to the output from the generators. If the test subject is able to exactly superimpose his dot on that of the test pattern, the net electrical output from the pursuit meter is 0 and a straight line is recorded on a biomedical recorder such as a Beckman R-411 Dynograph. If the subject's pattern deviates from the generated test pattern, a positive or negative voltage proportional to the deviation is then recorded on the oscillograph. Although an infinite variety of pursuit meter patterns can be used with this testing device, four different pursuit meter patterns were used in these particular tests and are illustrated in Fig. 2. Line A is the pattern displayed on the oscilloscope from the function generators. Pattern one is a simple sine wave of one cycle per second from one generator. The second pattern is a combination pattern from two generators, one operating in sine function and the

3. Motor and Mental Performance with Marijuana

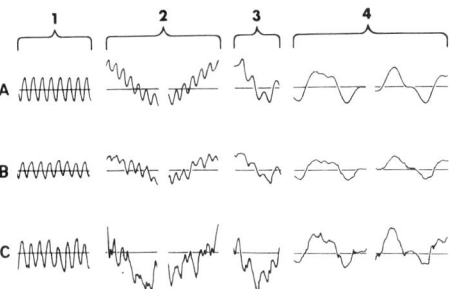

Fig. 2. Diagram of four different pursuit meter patterns used. A, programmed sweep; B, subject's response; and C, error signal.

other operating in triangular function. Patterns three and four are other more complex variations of mixed patterns. Line B represents the subject's response to the pattern; i.e., the pattern which he drew in an attempt to superimpose his dot on the test pattern dot. Line C is the error signal. It is impossible to exactly superimpose the operator's light beam on that from the test pattern, so an error pattern usually occurs. In order to calculate an error score in our studies, we measured the displacement of the error line from the center line in millimeters. Each distinct peak was measured individually and the total score was the sum from all the peaks.

B. Delayed Auditory Feedback

Mental performance was measured using delayed auditory feedback, a device designed to place the subject in a condition of self-induced anxiety. The subject spoke into a lavaliere microphone placed approximately 6 inches from the mouth. The subject's voice was recorded on a tape recorder operating at 3¾ inches/second. His verbal response was monitored into a pair of padded head phones from a playback head so located that a 0.28 second audio feedback delay resulted. Each of nine different tests was used for a duration of 2 minutes. Variations of the same tests were used for each experimental session to prevent familiarization with the testing material or problems. The nine tests used are described below. For test one, verbal output, the subject read a passage which was not completely comprehensible in itself since it was necessary to have read the full text in order to fully understand the meaning. For the next test, the subject read the same passage, but in reverse. For the third test, the subject was instructed to start counting at a number such as 10,000 and count in reverse. For the next test, the subject was given a number and instructed to add a specified number continually, e.g., the subject would start with 1 and add 3 each time and count 1, 4, 7, 10, etc. Next the subject was instructed to read aloud from a typed sheet of simple addition problems and provide the final answer, e.g., 5 plus 7 equals __?__. A subtraction test similar to the addition test, but using simple subtraction problems, was administered next in the examination sequence. The following two tests were modifications of the addition and subtraction test such that the subject was required to read the same problems aloud, but mentally add the number 7 before giving the final answer. For example, the subject would say 6 plus 2 equals 15 or 9 minus 7 equals 9. The final test used in the delayed audio feedback series was a color differentiation test. This was a modification of the Stroop Test and consisted of a board which had printed on it the names of colors: red, yellow, blue, green, orange, violet, and black. The names were printed in different colors and the subject was instructed to read the name of the first word and the color of the second printed word and to continue reading in this alternate pattern. Errors for all tests were enumerated as total output divided by the errors or as a percent error.

C. Static Equilibrium

Static equilibrium was measured by an apparatus designated as a "wobble board" which can measure quantitative changes in the stability of stance in man. It consists of four components, a platform assembly upon which the subject stands, an electromechanical sensing system that can provide a digital readout in arbitrary units as an index of the amount of swaying, a vibrator attached to the platform which can impart to it a horizontal nonrotating circular motion and an automatic timer that can be set for any period of time for a given test. By employing this apparatus, a measure in arbitrary "counts" of accumulated "unsteadiness" for a given time period can be obtained as an indication of the magnitude and frequency of the subject's balance seeking motion. One-hundred counts are generated when the platform is displaced through 2.4 minutes of arc. Each subject was requested to stand on the platform in stocking feet astraddle of the vibrator in a position within two shoe outlines (21 cm apart) painted on the platform. Four separate tests were made under these conditions. Test one was performed with the subject fixing his gaze on a small spot on a wall 9 feet in front of him. Test two was conducted in the same position, but with eyes closed. The same two tests were repeated with the vibrator turned on. Counts were taken for 20 seconds for each of the four conditions.

D. Subjective Tests

Each subject was also administered the Cornell Medical Index, a test which was developed at the Cornell University Medical College (1945) as a general symptom side-effect check list. Using this test, the physiological and psychological condition of an experimental subject can be quantified by the intensity of the symptomatology. The Marijuana Drug Correlation Scale reference developed by the Addiction Research Center at Lexington, Kentucky was also administered to each subject (Haertzen, 1966). The test was developed by observing individuals under the influence of marijuana and enumerating effects most commonly occurring and setting them forth in a questionnaire. Consequently, the more prominent the given responses, the more likely the individual is under the influence of marijuana. In addition, each subject was asked to guess whether he had smoked a placebo or an actual marijuana cigarette. They were also queried as to whether they felt capable of driving an automobile at that time. In experiments where the subject received both alcohol and marijuana, they were also asked to subjectively judge whether they had ingested alcohol or placebo alcohol. If they felt that they had received alcohol, they were asked to estimate the amount which they had consumed. They were also asked whether the alcohol antagonized or added to the marijuana effect.

E. Setting

All the experiments were conducted in a standard size, double bed hospital room located in the clinical research facility of the Eli Lilly Company. The room contained testing equipment, a hospital bed, table, and several chairs. There was one window which was kept completely draped throughout the experiment. The light level in the room was maintained constant, but indirect light was sufficiently bright to permit reading. The room was air conditioned and the temperature was maintained at 72°F. Prior to the actual test period, each subject was familiarized with experimental protocol without smoking in order to eliminate an instruction period on the day of testing. All subjects were either experienced cigarette smokers or had previous experiences with marijuana.

Thus, the smoking process was not unfamiliar to them. Each person was asked to refrain from intake of alcoholic beverages, coffee, tea, or cola on the evening prior to or the day of testing. Subjects were not permitted to smoke tobacco cigarettes or consume any beverage other than water during the experimental sessions.

F. Experimental Protocol

Our preliminary investigations indicated that the onset and duration of the marijuana effect are reasonably reproducible between individuals when the drug is administered by the standardized smoking method. The onset of symptoms generally occurred during the smoking period and reached a peak at about 30 minutes after smoking began. The "high" generally disappeared during the period up to 2 hours, although it occasionally persisted for as long as 3 to 4 hours. The performance tests were administered during the period when the test subject would be under the influence or subjected to the marijuana experience. Cornell Medical Index tests and the Addiction Research Center Inventory were administered at the period of peak high.

When marijuana was administered in combination with alcohol, each subject's breath was tested to determine if they had consumed alcohol prior to the testing period. All the subjects used in these experiments were males and ranged in age from approximately 20 to 29 years of age and were either medical or graduate students. All drugs were administered in a double-blind random block design. Several times throughout the experimental procedure, the subject's pulse rate was checked and the eyes were examined for dilatation of blood vessels of the conjunctiva. The eye scores were quantitated on an arbitrary 0 to 4 scale based on the amount of redness present in the eye. In the experiments with the combination of alcohol and marijuana, alcohol was administered to attain a blood alcohol concentration of 0.05%. This blood alcohol concentration is the minimum amount that will effect decrement in performance measurably by the pursuit meter and delayed auditory feedback tests. Blood alcohol of this concentration would be achieved if a 150-pound man drank 45 ml of ethanol contained in three bottles of beer or 3 oz. of 100 proof whiskey within one-half hour. The alcoholic beverage was consumed during the half-hour period prior to the subjects smoking the marijuana or placebo cigarette. When alcohol was administered to the subjects, it was mixed in a commercially available pineapple–grapefruit drink in an attempt to disguise its taste. The placebo alcohol was the same pineapple–grapefruit drink without any alcohol. Each person was permitted 30

3. Motor and Mental Performance with Marijuana

minutes in which to consume the entire drink which amounted to approximately 8 oz. of liquid. Thirty minutes after alcohol ingestion, the subject started smoking the marijuana cigarette. The smoking period lasted anywhere from 15 to 20 minutes, depending on the individual. Consequently, the maximum absorption of alcohol occurred during the smoking period (Manno et al., 1970). The onset of action of marijuana is rather rapid, usually occurring during the smoking period with the peak effect appearing within a few minutes after finishing the cigarette; therefore the maximum effects of marijuana and alcohol occurred together. The protocol used for the marijuana–alcohol investigation is illustrated in Table I. The protocol for the dose-response experiment is similar except that the alcohol drinking period was eliminated.

TABLE I

Protocol for Marijuana–Alcohol Investigation

Time	Event
0:00	Control pulse; eye check; breathalyzer test
0:00–0:30	Drinking period
0:30	Pulse check; eye check
0:30–0:50	Smoking period
0:50–0:60	Pulse check; eye check; Cornell Medical Index Test administered
0:60	Pulse check; eye check; breathalyzer test
1:05–1:25	Pursuit Meter Test
1:25	Pulse check; eye check; breathalyzer test
1:30–1:50	Delayed Auditory Feedback Tests
1:50	Pulse check; eye check; breathalyzer test

IV. MARIJUANA DOSAGE FORM

Approximately two-thirds of the recent clinical investigations into the actions of marijuana on human physiological and psychological functioning have been conducted utilizing the marijuana cigarette as a dosage form. Undoubtedly, these investigators realize that the variabilities of smoking can substantially alter the amount of THC available to their test subjects. The fact that marijuana is consumed as cigarettes appeared to have more importance to these investigators than the variability that they could possibly encounter because of the use of this unusual dosage form. We have determined in our investigations that the maximum amount of THC available to an individual smoking a marijuana cigarette is approximately 50% ± 10%. This computation is based on total consumption of the marijuana cigarette as well as maintaining inspiration so that at least 99% of the inhaled THC is not exhaled. Galanter et al. (1972) administered THC to three subjects by smoking and estimated the amount of the THC which was absorbed. After administering the same amount of THC to each subject, they found that between 14 and 41% of the THC originally present in the marijuana cigarette was absorbed, thereby demonstrating the enormous potential variability in the absorption of this drug among different people. Perhaps the only way to have absolute assurance of the amount of the administered dose of THC is by intravenous administration. This, of course, is not practical for most laboratory situations and the cigarette still is the preferred method of drug administration.

V. MOTOR PERFORMANCE

Data obtained from the four pursuit meter patterns are plotted in Fig. 3. The data are plotted as mean error scores for 12 subjects, with higher scores reflecting poorer performance. Smoking marijuana produced a significant decrement in performance for all four pursuit meter patterns. The combination of alcohol and marijuana had variable effects. There was a prominent subjective enhancement of the "marijuana high" when the subject consumed alcohol prior to smoking marijuana cigarettes. From these investigators' observations, the addition of alcohol intensifies the actions of marijuana. If an individual became "giddy" after smoking marijuana, he was more giddy when he consumed alcohol plus marijuana. If the individual, on the other hand, became quiet and reclusive, this was more prominent when alcohol was combined with marijuana. The effects on the pursuit meter performance showed significant additive effects between alcohol and marijuana only on the first pattern. Although there were slight differences in pursuit meter test scores for patterns 2 through 4, the difference in performance between the marijuana doses with and without alcohol was not significant.

The plateauing effect which occurred between the 2.5 and 5 mg doses of THC administered by smoking caused some concern in our laboratory because of the absence of a linear dose-response relationship. In an effort to further clarify a dose-response relationship, cigarettes were calibrated and THC was administered in another study so that each subject received a dose of THC proportional to his body weight. In addition to individ-

3. Motor and Mental Performance with Marijuana

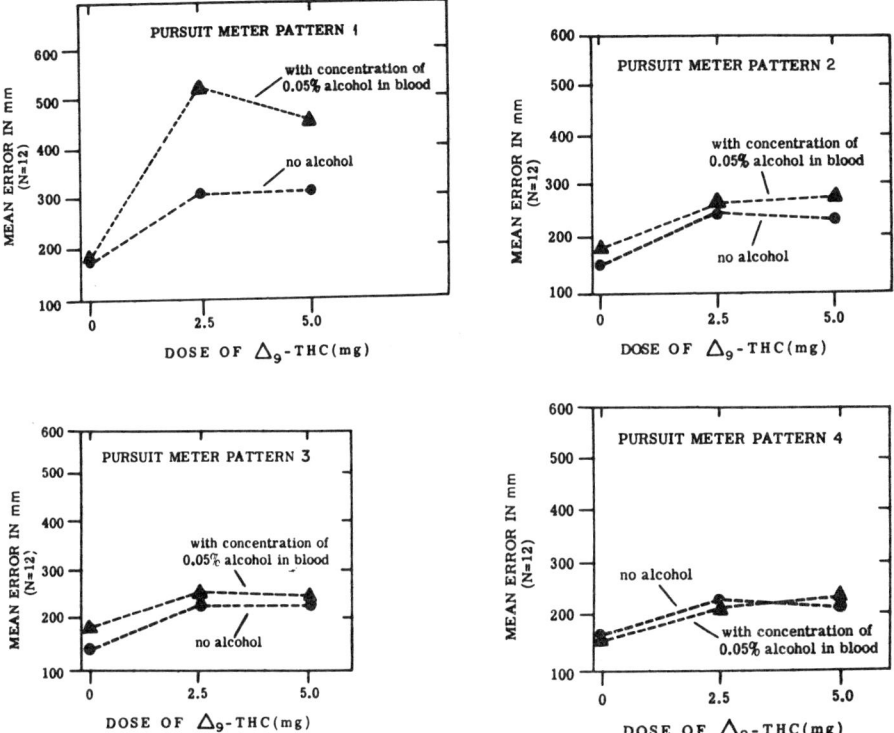

Fig. 3. Results from pursuit meter tests for alcohol–marijuana interaction study. Significant ($p < 0.05$) decrements in performance occurred with the 5 mg dose of THC for all four patterns. Significant additive effects between alcohol and marijuana occurred for pattern 1 only ($p < 0.05$).

ualizing the doses, we also extended the dose range over a wider area. The four doses selected were 6.25, 12.5, 25, and 50 µg/kg. The 25 and 50 µg/kg doses were approximately the same as the two doses used in the previous investigation where alcohol and 2.5 and 5.0 mg of marijuana were used in combination. The two lower doses were added in order to determine if there was a "minimal effect level." In other words, it was desirable to simulate the lower concentrations of THC which would be present in some of the weaker or decomposed samples that an individual might obtain. If one were to draw a comparison between the doses of THC administered in our studies and the percentage concentration of THC in marijuana, they would be as follows: The 6.25 µg/kg dose represents marijuana containing 0.25% THC, the 12.5 µg/kg dose corresponds to marijuana containing 0.5% THC, the 25 µg/kg dose equals 1% THC,

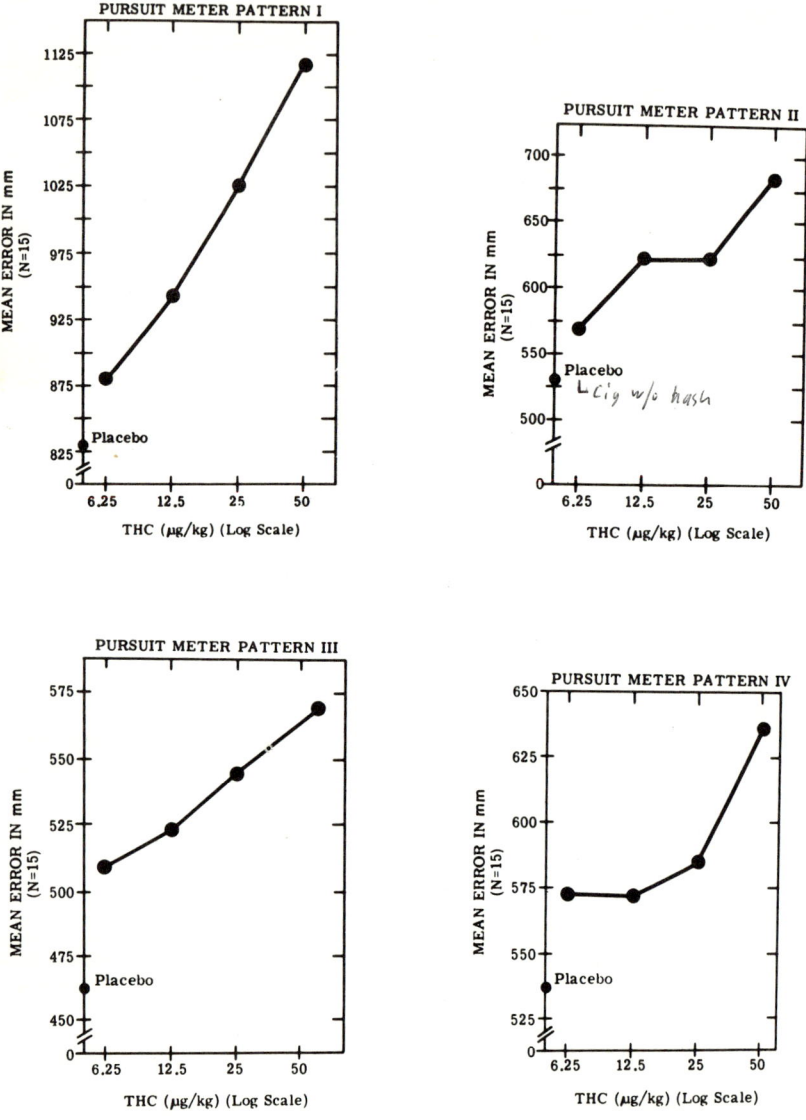

Fig. 4. Results from pursuit meter tests for several administered doses of THC. A linear dose-response relationship between increasing error score and increasing dose of THC occurred for all four test patterns ($p < 0.05$).

and the final and largest dose equivalent to marijuana containing 2% THC. The range of doses covered the gamut of marijuana which would normally be encountered in the street.

When THC was administered on a µg/kg basis, a dose-dependent decrement in performance occurred with all four pursuit meter patterns. The scores are represented in Fig. 4. The differences in responses between the four patterns probably can be accounted for by the manner in which these were graded. The first pursuit meter pattern, because it is a simple sine wave, necessitated more movement by the subject in order to superimpose his beam on the test pattern beam of the testing device. A larger score is involved and consequently there is in fact more chance of error with this pattern.

VI. MENTAL PERFORMANCE AND ATAXIA

When subjects were administered either 2.5 or 5 mg of THC, a significant decrement in performance occurred in 7 out of 9 delayed auditory feedback tests. The decrement was significant for verbal output, reversed verbal output, reversed count, progressive count, addition, addition plus seven, and subtraction ($p = < .05$). Again, there was no linear dose-response relationship between the 2.5 and 5 mg doses of THC. When the marijuana was combined with alcohol, a significant additive decrement occurred only in the reversed verbal output test. A linear dose-response relationship was found with some of the same delayed auditory tests after THC administration based on a µg/kg dose. The charts representing these tests are shown in Figs. 5 and 6. A significant linear dose-dependent decrement in performance occurred with the verbal output test, progressive count, color discrimination, and reversed count tests ($p < .05$).

VII. PHYSIOLOGICAL REACTIONS TO THC AND ALCOHOL

The physiological effects of smoking marijuana alone or in combination with ethanol occur in a dose-dependent fashion. Pulse rate increased in a linear manner depending on the dose of THC administered by smoking. The addition of alcohol to the marijuana produced a significant additive effect resulting in an increased pulse rate as shown in Fig. 7. This

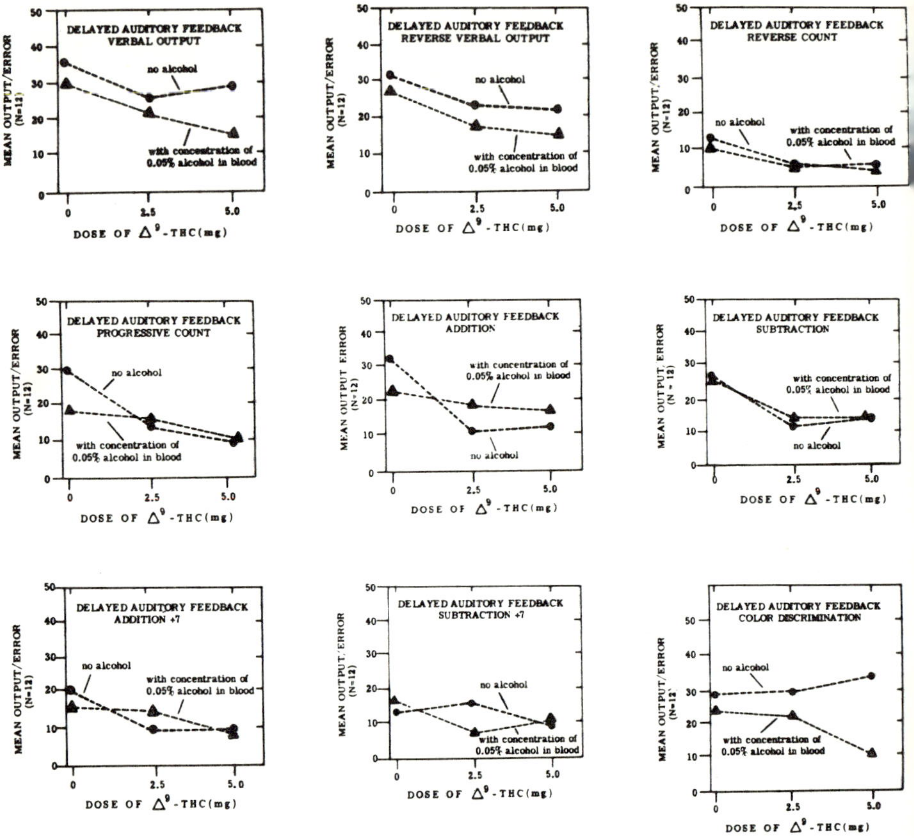

Fig. 5. Delayed auditory feedback data for the alcohol–marijuana interaction study. A significant decrement in performance occurred after the 5 mg dose for all tests *except* subtraction + 7 and color discrimination. Additive effects between THC and alcohol were significant only for reverse verbal output test.

relationship continued when the THC was administered on a µg/kg basis as shown in Fig. 8. Conjunctival injection also increased in a manner dependent on the administered dose of THC. The arbitrary score which we devised for grading conjunctival injections is described elsewhere (Manno *et al.*, 1970). As observed with the increase in pulse rate, the addition of alcohol to the marijuana produced a significant additive effect in conjunctival injection (Figs. 9 and 10). The increase in conjunctival injection was also a linear dose-dependent response after the THC was administered on a µg/kg basis.

Administration of THC on a µg/kg basis produced a significant in-

3. Motor and Mental Performance with Marijuana

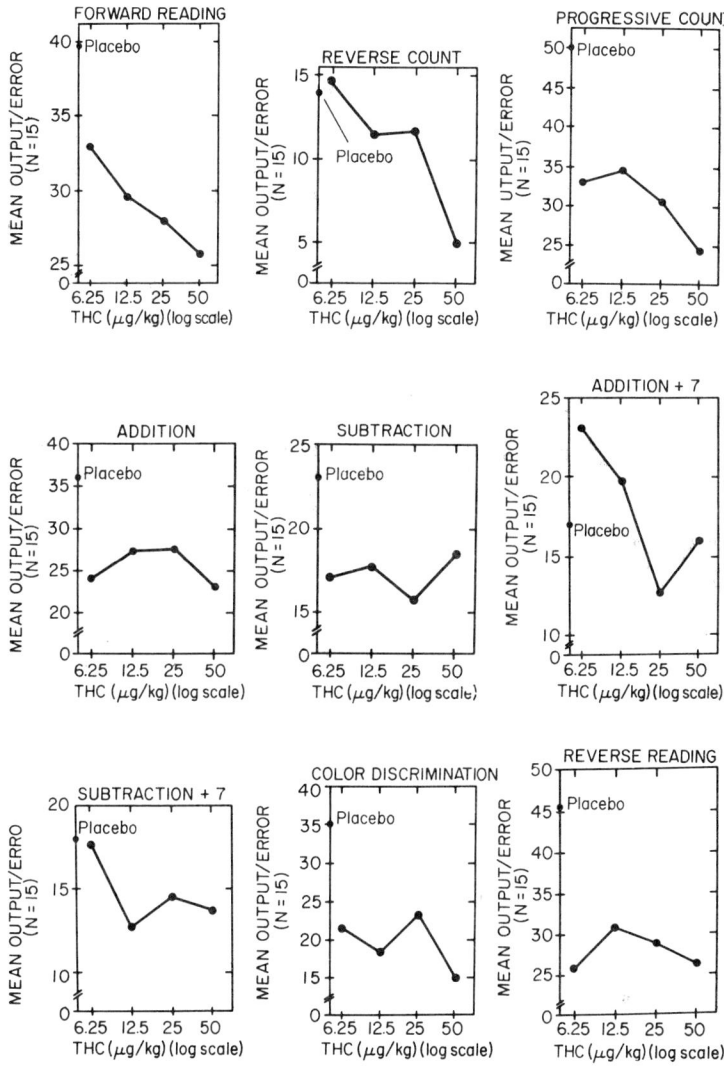

Fig. 6. Delayed auditory feedback results for several administered doses of THC. A significant decrement in performance occurred at the 50 μg/kg dose for verbal output, reserve count, progressive count and color discrimination. A linear dose-response relationship between output/error and administered dose of THC also occurred for these tests.

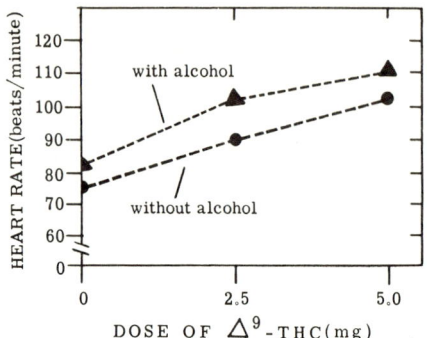

Fig. 7. Heart rate increases were highly correlated to administered dose of THC ($p < 0.001$). Additive effects between alcohol and marijuana were also significant ($p < 0.01$).

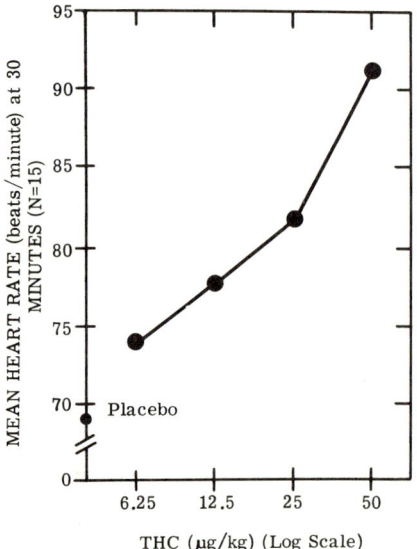

Fig. 8. A linear dose-relationship between administered dose of THC and heart rate occurred when THC was administered on a μg/kg basis ($p < 0.001$).

crease in "sway" or a decrease in stability as measured by the "wobble board." The data from this experiment are shown in Fig. 11. The ataxia produced by increased doses of THC as measured by the wobble board was significant ($p < .05$) and dependent on the administered dose of THC. It should be noted, however, that it is almost impossible to make gross observations of ataxia in subjects who have smoked marijuana and

3. Motor and Mental Performance with Marijuana

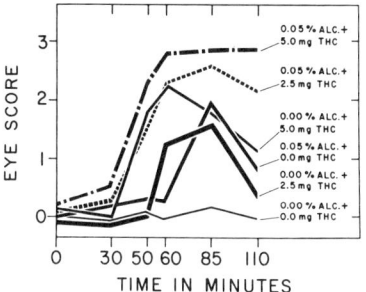

Fig. 9. Time course of heart rate increases after alcohol and/or THC.

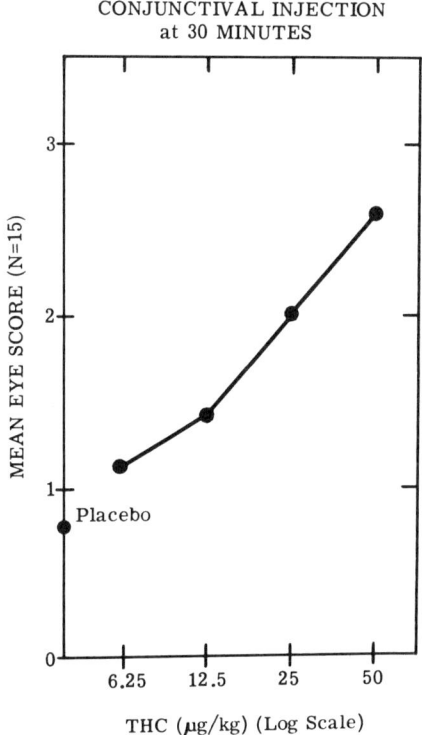

Fig. 10. Conjunctival injection increased with increasing doses of THC. The dose-response relationship was significant at $p < 0.001$.

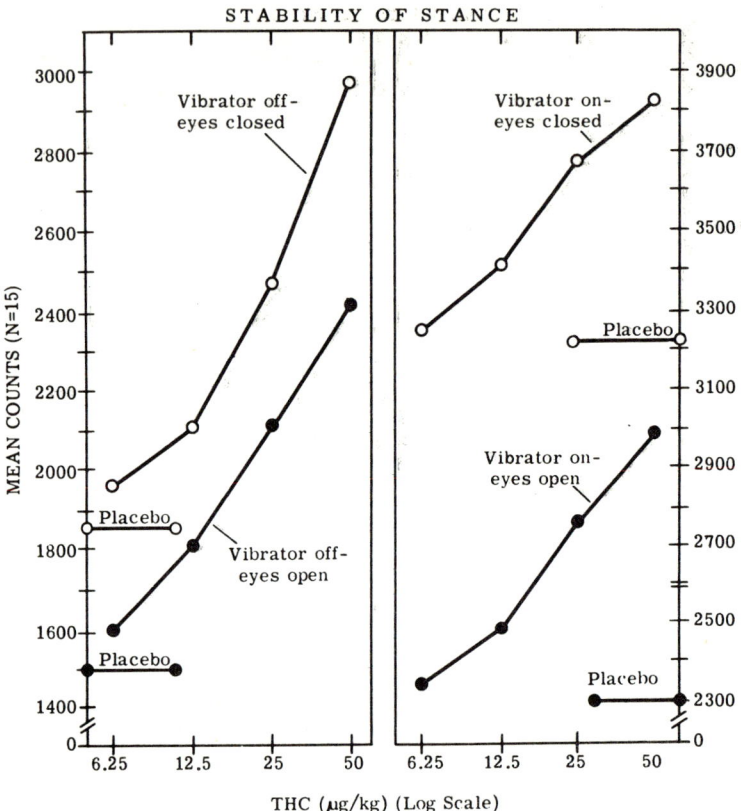

Fig. 11. Increased "sway" as measured by the wobble board occurred with increasing doses of THC. The response was linear ($p < 0.001$) for all four test conditions.

that this measurement was due to the extreme sensitivity of the testing equipment.

VIII. SUBJECTIVE REACTIONS

The subjective responses of our test subjects as measured by the Cornell Medical Index Test and Addiction Research Center Inventory (the Marihuana Drug Correlation Scale) indicated that the subject's response was intensified as the dose of THC increased. There was also a significant additive effect (in both the Cornell Index and the Addiction

3. Motor and Mental Performance with Marijuana

Research Center Inventory) when alcohol was used in combination with the marijuana. The data for both the Cornell Medical Index and Addiction Research Center Inventory are shown in Figs. 12 and 13.

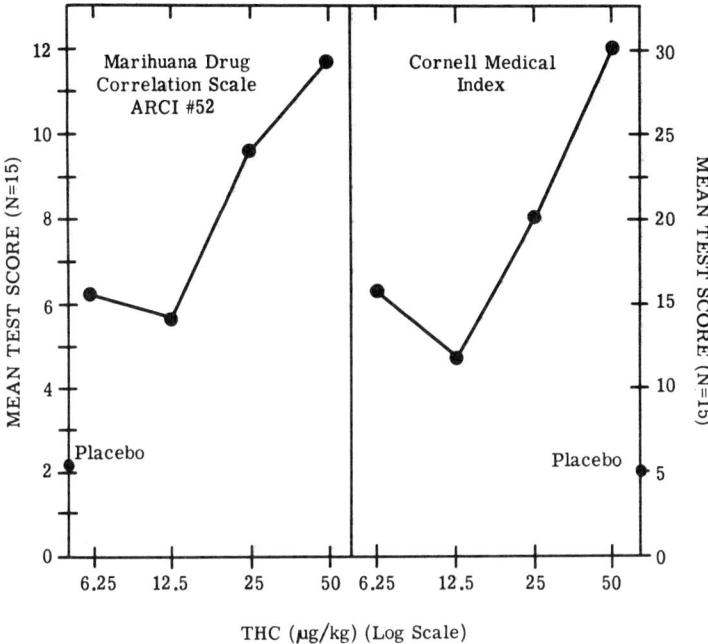

Fig. 12. Increased symptom scores occurred ($p < 0.001$) with increasing doses of THC for both the Cornell Medical Index test and the Addiction Research Center Inventory.

Our very earliest experiences with marijuana and placebo marijuana indicated to us quite dramatically that a substantial placebo response could be anticipated from our subjects. In these preliminary studies, each subject received either placebo or test marijuana, but was not informed that he would receive a placebo. In other words, each subject thought that he would receive two marijuana cigarettes. We used a total of eight subjects and the people who received placebo first reacted as if they had smoked test marijuana. They indicated that they were high and some actually became quite stimulated from the placebo marijuana cigarette. When these same individuals received the test marijuana cigarette in the next testing session, they commented that this marijuana was much more "potent" than that which they had received the first time. Several questioned whether they had received marijuana the first time, indicating

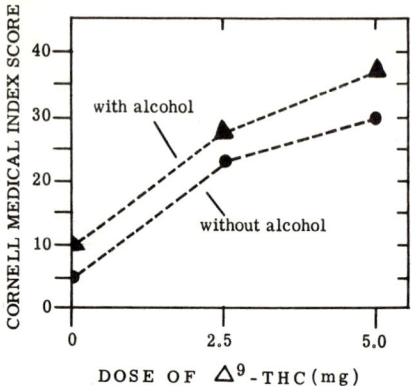

Fig. 13. Significant differences ($p < 0.05$) occurred between alcohol and marijuana as determined by increasing Cornell Medical Index test symptom scores.

that they had felt a distinct, subjective difference between the two smoking experiences. On the other hand, the subjects who received marijuana first and placebo second did not demonstrate reaction to the placebo cigarette and commented that they had probably received a placebo. This was also without the subjects having any prior knowledge or suspicion that a placebo was being administered in the study. When the scores of the subjects were computed, we found that they always performed better for the placebo run than they did during the marijuana run. In other words, the placebo effect, although it was a subjective high to marijuana, did not produce any decrements in the person's ability to perform the psychomotor function tests which we utilized for the studies.

The pursuit meter and delayed auditory feedback were developed in this laboratory. The sensitivity and flexibility which they permit in testing drug effects on human performance has been demonstrated with many compounds, e.g., alcohol (Hughes et al., 1963; Forney and Hughes, 1964a), tranquilizers (Bernstein et al., 1967; Hughes et al., 1963; Forney and Hughes, 1964a), barbiturates (Kaplan et al., 1968), antihistamines (Forney and Hughes, 1964b), mood elevators (Forney and Hughes, 1963), stimulants (Forney and Hughes, 1964c), and analgesics (Forney and Hughes, 1964d). Using these instruments, we were able to demonstrate that smoking marijuana cigarettes can produce significant decrements in both motor and mental performance in man. The decrements in motor performance can be attributed to several factors.

1. LOSS OF MOTIVATION

The pursuit meter tests were more boring to subjects after they had smoked marijuana. Some felt that the tests were lasting longer while they were under the influence of marijuana. Rather than continuing to do their best, subjects distracted themselves by making comments, or as with one subject "drawing patterns on the oscilloscope screen with the dot of light which he controlled." It appeared that their only interest was finishing the test. Performing well did not seem to be too important to the subject.

Description of the experience encountered with one subject can best describe the effects of marijuana on motivation. This individual particularly did not enjoy the feedback tests. However, when it was time to read the last test, color discrimination, he said that the colors on the chart intrigued him more while under marijuana and he enjoyed doing that part of the test. His performance after marijuana improved when compared to his performance after placebo.

2. INABILITY TO CONCENTRATE ON THE TEST

Several subjects remarked that it was more difficult to "mentally separate the two dots of light" while they were under the influence of marijuana. They would "track" the program beam for a while, then abruptly stop for a few seconds after the two dots became separated and start again. It seemed as though they had mentally lost contact with the task and were following the beam automatically until the two beams became separated, at which time they regained contact and returned to the assigned test. This situation was embarrassing to the subjects and many times they would laugh and comment about the "sneaky patterns."

3. LACK OF ABILITY TO COORDINATE MOVEMENTS

It was possible to track pursuit meter pattern 1 by establishing a rhythmical movement of the wheel which corresponded to the sine wave of the program pattern. While under the influence of marijuana, subjects would lose the rhythm of the pattern more easily, and once lost it appeared to be more difficult to recover. Whenever an individual would realize that he was doing poorly at operating the pursuit meter, he would make comments to that effect. It was as if the individuals were trying to explain that they were aware of their poor performance, but were unable to help it. This paranoid behavior occurred to some degree in almost every subject in all experiments in which active marijuana was smoked. In order to perform well on delayed auditory feedback, it was necessary for the experimental subject to ignore the feedback as much as possible. Medical and graduate students are suitable subjects as they have the ability to concentrate on what they are reading and thus are able to minimize the feedback effect. Under the influence of marijuana, it was more difficult for them to ignore the feedback. When they lost their place in the test, it would take longer to regain it after marijuana had been smoked than after the placebo. Some subjects were unwilling to put forth the extra effort after smoking marijuana and would distract themselves by blowing on the microphone or trying to make sound effects with the feedback. If they were urged to continue with the test, they would cooperate for a short while then revert to their previous behavior. The majority of subjects performed the entire series of tests on the feedback with few comments.

If the effects produced by alcohol or marijuana could easily be distinguished, the subjects should have had no problem guessing which drug they had received. When the subjects received alcohol plus placebo marijuana, the majority surmised that they had received both alcohol and marijuana. Apparently, the effects produced by marijuana and alcohol are sufficiently similar to account for this confusion. Individuals were reluctant to make a verbal comparison between the effects produced by marijuana and those produced by alcohol. Usually, the only comparison made was that the effect of the two drugs was somewhat comparable, but the marijuana was preferable because it did not produce a hangover or any other "undesirable effects" which could be produced by alcohol. The primary distinction observed by the investigators was that subjects did appear to be as high after 0.05% alcohol as they did after marijuana or marijuana plus alcohol. When individuals received the 2.5 mg dose of THC in combination with ethanol, many said that the effects produced were additive. When the high dose of THC (5 mg) was combined with alcohol, many stated that the marijuana effect was so much more powerful than the alcohol effect that the alcohol did not add on as much as it seemed to with the lower dose of THC (2.5 mg). The subjects appeared to be much more depressed when they consumed both alcohol and marijuana than after either one of the drugs alone. They were more quiet prior to the tests, demonstrated less paranoia, and volunteered fewer comments regarding their performance on the tests. One subject became very weak after smoking the high dose of marijuana in combination with alcohol and slept for 2 hours after the experiment. Four other subjects chose to remain in the laboratory after the testing sessions when they received alcohol and the high dose of THC. Even though none of these subjects slept for over one-half hour, it should be noted that nobody remained after the experimental sessions when they received either dose of THC alone or alcohol alone. When questioned if they thought that marijuana was a stimulant or depressant, the consensus was that it stimulated them "mentally" while depressing them "physically."

IX. SIGNIFICANCE AND CONCLUSION

Smoking marijuana cigarettes has been demonstrated to produce a decrement in human psychomotor performance (Casswell and Marks, 1973; Kielholz et al., 1973; Kiplinger et al., 1971; Manno et al., 1970, 1971; Tinklenberg et al., 1972; Weil et al., 1968). Generally, psychomotor function was tested using devices such as the pursuit rotor or the pursuit meter. The direct effects on psychomotor performance were slight when the pursuit rotor was used and tended to occur only when marijuana with a relatively high concentration of THC was used. Studies in our laboratory have indicated that significant changes in motor function do occur when subjects are tested with the pursuit meter. The significance of the changes is most likely related to the sensitivity of this particular type of instrumentation. Our previous experience has also indicated that medical and graduate students are preferable test subjects for psychomotor testing with our instrumentation. Generally, these individuals are more motivated and will expend more effort at the operation of the pursuit meter and also seem to possess better skills in their ability to concentrate. Consequently, it is easier to demonstrate changes in performance when a drug is administered to these persons. Production of a decrement in psychomotor performance after smoking marijuana was probably related to their own "high level" performance capabilities. Galanter et al. (1972) found that if a monetary reward was introduced as an inducement for errorless, rapid performance, the experimental subjects demonstrated a decreased reaction time after smoking marijuana. No change in reaction time was reported after marijuana administration when the monetary reward was not offered. This further substantiates the premise that incentive to perform at maximal output is adversely affected by the consumption of marijuana.

Although other investigators have compared the action of marijuana and alcohol (Cappell et al., 1972; Hollister et al., 1970; Tinklenberg et al., 1972) none have administered alcohol and marijuana and tested their combined effects on psychomotor performance. Manno et al. (1971) first demonstrated that an interaction occurred between these two drugs when they were administered concomitantly. However, an additive decrement in psychomotor performance occurred with the combination of alcohol and marijuana in only one of four pursuit meter test patterns. The test condition which was the simplest in nature, tracing a simple sine wave pattern, produced results which were the most significant. The most simple test permitted the subject the greatest opportunity to produce the largest error in performance because errors produced from this test pattern resulted in more "peaks" in the error signal than from the other patterns. Consequently, error score differences between several doses of a drug would be larger for pattern one than for the other three patterns. Perhaps, if the areas under error score curves could be computed, the "sensitivities" of the pursuit meter patterns might be increased also.

The delayed auditory feedback tests examined several components of the individual's mental capacity. These components were primarily concerned with visual and auditory perception, immediate recall of memory, and the ability to concentrate. The effects of marijuana on these same mental components have also been studied by others (Abel, 1970, 1971a,b; Casswell and Marks, 1973; Darley *et al.*, 1973; Melges *et al.*, 1971; Pearl *et al.*, 1973; Tinklenberg *et al.*, 1970) and in most instances it has been found that a diminished response in one or more of these functions occurred. Our data indicate that the decrements in mental performance, as demonstrated with the delayed auditory feedback, are significant in tests which require rapid vocalization and subsequently result in a total overall score so that decrements become more statistically significant with these tests.

Some correlation must now be drawn between these laboratory test conditions and actual human motor and mental performance tasks which can be affected by marijuana. One of the first tasks which can be questioned when one considers the effects of marijuana on psychomotor performance is that of driving an automobile. Driving will be discussed in greater detail in another chapter, therefore, we shall limit our comments to alterations in function related solely to driving after smoking marijuana. From our observations, smoking a single marijuana cigarette, especially if it contained a high quantity of THC, would probably have some detrimental effects on an individual's ability to operate a motor vehicle. Perhaps, after a single cigarette, this would not come into play until a time of crisis arose, for example, when a traffic light turns red a few seconds before the auto is at the intersection or when another car pulls into the path of the auto driven by the smoker. In a crisis situation requiring maximum concentrative ability resulting in the production of a maximum physical response, such as the turning of a steering wheel to prevent a collision, these functions are most likely to fail after smoking marijuana.

Consideration must also be given to the extrapolation of the psychomotor actions of marijuana in subjects in the laboratory to the effects which would be produced in the business and industrial environment. The actions of marijuana on performance can be grossly categorized into two primary areas of concern: safety and production. Industrial accidents occur many times with little or no warning. In order to protect himself, the worker must have full command of his reflexes, muscular coordination, and his thought processes. An individual smoking marijuana would be able to dodge a falling object. However, it may take him a fraction of a second longer to move from that object than a person who had not smoked marijuana. A machine operator or operator in a computer control room responsible for plant safety would probably require a longer time to turn off a machine if a malfunction developed. If this very small time delay did not produce significant compensation for the approaching dilemma, then an injury into the worker(s) or equipment damage would occur.

Many businesses have found that it is possible to increase their output of finished products by offering the employees a financial incentive for increased productivity. The effects of marijuana should be detrimental for two possible reasons: (1) If the individual is working at a capacity close to his maximum or at his maximum capacity, his total performance ability would be impaired regardless of promised remuneration or favor; and (2) the individual's receptiveness to the incentive would probably be diminished. In other words, he would not be as interested in earning the extra money as he would if he were not smoking the marijuana. Therefore, the effects of marijuana, not only on safety, but also on diminished productivity and work quality, would be most evident in those areas where concentration and judgment are involved.

REFERENCES

Abel, E. L. (1970). *Nature (London)* **227**, 1151–1152.
Abel, E. L. (1971a). *Nature (London)* **231**, 260–261.
Abel, E. L. (1971b). *Science* **173**, 1038–1040.
Bernstein, M. E., Hughes, F. W., and Forney, R. B. (1967). *J. Clin. Pharmacol. J. New Drugs* **7**, 330–335.
Cappell, H., Webster, C. D., Herring, B. S., and Ginsberg, R. (1972). *J. Pharmacol. Exp. Ther.* **182**, 195–203.
Casswell, S., and Marks, O. (1973). *Nature (London)* **241**, 61.
Cornell University Medical College. (1945). "Cornell Medical Index Health Questionnaire." Cornell University, New York.
Darley, C. F., Tinklenberg, J. R., Hollister, T. E., and Atkinson, R. C. (1973). *Psychopharmacologia* **29**, 231–238.
Forney, R. B., and Hughes, F. W. (1963). *J. Amer. Med. Ass.* **185**, 556–558.
Forney, R. B., and Hughes, F. W. (1964a). *J. Psychol.* **57**, 431–436.
Forney, R. B., and Hughes, F. W. (1964b). *Clin. Pharmacol. Ther.* **5**, 414–421.
Forney, R. B., and Hughes, F. W. (1964c). *Psychopharmacologia* **6**, 234–238.

Forney, R. B., and Hughes, F. W. (1964d). *Curr. Ther. Res.* **6,** 638–643.
Galanter, M., Wyatt, R. J., Lemberger, L., Weingartner, H., Vaughan, T. B., and Roth, W. T. (1972). *Science* **176,** 934–936.
Haertzen, C. A. (1966). *Psychol. Rep.* **18,** 163–194.
Hollister, L. E., Richards, R. K., and Gillespie, H. K. (1968). *Clin. Pharmacol. Ther.* **9,** 783–791.
Hollister, L. E., Moore, F., Kanter, S., and Noble, E. (1970). *Psychopharmacologia* **17,** 354–360.
Hughes, F. W., Forney, R. B., and Gates, P. W. (1963). *J. Psychol.* **55,** 25–32.
Isbell, H., and Jasinski, D. R. (1969). *Psychopharmacologia* **14,** 115–123.
Kaplan, H. L., Forney, R. B., Hughes, F. W., and Richards, A. B. (1968). *Arch. Int. Pharmacodyn. Ther.* **174,** 181–191.
Kielholz, P., Hobi, V., Lhdewig, D., Miest, P., and Richter, R. (1973). *Pharmakopsychiat./Neuro-Psychopharmakol.* **6,** 91–103.
Kiplinger, G. F., Manno, J. E., Rodda, B. E., and Forney, R. B. (1971). *Clin. Pharmacol. Ther.* **12,** 650–657.
Manno, J. E., Kiplinger, G. F., Haine, S., Bennett, I. F., and Forney, R. B. (1970). *Clin. Pharmacol. Ther.* **11,** 808–815.
Manno, J. E., Kiplinger, G. F., Scholz, N., and Forney, R. B. (1971). *Clin. Pharmacol. Ther.* **12,** 202–211.
Mayor's Committee on Marijuana. (1944). Jacques Cattell Press, Tempe, Arizona.
Mechoulam, R., ed. (1973). "Marihuana: Chemistry, Pharmacology, Metabolism and Clinical Effects." Academic Press, New York.
Melges, F. T., Tinklenberg, J. R., Hollister, L. E., and Gillespie, H. K. (1971). *Arch. Gen. Psychiat.* **24,** 564–567.
Pearl, J. H., Domino, E. F., and Rennick, P. (1973). *Psychopharmacologia* **31,** 13–24.
Tinklenberg, J. R., Melges, F. T., Hollister, L. E., and Gillespie, H. K. (1970). *Nature (London)* **226,** 1171–1172.
Tinklenberg, J. R., Kopell, B. S., Melges, F. T., and Hollister, L. E. (1972). *Arch. Gen. Psychiat.* **27,** 812–815.
Weil, A. T., Zinberg, N. E., and Nelsen, J. M. (1968). *Science* **162,** 1234–1242.

Chapter 4

MARIJUANA AND MEMORY

CHARLES F. DARLEY AND JARED R. TINKLENBERG

I. Introduction 73
II. Purposes of Marijuana–Memory Research 74
III. A Working Memory Model 76
IV. Experimental Tasks and Specific Experiments with Marijuana 78
    A. Experiment 1: Sternberg's Memory-Scanning Paradigm   78
    B. Experiments 2 and 3: Free Recall Memory Tasks 81
V. Locus of the Storage Deficit 88
VI. Evidence of State-Dependent Retrieval 92
VII. Alternative Interpretations of Experimental Results 94
VIII. New Directions and Promising Research 96
IX. Outlook for Marijuana–Memory Research 99
    References 100

I. INTRODUCTION

Reports from marijuana users such as "My memory span for conversation is shortened, so that I may forget what the start of a sentence was about even before the sentence is finished . . ." (Tart, 1971, p. 154) and "If I read while stoned, I remember less of what I've read hours later than if I had been straight" (Tart, 1971, p. 159) have led researchers to investigate the acute effects of marijuana on memory processes. Marijuana-intoxicated subjects have been called on to perform a great variety of experimental memory tasks, and, with some notable exceptions, they perform these tasks less efficiently in terms of accuracy and/or latency measures than nonintoxicated subjects.

II. PURPOSES OF MARIJUANA–MEMORY RESEARCH

There are three basic scientific contributions to be made by the study of acute effects of marijuana on human memory. The first is the determination of whether the effects of marijuana are sufficiently beneficial or harmful in terms of normal, everyday functioning to warrant taking special measures (educational, legislative, etc.) to either encourage or discourage its use in social situations. Drug research with this purpose is restricted in certain ways. Drug dosages must approximate those normally used in a social setting, and route of administration, experimental setting, and subjects' expectations must resemble their real-life counterparts. Perhaps most importantly, experimental tasks must be devised which are relevant to the requirements of daily life. With regard to memory research, relevancy means employing tasks such as story recall, picture recognition, or digit span that relate to ways in which people commonly use memory. Conclusions drawn from studies motivated by a desire for relevancy often take the form of statements relating drug state to performance on the experimental task with little regard for which specific memory function is impaired or enhanced by the drug. Often the tasks used are not amenable to such a component analysis. In other instances experimenters have chosen to obtain gross performance measures on a large sample of tasks in order to obtain an overall picture of behavioral effects rather than perform detailed analyses on a few tasks. Although such an approach maximizes the immediate relevancy of marijuana experiments, it minimizes the probability that the locus of marijuana's effect on memory will be identified.

A second approach to marijuana–memory research is to use the drug as a tool to extend and refine theories about memory. Although research on human memory has made little use of drugs, probably because of ethical considerations, the use of drugs in animal research has been vital in developing memory models (McGaugh, 1968; McGaugh and Dawson, 1971). With the recent emphasis on developing models of human memory containing precise mathematical and information-processing formulations, it has become important to find experimental variables which affect subsets of these models' parameters. If certain drugs were known to be selective in their effects, causing major alterations in some psychological mechanisms but not in others, they could be usefully applied in many areas of memory research. Of course, the potential value in combining the techniques of drug research with the insights into memory functioning provided by current models can only be realized if the experimental tasks used allow meaningful detailed analyses in terms of components defined by the models. Results from studies using tasks which allow componential analyses may not be as immediately socially relevant as those devised to mimic everyday uses of memory, but they may eventually be of greater value since they define more precisely the relation between a particular drug and specific memory mechanisms.

The third purpose of memory research with marijuana is to examine the nature of conscious, subjective experience. Human consciousness, although a topic of immense interest to philosophers, psychologists, scientists, and laymen, has received little attention in the laboratory. Owing to the recent advent of Cognitive Psychology (Miller et al., 1960; Neisser, 1967), greater stress has been placed on viewing much of human behavior as being under conscious control with the individual initiating and actively participating in perceptual, memorial, and inferential activities. Strategies and plans for the manipulation of environmental and internal events are formulated and then set into action via built-in processing mechanisms. The operation of these mechanisms may often be consciously monitored, allowing the individual to perceive and evaluate his ongoing experience and behavior. It is these directing and monitoring functions which most researchers have found not to be amenable to experimentation. Since the ingestion of centrally acting drugs appears to produce changes in such functions (Tart, 1972; Weil, 1972), information obtained via drug research about the mechanisms responsible for altering consciousness may provide insights into the nature of unaltered consciousness. It has been suggested that memory processes, particularly short-term or primary memory, may be strongly implicated in the functioning of consciousness (Atkinson and Shiffrin, 1971; James, 1890). If, as the research to be discussed here suggests, marijuana affects the short-term memory system, then the subjective changes noted by marijuana users may be partially explicable in terms of this effect. It is questionable whether changes in the way information is processed in short-term memory are sufficient to account for the wide range of subjective perceptual and cognitive effects reported by users (Tart, 1971), but any attempt at establishing relations between basic psychological functions and conscious experience is preferable to viewing consciousness as a phenomenon inaccessible to investigation.

In the succeeding sections we present first an outline of the model of the human memory system which has guided our research on the acute effects of marijuana on that system. The memory tasks used in the research will be described, followed by a discussion of the results of three experiments. Possible alternatives to the conclusions drawn from this data will then be presented. The chapter will conclude with a description of promising recent experimentation and suggestions concerning the direction of future marijuana–memory research.

III. A WORKING MEMORY MODEL

Most psychological research relies explicitly or implicitly on a particular theoretical framework to provide direction to experimental design and the analysis and interpretation of data. We use the model of human memory proposed by Atkinson and Shiffrin (1968, 1971), and expanded by Atkinson et al. (1974). In this model the activity of the memory system is viewed as involving a flow of information, largely directed by subject-initiated control processes, between three basic structural components—the memory stores of the system (see Fig. 1). The first of these

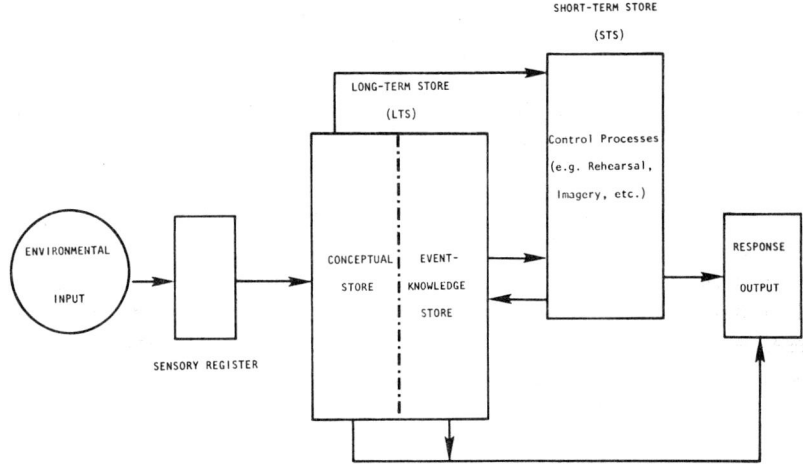

Fig. 1. Information from the environment is initially held for a brief period in the sensory register, while analysis by the perceptual system proceeds. An encoded representation of the stimulus, located in a portion of long-term store (LTS) called the conceptual store, is activated and entered into short-term store (STS), where it receives additional processing. Control processes allow information to be copied into a second portion of LTS, the event-knowledge store. Information about the context in which the stimulus occurred may be retrieved from the event-knowledge store and entered into STS. Depending on task requirements, a response may be initiated at nearly every stage of processing, utilizing information retrieved from the conceptual store, STS, or the event-knowledge store.

4. Marijuana and Memory

stores, the sensory register, maintains sensory information in a raw unprocessed form for a period of milliseconds as it is being analyzed, identified, and encoded (Sperling, 1960). Encoding involves the utilization of the individual's stored knowledge of his environment to obtain an internal representation or trace of the stimulus. Such knowledge is maintained in one partition of the second structural component, the long-term memory store (LTS). That portion of LTS which is responsible for stimulus encoding is the conceptual store. In most cases, the encoded representation of the stimulus is then entered into the third component of the memory structure, a short-term memory store (STS), at which point it may be said to have entered consciousness. The memory trace of the stimulus may be displaced from STS by newly arriving items (Reitman, 1971), or maintained indefinitely by means of certain control processes including rehearsal (rote repetition), the formation of mnemonics or visual images, and other complex coding schemes. The subset of items* on which such control processes act reside in a partition of STS called the rehearsal buffer. Depending on the complexity of the control process chosen, some variability exists in the number of items which can be maintained in the rehearsal buffer, but usually this number is small, say 4 or 5 items. Maintaining an item in the rehearsal buffer not only increases its length of stay in STS, but also increases the chance that information concerning its occurrence as an environmental event will be registered in a second partition of LTS, the event-knowledge store. In contrast to the short length of time an unrehearsed item may be maintained in STS, and the small number of different items which may reside there, the event-knowledge partition of LTS is a permanent memory store of unlimited capacity.

Since transfer of information occurs continuously between STS and LTS, an item may be thought of as residing at any moment in time in either STS, LTS or both. Information passes not only from STS to the event-knowledge partition of LTS, but in the opposite direction as well. In some memory tasks it may be a useful strategy to relate recent events residing in STS to earlier events already stored in LTS. Thus, information may be retrieved from LTS for further processing in STS. In other cases, information currently held in STS must be compared with sensory input; this requires the items in STS to be accessed via some retrieval scheme. Since all such information-retrieval, transfer, and storage processes may be directed by the subject, they are termed control processes. Depending on the nature of the task to be performed, particular control processes and particular memory stores may be utilized more than others.

---

* Whenever reference is made to processing performed on an "item" or "event" residing in memory, these terms refer to the memory traces containing information about the occurrence of that item or event in a particular environmental context.

It should be noted, however, that even tasks classically referred to as short-term memory tasks, involving memory for relatively few items over a short period of time, usually involve the utilization of LTS as it is defined here. So, by the model presented here, marijuana's impairment of digit span may result from the drug's effects on the operation of either STS or LTS, or on the transfer of information between the memory stores. This conception of a rapidly decaying STS trace from which information is immediately transferred to LTS contrasts with the dual-trace notions arising from animal memory research (McGaugh and Dawson, 1971). In some cases those models postulate that information may reside in STS from seconds to hours during which time it is transferred to, i.e., consolidated in, LTS. The problems in synthesizing the results of human and animal memory research are discussed in detail by Norman (1972). We believe that the above model, with its emphasis on conscious processes which control the flow and maintenance of information within the memory system, provides a clear, detailed, and intuitively reasonable vehicle by which we may examine the effects of marijuana on memory.

IV. EXPERIMENTAL TASKS AND SPECIFIC EXPERIMENTS WITH MARIJUANA

Two tasks which we have used in our recent research, memory scanning and free recall, meet the criterion of being analyzable into components which are meaningful in terms of our working memory model. These tasks used in concert allow each phase of processing in the memory system to be examined: STS storage, STS retrieval, transfer from STS to LTS, and LTS retrieval.

A. Experiment 1: Sternberg's Memory-Scanning Paradigm

The first paradigm, short-term memory scanning, was developed by Sternberg (1966, 1969) to study the processes involved in accessing (retrieving) information residing in STS. In this paradigm the subject is presented, on each trial of the experiment, a set of items, called the memory set, which contains few enough items that they may all be held in the rehearsal buffer. The subject is asked to hold these items in memory until a single item, the test stimulus, is presented. The test stimulus

4. Marijuana and Memory

may or may not be a member of the memory set; the subject is instructed to make a positive response if it is a member and a negative response if it is not. Since subjects are nearly always correct in their responses, the principal measure of performance is reaction time (RT) which is defined as the interval between presentation of the test stimulus and the response. Thus, the latency measure of performance allows the retrieval process to be studied in a task where the correct response is made on virtually every trial. Because the size of the memory set varies from trial to trial, functions may be plotted relating RT to memory-set size for both positive and negative responses. These functions typically are linear and increasing with memory-set size. Sternberg proposes that a subject performs this task in three independent stages, each of which relates to either the 0-intercept or slope values of the RT functions. When the test stimulus is presented the subject must first encode it, as described earlier. Stage 1 of the task is completed when a representation of the test stimulus has been retrieved from the conceptual store in LTS. During Stage 2 of the task the subject must compare this encoded representation of the test stimulus with representations of each of the memory-set items residing in STS. Thus, this second stage represents the process of accessing information already stored in STS. After having completed this comparison stage, the subject must decide whether or not a match occurred between the test stimulus and one of the memory set items and make the appropriate response. Sternberg has shown that the slope of the RT function is an estimate of the time to compare the test stimulus with a memory-set item (Stage 2) and the intercept is an estimate of encoding plus response time (Stages 1 and 3).

The usefulness of this paradigm for marijuana research lies in the opportunity to interpret the data in terms of Sternberg's component analysis. By comparing slope and intercept values for drug and placebo subjects we hoped to be able to isolate possible drug effects. The drug's effects on Stage 2 comparison processes were of particular interest, since there were strong indications in the literature that marijuana affected the processing of recently presented information.

In Experiment 1 we used this Sternberg memory-scanning task (Darley *et al.*, 1973a). We presented subjects memory sets of two-syllable English words, varying in size from 1 to 4 items. On Day 1 of the experiment, 12 subjects performed a series of 128 trials on the task and all 12 were then administered a 20 mg oral dose of THC followed by another 128 trials. In Fig. 2, mean combined positive and negative trial RT's for each memory-set size are plotted for both before and after drug-challenge sessions, and best-fitting straight lines obtained by the method of

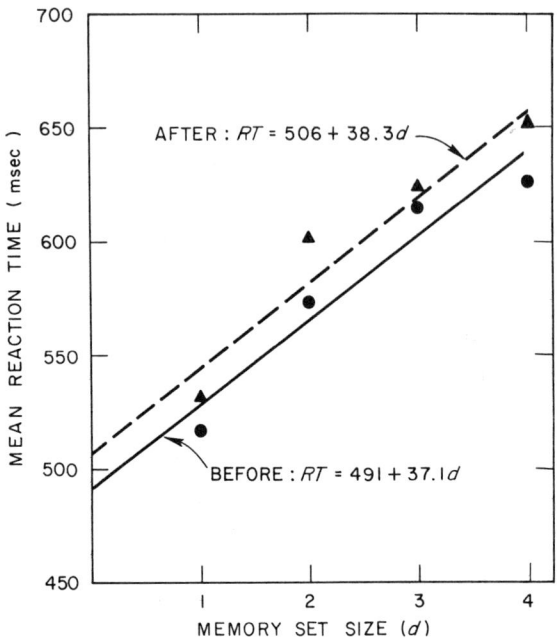

Fig. 2. Memory-scanning performance on Day 1 for before- and after-challenge sessions. Mean reaction time for combined data from positive and negative responses is plotted as a function of memory-set size (d) (Experiment 1). (Reprinted with permission from Darley et al., 1973a.)

least squares are shown.* If the drug had no effect on performance we would have expected any differences in the two sessions to be in favor of after drug-challenge trials due to practice effects. However, the results show overall RT on after drug-challenge trials to be slower, so there is a drug effect. The slopes of the two RT functions are virtually identical; the drug effect is entirely on the intercept value. Data from a second testing session 3 days later, in which half the subjects received placebo between blocks of 128 trials and the other half again received drug, confirm the results from the first testing day. The data are displayed in Fig. 3. Placebo subjects (right panel) show no change in performance, probably since practice effects have asymptoted by this time. Drug subjects (left panel) again show a slowing of RT from before- to after-challenge sessions, with the effect entirely accounted for by an increase in the intercept. We conclude that if Sternberg's model accurately describes the processes involved in the memory-scanning task, our results indicate that

---

* "Challenge" refers to the administration of either drug or placebo.

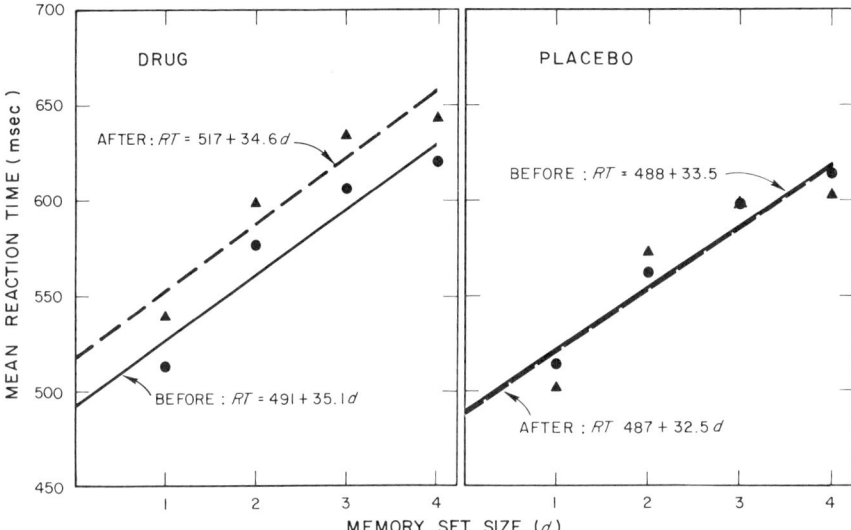

Fig. 3. Memory-scanning performance of drug and placebo subjects on Day 5 for before- and after-challenge sessions. Mean reaction time for combined data is plotted as a function of memory-set size (d) (Experiment 1). (Reprinted with permission from Darley et al., 1973a.)

marijuana slows the encoding and/or the response process, but not the comparison process. We are not able to state which component, encoding or response, is affected, but we are able to conclude that accessing information in STS is not disrupted.

B. Experiments 2 and 3: Free-Recall Memory Tasks

Requiring a person to write down in any order as many words as possible from a list which he saw or heard a short time earlier provides another useful method of investigating how his memory system functions. In the experiments to be described shortly, subjects were read several lists of 20 words each. Subjects were instructed that while the words were being read they were to memorize them, since following each list they were to write down in any order as many words as they could remember from that list.

1. A THEORETICAL ANALYSIS OF FREE RECALL

In terms of our working memory model, this free-recall task involves a complex flow of information between the memory stores. During the presentation phase of the task, the processing of the list items proceeds as follows. Each of the first few items in the list is encoded, enters the rehearsal buffer, and is operated on by control processes in order that a trace in LTS is established, signifying its occurrence in the list. At some point during list presentation the rehearsal buffer reaches its capacity and old items begin to be dropped as new items enter. At this point newly entered items receive less processing than did initial items since the average length of time an item stays in the rehearsal buffer decreases once the buffer is full. During list presentation items lost from the rehearsal buffer may reenter it, if related in some sense to a newly presented word.

At the time of the test, the following analysis applies. Subjects first retrieve the set of items still residing in the rehearsal buffer; this set usually consists of terminal items since earlier items are likely to have been replaced in the buffer by these recently presented items. The LTS is then searched for information regarding the occurrence of other items. Those which received the most processing, and consequently the most increase in strength in LTS, are most easily retrieved. Thus, the set of items recalled includes items retrieved from STS, those retrieved from LTS, and those which have traces present in both memory stores. Since items residing in the rehearsal buffer are easily retrieved, words presented at the end of a list show a high probability of recall. Since probability of retrieval from LTS is a function of strength in LTS, early list items are recalled better than other nonrehearsal-buffer items.

Evidence for this description of how items are studied, stored, and retrieved in the free-recall task is available in the serial position curve, which plots the probability of free recall against list positions. This function is invariably U-shaped, showing a primacy effect, representing the high probability of retrieval for early items, and a recency effect, representing high-probability retrieval of late items from STS. When recall testing is delayed following list presentation, the primacy effect is maintained, but the recency effect is eliminated (Glanzer and Cunitz, 1966; Craik, 1970); presumably recency disappears because items are lost from STS during the period between list presentation and test.

Further evidence for this conception of list-learning performance is provided by Rundus and Atkinson (1970) who investigated directly the relation between the active processing items received while residing in the rehearsal buffer and recall test performance. Rundus and Atkinson instructed subjects to externalize the rehearsal process by saying list items aloud whenever they thought about them during list presentation. When performance on an immediate test was plotted as a function of the number of overt rehearsals items received, they found that, except for terminal items, there was a direct relationship. In other words, the length of stay of an item in STS, as reflected by the number of overt rehearsals it received, was an accurate predictor of the probability the item would be recalled, provided the item was not in STS at the time of test.

The free-recall task is an excellent one for drug research for at least two reasons. First, since the serial position function is a statistic which yields information about theoretical components of the task, it is possible to assess drug effects on each of those components. Second, because the presentation phase of the task allows subjects to intensively memorize items and thereby register them in LTS, a delay in testing does not produce a precipitous drop in performance as might be expected in a task allowing less study time, such as the Sternberg task. For this reason drug administration may be interposed between study and test so that drug effects on storage, defined here as those processes operating during the presentation of to-be-remembered information, can be separated from effects on retrieval, i.e., those processes which permit a subject to access memory and produce an appropriate response at the time of the test.

2. EXPERIMENT 2: MEMORY STORAGE AND RETRIEVAL UNDER MARIJUANA

In the two free-recall experiments to be described here we used a delayed-testing procedure similar to that employed by Craik (1970). A summary of our procedure for Experiment 2 is presented in Table I (see

TABLE I

Experiment 2: Sequence of Experimental Procedures

Elapsed time since drug administration[a] (hours)	Experimental procedures
	Presentation and immediate recall of first 10 lists
1	Delayed tests on first set of lists
2	Presentation and immediate recall of second 10 lists
2½	Delayed tests on second set of lists

[a] Elapsed times indicate the number of hours from drug administration to the beginning of each procedure. (Reprinted with permission from Darley et al., 1973b.)

Darley et al., 1973b, for further details of the procedure). Subjects were first presented 10 lists of 20 words each, each list followed by an immediate-recall test. Immediately following the test on the last list, half the subjects received 20 mg of THC orally and half received placebo. One hour after drug administration a delayed-recall test was presented in which subjects were to write down as many words as they could recall from all 10 lists. A delayed-recognition test, containing each word from the pool of 10 lists as well as two nonlist items per list word, was then presented. Subjects were required to choose which word of each group of three had been a list item. This sequence of list presentation, immediate tests, delayed recall, and delayed recognition was then repeated with a second group of lists constructed from 200 new words. In the second sequence the immediate-recall test on the final list was not followed by drug administration, but instead the delayed-recall test was administered immediately.

Serial position curves for the immediate-recall data from the first set of lists are shown in the left panel of Fig. 4. The typical primacy and

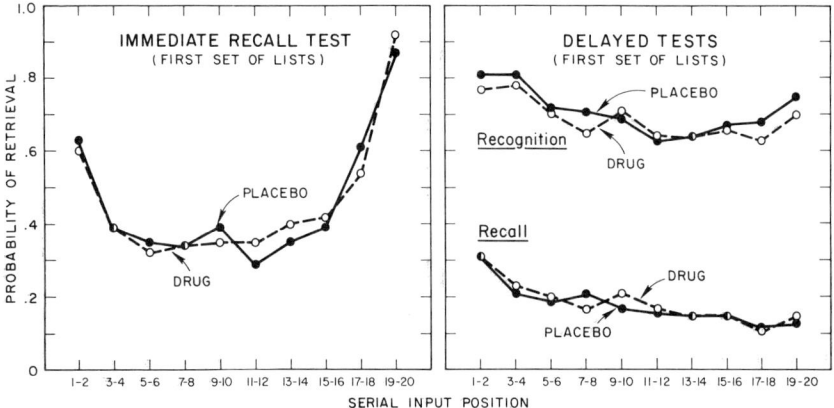

Fig. 4. The probability of immediate recall (left panel) and delayed recall and recognition (right panel) as functions of the serial input position of items from the first set of lists. Separate functions are plotted for drug and placebo subjects (Experiment 2). (Reprinted with permission from Darley et al., 1973b.)

recency effects are apparent. The virtually identical curves for placebo and drug subjects were expected, since subjects became differentiated as to drug group after presentation of the lists and immediate-recall testing had occurred. The delayed-test data for this first set of lists, presented in the right panel of Fig. 4, show that drug and placebo subjects recall and recognize list items equally well when drug administration follows list presentation and precedes delayed testing. That is, the ability of subjects to retrieve information from LTS was not impaired by marijuana.

The finding that marijuana does not disrupt retrieval processes is fortuitous because it allows us to conclude that any group differences in performance on the second set of lists result from effects on storage processes. The nature of these group differences for immediate recall is shown in the left panel of Fig. 5. Again, the shapes of the serial position curves are similar for the two groups, but performance for drug subjects is significantly depressed for all items except those in terminal list posi-

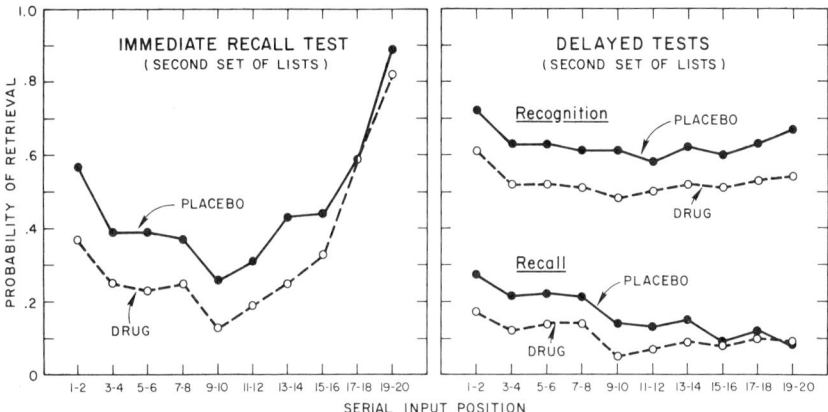

Fig. 5. The probability of immediate recall (left panel) and delayed recall and recognition (right panel) as functions of the serial input position of items from the second set of lists. Separate functions are plotted for drug and placebo groups (Experiment 2). (Reprinted with permission from Darley et al., 1973b.)

tions. The overall deficit for drug subjects indicates that some phase of information storage is disrupted by marijuana. The convergence of the serial position curves for terminal positions suggests that drug subjects enter items into and retrieve items from the rehearsal buffer as well as do placebo subjects. This finding adds support to our conclusions from Experiment 1 that accessing items in STS is performed equally well by placebo and drug subjects. An additional finding from Experiment 1 that response error rates were equivalent for the two groups strengthens our belief that entry into the rehearsal buffer is not affected by marijuana. The conclusion that the drug impairs entry of information into LTS is verified by the results for delayed testing shown in the right panel of Fig. 5. In this case, retrieval is entirely from LTS, and the deficit at nearly all positions for both delayed recall and recognition reflects the weaker traces in LTS for information presented in the drug state. The convergence for terminal items in delayed recall is puzzling, but may simply result from performance on items of minimal LTS strength approaching an asymptote for both groups.

Abel (1971a) also utilized a delayed-testing procedure to investigate marijuana's effects on storage and retrieval processes. Despite flaws in his procedures for subject assignment and his use of unknown dosages of marijuana, Abel's findings for drug vs. placebo immediate- and delayed-recall performance were similar to ours. He concluded that drug subjects engage in less rehearsal so that less information is entered into LTS. The conclusion we drew (Darley et al., 1973b) was similar in that we pinpointed the drug deficit at the stage of transferring information from STS to LTS; however without additional information it is not possible to state that the application of control processes causes the deficit. It is conceivable that drug subjects consciously process information as vigorously as placebo subjects, but that some other impairment in the system reduces the efficiency with which these processes operate.

3. EXPERIMENT 3: EFFECTS OF REHEARSAL PROCEDURE ON THE STORAGE DEFICIT

In order to precisely identify the effect of marijuana on memory storage, we employed a procedure which others have found useful in studying control processes and the functioning of the memory stores. A fixed-rehearsal procedure requires subjects to rehearse a well-defined subset of items between presentations of items in the list (Fischler et al., 1970; Palmer and Ornstein, 1971; Waugh and Norman, 1965). The fixed-rehearsal procedure is useful for our purposes because it allows us to equate the degree to which drug and placebo subjects utilize control processes. If properly applied, the procedure serves to focus subjects' attention on the production of rehearsals and prevents rehearsal or coding of items other than those most recently presented. Thus, if the effect of marijuana on storage results from only rehearsal or coding difficulties this fixed-rehearsal procedure should eliminate the effect. We utilized the fixed-rehearsal procedure in Experiment 3 (Darley et al., 1974). As in Experiment 2, all subjects were first presented 10 lists, each list followed by an immediate-recall test; however, in this case subjects studied half the lists using the normal free-rehearsal procedure and half using the fixed procedure. Subjects were tested in groups, so in the fixed procedure subjects rehearsed aloud, repeating in unison the two most recently presented items. In order that the inter-item interval be completely filled by the production of their rehearsals, they alternatively pronounced each of the two most recent items three times between item presentations. Following the presentation of the initial item in the list, subjects repeated that item 6 times, so that it received 3 more rehearsals over the course of the list than all other items except the last (which received a total of only 3 rehearsals). After presentation of the first 10 lists, all subjects received a 20 mg oral dose of THC, followed 1½ hours later by presentation and immediate-recall testing of 10 more lists, half studied under the free-rehearsal procedure and half under the fixed procedure. Subjects returned

4. Marijuana and Memory

3 days later and, following administration of either drug or placebo, received delayed-recall, -recognition, and -order tests (results from the order test will not be discussed here). The schedule of list presentation and testing is summarized in Table II.

TABLE II
Experiment 3: Sequence of Experimental Procedures, Day 1 and Day 4

Elapsed time since drug administration[a] (hours)	Experimental procedures
Day 1	Presentation and immediate recall of first 10 lists
	All subjects received marijuana
$1\frac{1}{2}$	Presentation and immediate recall of second 10 lists
Day 4	
	Subjects received marijuana or placebo
$1\frac{1}{2}$	Delayed-recall test
2	Delayed-recognition test
$2\frac{5}{6}$	Delayed-order test

[a] Elapsed times indicate the number of hours from drug administration to the beginning of each procedure. (Reprinted with permission from Darley et al., 1974.)

The crucial data bearing on the problem of locating the drug-induced deficit in storage were obtained on Day 1 and are displayed in Fig. 6 in the form of serial position curves. The functions for lists presented under the free-rehearsal procedure, where subjects were allowed to covertly study the list however they chose, show the primacy and recency effects seen for immediate recall in the first free-recall experiment. There is again a substantial difference in recall performance between lists learned during drug intoxication and those learned in the no-marijuana state. We ascribe the difference to drug state and not order of list presentation (although the two factors are confounded) since over a series of lists, recall performance has been found to neither increase nor decrease significantly (Keppel and Mallory, 1969; Dallet, 1963). The overall drug deficit is largely due to inferior recall of nonterminal list items, although in this case a slight deficit is present for terminal items. The fact that the difference in performance for positions 19 and 20 is the smallest difference between the curves confirms that drug effects on buffer entry and access are at least minimal and probably nonexistent.

Turning to the curves for fixed-rehearsal lists, an immediate observation is that controlling rehearsal in this way radically alters the shape of the serial position function. The two fixed-rehearsal curves show the

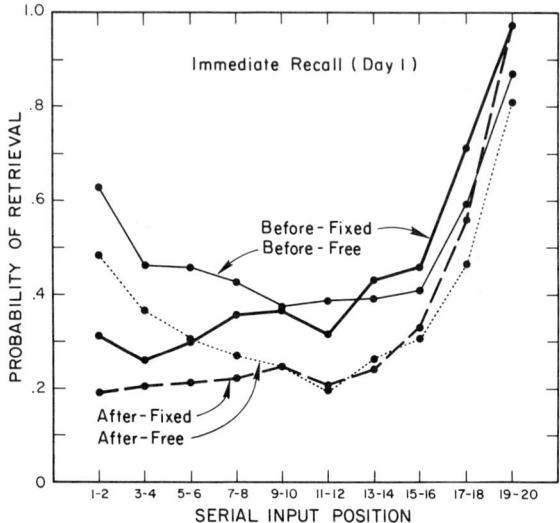

Fig. 6. The probability of immediate recall on Day 1 as a function of serial input position. Separate functions are plotted for lists presented before or after drug administration for which either fixed- or free-rehearsal study procedures were used (Experiment 3). (Reprinted with permission from Darley et al., 1974.)

recency effect, but no primacy effect is present. This is an encouraging result; it indicates the success of the procedure since subjects did not, as on free-rehearsal lists, spend more time processing early items. The effectiveness of the fixed-rehearsal procedure is also demonstrated by the nearly perfect performance for terminal items, both before and after drug administration. At the time of test these items were apparently in the rehearsal buffer, as they should have been, and were retrieved accurately both in the drug and no-drug state. Given this assurance that subjects rehearsed as instructed, the striking contrast between before- and after-drug performance is noteworthy. Although subjects were equally diligent in processing list items in the two states, there is still a substantial deficit in the recall of nonrehearsal-buffer items due to drug intoxication.

V. LOCUS OF THE STORAGE DEFICIT

Experiment 3 shows that at least a portion of and perhaps the entire storage deficit induced by marijuana results from some factor other than inferior use of active study procedures by drug subjects. One possible alternative explanation for the deficit is that for each unit of time an item resides in the buffer, or for each rehearsal or coding operation applied to it while it is there (whichever is crucial in information transfer) there is a greater increase in LTS strength in the nonintoxicated state. If this were the case, there would be interesting implications for memory theory, particularly with regard to the relation between attentional processes and memory performance. It has generally been assumed that the chief determinants of the degree of transfer of information from STS to LTS are the type and quantity of control processing performed on an item. For example, it has been shown that the seemingly powerful variable of intention to learn is only effective in enhancing performance to the extent that it causes optimal learning strategies to be applied efficiently to to-be-remembered material (Hyde and Jenkins, 1969; Postman, 1964). We have assumed that a behavioral indicator, the overt repetition of list items, accurately reflects the degree of internal processing items receive. It may be that this assumption is invalid. Perhaps in the no-drug state subjects give full attention to the items while repeating them, whereas in the drug state they attend only enough to satisfy the requirements of the fixed-rehearsal procedure. This reduced level of attention to list items, possibly caused by increased competition during drug intoxication from the subject's own thoughts, might be sufficient to hold items in STS but inadequate for optimal transfer to LTS. The fact that a variable such as drug state may alter the effectiveness of control processes without creating any behavioral sign that it has done so suggests that memory researchers should be alert for other factors which reduce processing capacity without seeming to disrupt the operation of control processes.

Another explanation for the storage deficit is that transfer to LTS is impaired for items residing in the nonrehearsal-buffer portion of STS; i.e., in the drug state less information about an item's occurrence is transferred to LTS between the time it is removed from the buffer and the moment it is lost from STS. Using the distractor paradigm developed by Brown (1958) and Peterson and Peterson (1959), Dornbush et al. (1971) showed that information is lost from STS more quickly than normal during marijuana intoxication. Dornbush et al. presented subjects a new trigram of consonants on every trial. Following trigram presentation the subjects engaged in rehearsal-preventing activity for a period of either 0, 6, 12, or 18 seconds. At the end of the interval they received a cue to recall the trigram. As shown in Fig. 7, the rate of forgetting was the same for placebo and low dose (7.5 mg THC smoked) but greater for the high dose (22.5 mg smoked).

Increased forgetting from STS might be sufficient to explain inferior performance during marijuana intoxication when subjects use a free-

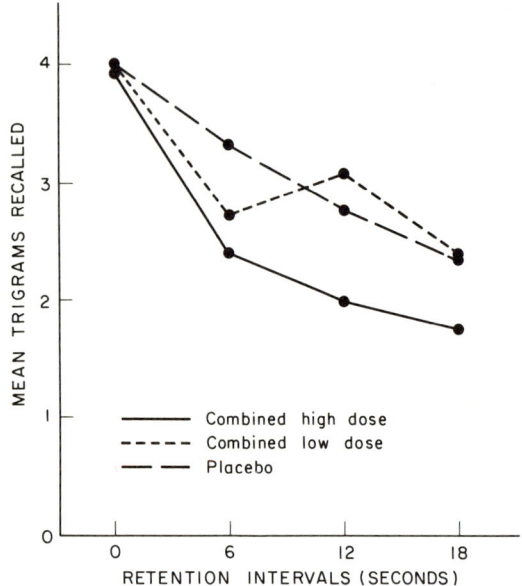

Fig. 7. Effects of marijuana on the Brown-Peterson task. Mean trigrams recalled is plotted as a function of retention interval for three conditions: placebo, low dose (7.5 mg THC smoked), and high dose (22.5 mg THC smoked). (Reprinted with permission from Dornbush et al., 1971.)

rehearsal strategy. The free-rehearsal strategy allows items which have been dropped from the rehearsal buffer to be retrieved from STS or LTS and reenter the buffer (Rundus and Atkinson, 1970). If forgetting from STS is accelerated by marijuana, it is conceivable that fewer reentries of items retrieved from STS would be made. This would particularly hamper complex coding operations in which list words are associated with one another.

On fixed-rehearsal lists, items which have left the rehearsal buffer do not reenter. In order to show that increased forgetting of unrehearsed information in STS causes poorer recall on fixed-rehearsal lists, it must be demonstrated that information is transferred to LTS while an item resides in STS, even if it has been dropped from the rehearsal buffer. If unrehearsed information is transferred to LTS, then loss of that information from STS would prevent transfer.

Using a variation of the Brown-Peterson procedure, Atkinson and Shiffrin (1971) showed that the memory trace of an item must be maintained in STS for a short time following its removal from the buffer if transfer to LTS is to be optimal. Subjects were presented a consonant pentagram on each trial. They then performed a nonverbal signal-detection task of 1, 8, or 40 seconds duration, followed by 30 seconds of difficult rehearsal-preventing arithmetic. Recall of the pentagram was then required. Unlike arithmetic or counting tasks, engaging in a nonverbal detection task does not cause information to be lost from STS (Reitman, 1971). Presumably this is because forgetting of verbal information from STS is due to interference from subsequent verbal input rather than time-dependent decay. Consequently, in Atkinson and Shiffrin's experiment the three durations of signal detection allowed subjects to hold strong memory traces of pentagrams in STS for relatively short, intermediate, or long periods of time. The arithmetic was added to ensure that retrieval would be from LTS. Although retrieval is largely from STS in the Brown-Peterson task, some information is transferred to LTS during stimulus presentation (Hellyer, 1962), and this information is particularly useful for recall during early trials of the task (Keppel and Underwood, 1962) and after long retention intervals on later trials (Peterson and Peterson, 1959). Executing 30 seconds of arithmetic causes virtually all information to be lost from STS, so retrieval following arithmetic must be from LTS. Atkinson and Shiffrin's results showed that holding unrehearsed information in STS for 8 seconds during signal detection increased recall probability following arithmetic above the level for 1 second, but there was no additional increase for the 40 second condition. In other words, engaging in the interfering arithmetic task 1 second after stimulus presentation in some way suppressed the transfer of unrehearsed information to LTS, a process which is completed some time between 1 and 8 seconds.

Combining the results of Dornbush *et al.* and Atkinson and Shiffrin, it appears that marijuana may impair storage in LTS by increasing the probability that unrehearsed information is lost from STS before transfer to LTS is complete. Whether marijuana causes accelerated forgetting from STS or reduced attention during rehearsal, the drug's effects on a variety of experimental tasks is understandable. Incomplete storage of past events during drug intoxication is likely to reduce an individual's ability to link these events with current input in order to perform higher level operations such as the understanding of and memory for narrative material (Drew *et al.*, 1972; Miller *et al.*, 1972) or problem solving and concept formation (Klonoff *et al.*, 1973). Drug-induced deficits in less complex tasks such as digit span (Melges *et al.*, 1970a; Tinklenberg *et al.*, 1970), goal-directed serial alternation (Melges *et al.*, 1970a,b), and digit code (Clark and Nakashima, 1968; Clark *et al.*, 1970; Jones and Stone, 1970) probably result from the reduced availability of information in STS and/or inefficient transfer to LTS. As Melges *et al.* (1971) have suggested, it may also be the case that the impairment in memory functioning during marijuana intoxication reduces the saliency of past events, thereby accounting for subjective drug effects such as isolation or timelessness of present experiences, euphoria, and an increased vividness of perceptions.

VI. EVIDENCE OF STATE-DEPENDENT RETRIEVAL

It is clear that for material learned in the no-drug state, recall performance does not vary as a function of drug state during delayed testing. This finding indicates that for marijuana, retrieval may not be state dependent; i.e., optimal retrieval of information stored in memory while the system was in a particular state may not depend on the existence of that same state at the time of retrieval (Overton, 1968). However, since retrieval has been shown to be asymmetrically state dependent for other drugs (Barnhart and Abbott, 1967; Berger and Stein, 1969; Gardner et al., 1972) we decided to determine if retrieval of information originally presented during marijuana intoxication is state dependent. Experiment

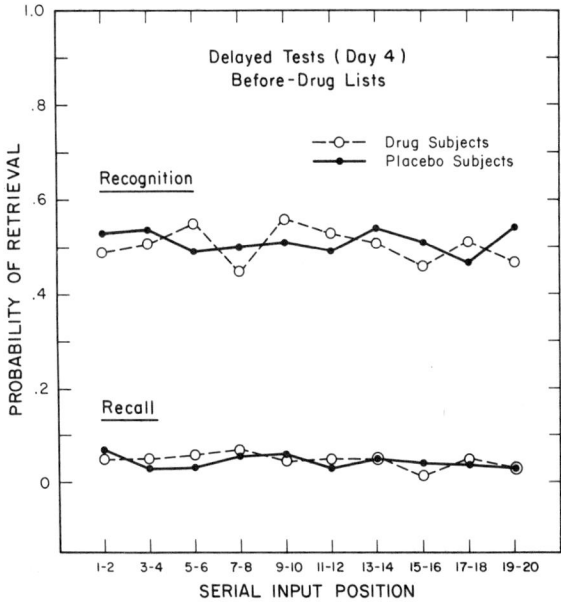

Fig. 8. The probability of delayed recall and recognition on Day 4 as functions of the serial input position of items from pre-drug lists on Day 1. Separate functions are plotted for drug and placebo groups (Experiment 3). (Reprinted with permission from Darley et al., 1974.)

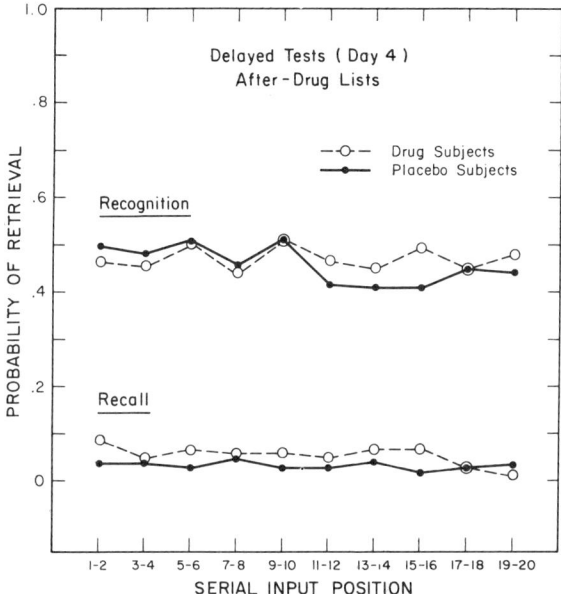

Fig. 9. The probability of delayed recall and recognition on Day 4 as functions of the serial input position of items from post-drug lists on Day 1. Separate functions are plotted for drug and placebo subjects (Experiment 3). (Reprinted with permission from Darley et al., 1974.)

3 (Section IV,B,3) was designed so that in addition to examining immediate-recall performance for the fixed- and free-rehearsal procedures, we could compare drug and placebo retrieval for words learned in either the drug or no-drug states. Figures 8 and 9 show serial position curves for delayed recall and recognition on Day 4. Separate curves are plotted for subjects who received marijuana on Day 4 and those who received placebo, but data are pooled for fixed- and free-rehearsal lists. We had hoped that performance levels would be higher than those shown, but apparently the relatively long interval between presentation and delayed test (necessitated by a desire to avoid carry-over effects from Day 1 drug administration) made list words difficult to retrieve on Day 4. These low performance levels for both recall and recognition (chance recognition performance is 0.33) probably account for the unexpected absence of a strong primacy effect. Combining across serial positions, the data show that words presented before drug administration on Day 1 (Fig. 8) were recalled and recognized equally well by drug and placebo subjects on Day 4. This confirms our previous results (Darley et al., 1973b) and those of Abel (1971a). On the other hand, drug subjects were significantly better at recalling words presented in the drug state on Day 1 (Fig. 9).

We conclude that for word recall, retrieval is asymmetrically state dependent for marijuana. The absence of a state-dependent effect for recognition testing, the finding by others that retrieval is symmetrically state dependent for marijuana, and problems in interpreting our results are discussed below.

VII. ALTERNATIVE INTERPRETATIONS OF EXPERIMENTAL RESULTS

We have attempted to present a straightforward discussion of our research in terms of a particular theoretical framework; therefore, we have avoided mentioning alternative interpretations of the data not consistent with that framework. Also, certain features of the data have not been mentioned so that our conclusions could be presented as clearly as possible. These alternative interpretations and additional data are discussed below.

Shallice and Warrington (1970), Wickelgren (1970), and Kesner (1973) have proposed models of the human memory system in which STS and LTS are not only structurally or functionally separate memory stores but may operate independently. The strongest evidence for this point of view is provided by observations of an individual whose performance on memory tasks indicates a sharply reduced rehearsal-buffer capacity for auditorily presented materials, but normal levels of retrieval from LTS (Shallice and Warrington, 1970; Warrington and Shallice, 1969). If entry into LTS depends on processing in STS, then it is difficult to understand how storage into LTS can proceed normally in the presence of impaired STS functioning. While we still ascribe to the notion of a sequentially operating memory system, it is probably important to mention that the results from our experiments can be explained by the alternative model in which information enters STS and LTS in parallel. Drug-induced storage deficits would occur because of inefficient direct entry of encoded information into LTS.

Those studying drug effects on learning in animals are particularly sensitive to "nonspecific" effects of drugs (e.g., increased arousal) which may be confounded with memory effects in some tasks (McGaugh, 1973). It might be argued that the drug effects observed in our experiments are motivational effects; placebo subjects may simply try harder on the memory tasks. Immediate free-recall performance could be affected in two ways by such a motivational factor. First, drug subjects might perform less processing on list items. We showed that when the number of overt rehearsals is equated in the drug and no-drug states the storage deficit persists. It is clear, therefore, that decreased willingness to rehearse items is not responsible for the deficit. We proposed that in the drug state subjects may attend less while rehearsing; although competition from thought processes could explain this deficiency in attention, decreased motivation to attend cannot be ruled out.

A second possible result of decreased motivation is that drug subjects might put less effort into writing responses on the immediate-recall test. Such an effect would be indistinguishable from a retrieval deficit and is therefore refuted by the same data used to show that marijuana does not impair retrieval. If motivation were a factor in word recall, then for words learned in the no-drug state, placebo subjects should show better delayed-recall performance than drug subjects. In Experiments 2 and 3 no such group difference was obtained.

Abel (1971b) has provided evidence which suggests that decreased motivation during either rehearsal or recall is an unsatisfactory explanation of the effect of marijuana on storage. He administered the Jackson Personality Research Form to subjects in order to obtain a measure of "achievement motivation." Based on this test he concluded that drug subjects were no less willing than placebo subjects to "put forth effort to obtain excellence."

Although marijuana-intoxicated subjects apparently suffer no deficiencies in retrieval capabilities or motivation at the time of test, there may be another nonstorage factor which combines with a peculiarity in the way information is stored in the drug state to produce the observed group differences in immediate recall. In order to accurately recall words presented on a list, a subject must have access to stored information telling him on which list a particular item had been presented (Anderson and Bower, 1972). Drug subjects appear less able to make list discriminations than placebo subjects. In Experiment 2 drug subjects produced many more incorrect responses in immediate recall than did placebo subjects. These intrusion errors included both prior-list and nonlist items. This fact does not necessarily lead to the conclusion that the immediate-recall deficit is produced by inefficient storage of list-membership information rather than poorer storage of item information. In order to make this argument one must assume that at the time of test subjects attempt to retrieve items until a criterion point is reached such as a limit on total number of items output or time spent on retrieval. Given that subjects emit more intrusions and assuming that drug and placebo subjects maintain equivalent total-item or total-time criteria for determining retrieval attempts, then drug subjects will recall fewer correct items. On the other hand, if the termination of recall is controlled by a limit on the number of unsuccessful retrieval attempts (which will depend on the availability of stored memory traces), then an inability to edit intrusions will not affect the probability of recall of correct list items. We are convinced that if subjects do use a criterion for the termination of memory search, in our experiments it is probably of the latter type. In Experiment 2, data from the delayed-recall test on the first set of lists showed that although drug subjects produced twice as many intrusions as did placebo subjects, the output of these words that did not appear on any list did not cause drug subjects' recall of list words to decline. It could be argued that the chance that list items might be omitted from recall is reduced in delayed recall because time and item constraints are not as strict. The fact that subjects were allowed sufficient time for immediate recall (2 minutes) and were urged to use the entire time to search memory for list items leads us to believe that relative to the size of the pool of possible correct responses the criterion for termination of search was not likely to be more strict for immediate recall than delayed recall. We conclude that while the drug subjects' propensity for committing intrusion errors is worthy of further investigation, drug-induced immediate recall deficits are probably not caused by intrusion-producing processes acting at the time of response.

It could be argued that the delayed-recall data from Experiments 2 and 3 result from a marijuana-induced enhancement of retrieval processes combined with a symmetric state-dependency effect. A paired-associate learning study by Rickles et al. (1973) in which retrieval was found to be symmetrically state dependent for marijuana supports this view. The limitations of a 2 × 2 design such as that used by Rickles et al., or a modification of that procedure such as we used in Experiment 3, have been described in detail by Overton (1972). In most cases, it is simply not possible using such designs to arrive at a single irrefutable interpretation of the data. Nevertheless, we prefer our original conclusion. First, there is no evidence in the literature that marijuana facilitates retrieval. Second, it seems unlikely that in both Experiments 2 and 3 and in Abel's study (1971a) the effects of enhanced retrieval under drug and state dependency would balance one another so as to produce equal drug and placebo delayed-recall performance for words originally presented in the no-drug state.

VIII. NEW DIRECTIONS AND PROMISING RESEARCH

While the research presented here hopefully provides a more detailed description of the interaction between marijuana and memory processes than has been available heretofore, it is limited in certain ways. The effects of marijuana on certain interesting complexities of list-learning performance have not been considered. Much recent psychological research deals with organizational procedures used by subjects in order to maximize later recall and recognition performance (Tulving and Donaldson, 1972). These procedures involve grouping lists of items together on the basis of one or more common features, with the result that the list is stored in memory as a series of higher order units, each composed of several elementary units (Tulving, 1968). At the time of recall test the probability that a particular item will be retrieved may depend on whether the higher order unit to which it belongs is retrieved. In some cases, information regarding an item's occurrence on a list may be *available* in memory, having been registered there during list presentation, but it may not be *accessible* for recall (Tulving and Pearlstone, 1966). Optimal access to higher order units and their elementary unit members is contingent on the formation during presentation and presence at the time of test of retrieval cues. These cues direct the search of memory to appropriate locations. Thus, to understand the effects of marijuana on list learning, one must not only examine the drug's effects on item recall, but also its effects on the organization of recall and the utilization of retrieval cues.

An effective means of studying organization in free recall is to present lists containing items from a small set of conceptual categories. This procedure allows recall to be analyzed in terms of number of words per category recalled, as well as the total number of items recalled. Subjects' responses may also be examined for evidence of category clustering. Pearl *et al.* (1973) presented subjects categorized lists and found that marijuana subjects both recalled less total items and clustered items from the same category less often in recall than did placebo subjects. Eich *et al.* (1974) found that on a delayed-recall test subjects intoxicated with marijuana before list presentation and testing recalled fewer categories and fewer total words than did subjects who received placebo before both presentation and test. However, the number of words recalled per category was the same for both groups. Thus, it may be that the storage deficit for marijuana results from the inefficient formation during list presentation of retrieval cues such as category names.

Eich *et al.* also examined state-dependent retrieval in their study. They suggested that state-dependent learning may result from the inaccessibility of information during retrieval due to state change rather than to its unavailability. They reasoned that if information learned in a particular drug state were merely inaccessible due to a state change, the presentation during test of potent retrieval cues like category names might eliminate the effect. They presented subjects categorized lists in either the marijuana or placebo state and tested them 4 hours later in either the same or a changed state. Testing was either free recall or cued recall. In cued recall, subjects were provided at the time of test the names of the categories present in the list. Eich et al. found that while free recall was asymmetrically state dependent for marijuana, cued recall showed no state-dependent effects, a result that supported their hypothesis. The results of this study show that for human subjects the appearance of state-dependent effects is sensitive to the nature of the memory task and the method of testing. Our finding that retrieval was asymmetrically state dependent for recall testing, but not state dependent for recognition, and the Rickles et al. (1973) result that retrieval was symmetrically state dependent for a paired-associate learning task further emphasize this point. The next step is to try to understand these varied results in terms of what we know about the memory mechanisms involved in the tasks used and how marijuana affects such mechanisms. A satisfactory result would be the explanation of all state-change effects in terms of existing concepts of human memory. The research of Eich et al. is a promising step in this direction. On the other hand, if new conceptions must be introduced, the drug will have been a valuable implement for increasing the precision of memory models.

While it would be desirable for drug researchers to use marijuana as a tool to examine encoding, organization, and retrieval of list information in greater depth, possible drug effects on memory of a less verbal and/or less temporally defined nature should not be ignored. For example, except for some work by Klonoff et al. (1973) we know little about how marijuana affects the storage and retrieval of pictures, shapes, patterns, tones, complex sounds, smells, or tactile and kinesthetic sensations. Also, no information is available concerning the accessibility during marijuana intoxication of semantic information, i.e., that information which infuses words with meaning and allows concepts to be manipulated and related to one another (Tulving, 1972). As an example, it would be interesting to know if marijuana facilitates or impairs the speed or accuracy of response to such questions as "Do penguins have wings?" Marijuana users report that the drug commonly alters perceptions of, associations with, and conceptions about even simple objects. If such effects reflect changes in the process of retrieving semantic information, the application to drug research of methods used to study semantic memory (Collins and Quillian, 1969; Meyer, 1970; Landauer and Freedman, 1968; Rips et al., 1973) could provide explanations for some subjective drug effects as well as insight into the structure and functioning of semantic memory.

We mentioned early in this chapter (Section II) the potential value of drugs for examining the conscious monitoring process by which the individual perceives and appraises his own ongoing behavior. During task performance the individual is able to assess the progress of his efforts at converging on a specified goal (Miller et al., 1960). This monitoring process allows inefficient strategies to be discarded and potentially useful strategies to be initiated. Covert mental operations such as memory control processes may be subject to such monitoring just as overt motor acts are perceived and evaluated. Hart (1965) has shown that subjects are able to examine their memories in order to determine with some accuracy whether currently irretrievable information is potentially available for recall. Specifically, when confronted with a common knowledge question they could not immediately answer, subjects often correctly predicted whether or not they would be able to select the correct answer from a list of alternatives. The subjective experience of this "memory monitoring process" Hart calls one's "feeling of knowing." The existence of such a process enables the individual to decide whether, after a series of retrieval failures, further similar attempts should be made, retrieval strategies should be altered, or retrieval efforts should be abandoned altogether. We are currently examining the effects of marijuana intoxication on the accuracy of memory monitoring. Hopefully, Hart's paradigm will serve as a prototype for further investigations into the subjective aspects of the drug experience.

IX. OUTLOOK FOR MARIJUANA–MEMORY RESEARCH

We conclude by expressing optimism about the heuristic value of emerging drug research as it applies to human memory. It appears that drugs are being used incisively in order to explore questions which may be unanswerable by other means. Hopefully, marijuana will continue to be used for this purpose, since its unique effects on objective performance and subjective experience, as well as the apparent absence of harmful long-term effects from its use, make it an interesting and safe tool from the standpoint of experimenter and subject.

ACKNOWLEDGMENTS

The authors thank Richard C. Atkinson for his helpful suggestions and Cynthia Demos, Patricia Murphy, and Peggy Murphy for their assistance in preparing the final draft of this chapter.

The authors' research reported in this chapter was supported in part by the van Ameringen Foundation.

REFERENCES

Abel, E. L. (1971a). *Science* **173**, 1038–1040.
Abel, E. L. (1971b). *Nature (London)* **231**, 58.
Anderson, J. R., and Bower, G. H. (1972). *Psychol. Rev.* **2**, 97–123.
Atkinson, R. C., and Shiffrin, R. M. (1968). In "The Psychology of Learning and Motivation" (K. W. Spence and J. T. Spence, eds.), Vol. 2, pp. 89–195. Academic Press, New York.
Atkinson, R. C., and Shiffrin, R. M. (1971). *Sci. Amer.* **224**, 82–90.
Atkinson, R. C., Herrmann, D. J., and Wescourt, K. T. (1974). In "Theories in Cognitive Psychology: The Loyola Symposium" (R. L. Solso, ed.), pp. 101–146. V. H. Winston, Washington, D. C.
Barnhart, S. S., and Abbott, D. W. (1967). *Psychol. Rep.* **20**, 520–522.
Berger, B. D., and Stein, L. (1969). *Psychopharmacologia* **14**, 351–358.
Brown, J. (1958). *J. Exp. Psychol.* **10**, 12–21.
Clark, L. D., and Nakashima, E. N. (1968). *Amer. J. Psychiat.* **125**, 379–384.
Clark, L. D., Hughes, R., and Nakashima, E. N. (1970). *Arch. Gen. Psychiat.* **23**, 193–198.
Collins, A. M., and Quillian, M. R. (1969). *J. Verb. Learn. Verb. Behav.* **8**, 240–247.
Craik, F. I. M. (1970). *J. Verb. Learn. Verb. Behav.* **9**, 672–678.
Dallet, K. M. (1963). *J. Exp. Psychol.* **66**, 65–71.
Darley, C. F., Tinklenberg, J. R., Hollister, L. E., and Atkinson, R. C. (1973a). *Psychopharmacologia* **29**, 231–238.
Darley, C. F., Tinklenberg, J. R., Roth, W. T., Hollister, L. E., and Atkinson, R. C. (1973b). *Memory & Cognition* **1**, 196–200.
Darley, C. F., Tinklenberg, J. R., Roth, W. T., and Atkinson, R. C. (1974). *Psychopharmacologia* **37**, 139–149.
Dornbush, R. L., Fink, M., and Freedman, A. M. (1971). *Amer. J. Psychiat.* **128**, 194–197.
Drew, W. G., Kiplinger, G. F., Miller, L. L., and Marx, M. (1972). *Clin. Pharmacol. Ther.* **13**, 526–533.
Eich, J., Weingartner, H., and Stillman, R. C. (1974). Submitted for publication.
Fischler, I., Rundus, D. E., and Atkinson, R. C. (1970). *Psychon. Sci.* **19**, 249–250.
Gardner, E. L., Glick, S. D., and Jarvick, M. E. (1972). *Physiol. & Behav.* **8**, 11–15.
Glanzer, M., and Cunitz, A. R. (1966). *J. Verb. Learn. Verb. Behav.* **5**, 351–360.
Hart, J. T. (1965). "Recall, Recognition and the Memory-monitoring Process." Unpublished Ph.D. Thesis, Stanford University, Stanford, California.
Hellyer, S. (1962). *J. Exp. Psychol.* **64**, 650–651.
Hyde, T. S., and Jenkins, J. J. (1969). *J. Exp. Psychol.* **82**, 472–481.
James, W. (1890). "The Principles of Psychology." Dover, New York (reprinted, 1950).
Jones, R. T., and Stone, G. C. (1970). *Psychopharmacologia* **18**, 108–117.
Keppel, G., and Mallory, W. A. (1969). *J. Exp. Psychol.* **79**, 269–275.
Keppel, G., and Underwood, B. J. (1962). *J. Verb. Learn. Verb. Behav.* **1**, 153–161.
Kesner, R. (1973). *Psychol. Bull.* **80**, 177–203.

Klonoff, H., Low, M., and Marcus, A. (1973). *Can. Med. Ass. J.* **108**, 150–157.
Landauer, T. K., and Freedman, J. L. (1968). *J. Verb. Learn. Verb. Behav.* **7**, 291–295.
McGaugh, J. L. (1968). *U.S., Pub. Health Serv., Publ.* **1836**.
McGaugh, J. L. (1973). *Annu. Rev. Pharmacol.* **13**, 229–241.
McGaugh, J. L., and Dawson, R. G. (1971). *Behav. Sci.* **16**, 45–63.
Melges, F. T., Tinklenberg, J. R., Hollister, L. E., and Gillespie, H. K. (1970a). *Science* **168**, 1118–1120.
Melges, F. T., Tinklenberg, J. R., Hollister, L. E., and Gillespie, H. K. (1970b). *Arch. Gen. Psychiat.* **23**, 204–210.
Melges, F. T., Tinklenberg, J. R., Hollister, L. E., and Gillespie, H. K. (1971). *Arch. Gen. Psychiat.* **24**, 564–567.
Meyer, D. E. (1970). *Cog. Psychol.* **1**, 242–300.
Miller, G. A., Galanter, E., and Pribram, K. H. (1960). "Plans and the Structure of Behavior." Holt, New York.
Miller, L., Drew, W. G., and Kiplinger, G. F. (1972). *Nature (London)* **237**, 172–173.
Neisser, U. (1967). "Cognitive Psychology." Appleton, New York.
Norman, D. A. (1972). *In* "The Physiological Basis of Memory" (J. A. Deutsch, ed.), pp. 397–414. Academic Press, New York.
Norman, D. A., and Waugh, N. C. (1965). *Psychol. Rev.* **72**, 89–104.
Overton, D. A. (1968). *U.S., Pub. Health Serv., Publ.* **1836**.
Overton, D. A. (1974). *Fed. Proc.* **33**, 1800–1813.
Palmer, S. E., and Ornstein, P. A. (1971). *J. Exp. Psychol.* **88**, 60–66.
Pearl, J. H., Domino, E. F., and Rennick, P. (1973). *Psychopharmacologia* **31**, 13–24.
Peterson, L. T., and Peterson, M. J. (1959). *J. Exp. Psychol.* **58**, 193–198.
Postman, L. (1964). *In* "Categories of Human Learning" (A. W. Melton, ed.), pp. 145–201. Academic Press, New York.
Reitman, J. S. (1971). *Cog. Psychol.* **2**, 185–195.
Rickles, W. H., Jr., Cohen, M. J., Whitaker, C. A., and McIntyre, K. E. (1973). *Psychopharmacologia* **30**, 349–354.
Rips, L. J., Shoben, E. J., and Smith, E. E. (1973). *J. Verb. Learn. Verb. Behav.* **12**, 1–20.
Rundus, D. J., and Atkinson, R. C. (1970). *J. Verb. Learn. Verb. Behav.* **9**, 684–688.
Shallice, T., and Warrington, E. K. (1970). *J. Exp. Psychol.* **22**, 261–273.
Sperling, G. (1960). *Psychol. Monog.* **74**, No. 498.
Sternberg, S. (1966). *Science* **153**, 652–654.
Sternberg, S. (1969). *Amer. Sci.* **57**, 421–457.
Tart, C. T. (1971). "On Being Stoned." Science and Behavior Books, Palo Alto, California.
Tart, C. T., (ed.) (1972). "Altered States of Consciousness." Doubleday, Garden City, New York.
Tinklenberg, J. R., Melges, F. T., Hollister, L. E., and Gillespie, H. K. (1970). *Nature (London)* **226**, 1171–1172.
Tulving, E. (1968). *In* "Verbal Behavior and General Behavior Theory" (T. R. Dixon and D. L. Horton, eds.), pp. 2–36. Prentice-Hall, Englewood Cliffs, New Jersey.
Tulving, E. (1972). *In* "Organization of Memory" (E. Tulving and W. D. Donaldson, eds.), pp. 381–403. Academic Press, New York.
Tulving, E., and Donaldson, W. D., eds. (1972). "Organization of Memory."

Academic Press, New York.
Tulving, E., and Pearlstone, Z. (1966). *J. Verb. Learn. Verb. Behav.* **5**, 381–391.
Warrington, E. K., and Shallice, T. (1969). *Brain* **92**, 885–896.
Waugh, N. C., and Norman, D. A. (1965). *Psychol. Rev.* **72**, 89–104.
Weil, A. T. (1972). "The Natural Mind." Houghton, Boston, Massachusetts.
Wickelgren, W. A. (1970). *In* "Models of Human Memory" (D. A. Norman, ed.), pp. 65–102. Academic Press, New York.

Chapter 5

A MODEL OF ATTENTION DESCRIBING THE COGNITIVE EFFECTS OF MARIJUANA

FONYA LORD DELONG AND BERNARD I. LEVY

I. Introduction 103
II. A Model of Attention 104
   A. Experimental Studies of Acute Effects 104
   B. Experimental Studies of Chronic Effects 113
   C. Clinical Studies of Chronic Effects 115
   D. Studies of the Relationship of Marijuana Use to Motivation and Academic Achievement 115
III. Summary 117
   References 117

I. INTRODUCTION

Recently much research has focused on the effects of marijuana use on cognition. Most research has been performed on acute effects since testing soon after use is easy to accomplish. Relatively little data are available for chronic or long-term effects even though this is where the greatest concern is.

This chapter will present a model of attention which can be used to organize the research findings to date reasonably well. Both acute and chronic effects will be discussed in terms of this model since it is possible that chronic effects will turn out to be similar to the acute effects.

II. A MODEL OF ATTENTION

Sack and Rice (1974) have isolated three separate processes of attention: *degree of selectivity, resistance to distraction,* and *shifting.* Degree of selectivity is defined operationally in terms of performance on any of the several embedded figure tests and has also been called field articulation (Gardner and Moriarity, 1968). It is a continuum ranging from very sharp distinctions between what is relevant and what is not, to considerably less sharp distinctions—a way of attending in a much less differentiated way. This process of attention has actually generated considerable interest for a number of years, but it has usually been conceptualized as an indicator of cognitive style or personality (Witkin *et al.*, 1954, 1962). Those who make sharp distinctions are said to be field independent, while those who do not are termed field dependent.

The second process is resistance to distraction, which is seen as a continuum ranging from great concentration to extreme inability to maintain a focus of attention. Distraction is an involuntary change in an established focus of attention, thus occurring later in time than selectivity, which is the act of establishing a focus.

Shifting is the third process and refers to the ability to voluntarily shift the focus of attention. It requires the cessation of the current focus and the establishment of a new one. It is measured along a continuum ranging from perfect voluntary control to perseveration, the inability to stop focusing despite the desire to do so.

A. Experimental Studies of Acute Effects

Briefly, the work done on acute effects shows various cognitive impairments which increase as dosage increases. Dose-related decrements have been found in a complex calculating task, goal-directed serial alternation (Melges *et al.*, 1970), delayed auditory feedback (Kiplinger *et al.*, 1971), and visual-motor tasks (Weil *et al.*, 1968; Kiplinger *et al.*, 1971). It seems reasonable to suppose that other cognitive decrements found in the literature are related to dosage, although specific studies for each one have not been performed.

In general, it has been found that naive subjects and casual users show more decrements in performance when intoxicated than do chronic users (Weil *et al.*, 1968; Meyer *et al.*, 1971). This effect seems to be an example of state-dependent learning—learning that occurs when in a drugged state and is accessible only again in the drugged state.

1. DEGREE OF SELECTIVITY OR FIELD ARTICULATION

The evidence that marijuana affects the first process, *degree of selectivity*, is equivocal. Only one study of acute effects found that marijuana made a significant difference in performance. Pearl (1972) found that experienced users when intoxicated performed significantly less well on Witkin's Embedded Figures Test and the Closure Speed Test. In other words, they were more field dependent. Another study found a trend in the same direction, but the difference was not significant. Meyer et al. (1971), using an embedded figures test and the Stroop Color Word Test,* found that subjects (6 casual and 6 daily users) when intoxicated tended to do less well. Two studies have found no effect. Miller et al. (1972), using relatively naive subjects, found no differences between intoxicated and placebo control subjects using the Stroop Color Word Test. Furthermore, Jones and Stone (1970), using the Rod and Frame Test (which correlated highly with the Embedded Figures Test) found no differences in performance under marijuana. These subjects had used marijuana daily for several years.

More research is obviously needed. The idea of change in figure-ground relationships makes sense, however, in terms of the subjective effects of the drug. Visual and auditory details (and others) which would usually be overshadowed become noticed and are more distinct.

2. RESISTANCE TO DISTRACTION

Good concentration is necessary in order to accomplish many cognitive tasks, and this seems to be the crucial factor in many of the decrements in cognition that have been found in the acute marijuana state. Three studies have attempted to measure resistance to distraction directly. All used delayed auditory feedback which functions as a distracting external stimulus on various cognitive tasks. (It should be noted here that many of the tests discussed in this article are different from those used by Sack and Rice in developing their model, and that there is no guarantee that the tests actually measure the factors of attention that they are said to measure. Analysis of the underlying processes, though, suggests that they do.)

The cognitive tasks used in the delayed auditory feedback studies

---

* According to Sack and Rice (1973), this test measures both selectivity and shifting.

consisted of reading Aristotle forward and backward, counting, counting backward from 10,000, addition and subtraction, adding or subtracting seven from the answers to arithmetic problems, and color discrimination. Manno et al. (1970) found that marijuana significantly impaired performance on five of the nine tasks, while Kiplinger et al. (1971) found that four of the nine tasks were significantly impaired. A third experiment, however, using low doses, found no effect using three tasks: progressive count, color discrimination, and addition (Evans et al., 1973). Two tasks were significantly impaired in two experiments: reading forward and counting backward from 10,000. However, the important thing here is not which tasks were most impaired, because that will vary somewhat with different groups of subjects when the groups are small (8 and 12), but rather the fact that subjects engaged in cognitive tasks are more easily distracted by delayed auditory feedback and probably other external stimuli when they are intoxicated. Lowered resistance to distraction is also probably at least partly responsible for the decrements found in arithmetical ability, visual-motor tasks, including reaction time, verbal behavior, and memory.

Rapaport et al. (1970) have pointed out that arithmetical ability measures concentration or resistance to distraction, among other things. Subjects under the influence of marijuana have been found to show impairment of accuracy in serial addition (Hollister, 1971; Waskow et al., 1970) and on the numerical subtests of the Army Alpha (Halpern, 1944). Hollister (1971) found that performance on an arithmetic test was slowed, although accuracy was maintained. L. Rafaelsen et al. (1973) found identical results for addition but found a slight increase in errors for subtraction. Melges et al. (1970), using a complex calculating task called goal-directed serial alternation (GDSA), found that marijuana caused a significant decrement in performance. Tinklenberg et al. (1972), using the same task with different subjects, found a decrement, but it was not significant. Intoxicated subjects were described as losing their places more often, forgetting whether to add or subtract, and forgetting the goal number; in short, they were distracted. Butler (1973), studying chronic users, found no effect on GDSA, however; and Melges et al. (1970) found no effect on the subtraction of serial sevens.

On visual-motor performance tasks, the evidence for a performance decrement caused by poor concentration is more equivocal, although decrements have been shown often enough to warrant the conclusion that they are real, not artifacts. Clark et al. (1970), using the Digit Symbol test, a measure of psychomotor speed, found impairment of performance, as had Clark and Nakashima in 1968. The impairment, however, was not significant, and the presence of marked individual differences was noted. Meyer et al. (1971) noted that impairment was more evident in casual than heavy users but that the differences were not significant. Weil et al. (1968) found a decrement for naive users but noted a slight improvement for chronic users. Butler (1973), using 60 chronic subjects, also found no significant decrement when they were intoxicated. Halpern (1944) found a decrement in visual-motor performance using the larger of two doses but no effect with the lower dose. Two studies found no effects (Hollister and Gillespie, 1970; Jones and Stone, 1970). Jones and Stone's study employed very heavy users as subjects, however, and they would be expected to compensate for the effect of the drug better than anyone else. Halpern (1944) also found that intoxicated subjects did more poorly on Koh's Block Design and the Cancellation Test.* L. Rafaelsen et al. (1973), using Bourdon's cancellation test, however, found no differences.

Several studies have been done using the continuous performance test, which involves pressing a key every time an X flashes on a screen on which letters continually flash. Meyer et al. (1971) found a significant increase in errors for casual users but no increase for heavy users. Other studies have found no effect on this type of task (Weil et al., 1968; Weingartner et al., 1972).

Rodin et al. (1970) found that ten intoxicated users displayed significantly poorer performance on the Bender-Gestalt test, a pencil-and-paper task of copying designs. Using the Halstead-Reitan, a test involving many different visual-motor tasks, Klonoff et al. (1973) found 7, 9, and 11 out of 13 tests affected, depending on the dosage and timing of sessions (the difference due to timing was not significant).

Several studies have investigated the effect of marijuana on reaction time. Dougherty (1972) found a significant impairment as did Dornbush et al. (1971) with a high dose but not for a low one. In their study of complex reaction time, Clark and Nakashima (1968) found impairment but marked individual differences. Clark et al. (1970) found a sporadic impairment, while Hollister and Gillespie (1970) and Moskowitz et al. (1972) found no significant effect of marijuana on reaction time. Butler (1973), using 60 chronic users, also found no significant difference on a test of multichoice reaction time.

While marijuana seems to have an effect on reaction time, it is possible

---

* It consists of crossing out a specific geometric figure every time it appears on a sheet of figures. It probably also measures the third factor, shifting, since it is similar to a test that, according to Sack and Rice (1974), measured both distraction and shifting.

that, as Dougherty (1972) points out, the most important effect is the increase in the number of very long reaction times. This shows that the subject is having trouble both in resisting distraction and in shifting, the third factor. What may happen is the subject becomes unable to sustain a focus of attention, involuntarily establishes a new and probably irrelevant focus, and then has a hard time shifting his focus of attention voluntarily back to the task; he tends to perseverate slightly.

Those tasks used in some of the studies of driving seem most analogous to reaction time and thus probably measure distraction primarily. O. J. Rafaelsen et al. (1973) found that intoxicated subjects were significantly slower in both braking and starting. Crancer et al. (1969) did not find a significant difference in total errors except speedometer errors, which were not correlated with accidents. However, this latter study should not be seen as conclusive because of various methodological problems such as lack of dose response data (Kalant, 1969).

Verbal behavior is another cognitive function affected by marijuana. This is the one area in which chronic users when intoxicated perform more poorly than naive or casual users. Weil and Zinberg (1969) found that chronic users had a greater tendency to forget what they were going to say, to go off on tangents, and to talk about subjects that were either irrelevant or not directly related to the topic under discussion. They also had a hard time remembering their train of thought from moment to moment and showed a definite tendency to be distracted by various objects in the room. Barratt et al. (1972) found that when intoxicated subjects were asked to discuss a topic for 5 minutes, they lost their train of thought in 9 out of 10 instances. Zeidenberg et al. (1973) also found evidence that could be interpreted to show that intoxicated subjects were constantly struggling to maintain a focus of attention; they found a decrease in phrase length combined with an increase in pause and vowel length.

Although Weil and Zinberg (1969) noted that there was an increased free associative quality to verbalizations under marijuana, they did not find any distortion on the level at which words are combined into sentences. Weingartner et al. (1972) report a similar finding that marijuana has no effect on the frequency of associations; in short, associations formed during the intoxicated state are not more unusual or bizarre.

These experiments are also relevant to memory, another cognitive function affected by marijuana. There has been considerable discussion as to whether it is storage or retrieval of information that is affected, and the evidence on both sides will be reviewed. While only future research can completely clarify this issue, it seems likely that both are affected to some degree. In any event, the model of attention can encompass both. Poor

5. Cognitive Effects of Marijuana 109

concentration would affect the storage of information, and difficulty in shifting would affect retrieval.

Since it was found that learning of new visual-motor tasks was affected under marijuana but that Cloze analysis of sentence structure was not, Weil and Zinberg (1969) decided that there was interference with retrieval of information while in immediate memory storage; once it passes into the next (recent-memory) storage, it again seems easily accessible to consciousness. The data of Weingartner et al. (1972) suggest that when something is in long-term storage it is accessible, since the subjects are able to remember their associations as well when intoxicated as when not. These investigators are in agreement with Abel (1971b) who, using delayed free recall as the memory task, found that marijuana affects storage rather than retrieval. He noted that the inability to concentrate is presumably the cause. Darley et al. (1973), using free recall, have confirmed his results. *Marihuana and Health* (National Institute of Mental Health, 1972), summarizing the work on memory, notes that information needs to be rehearsed before it can enter storage, and marijuana prevents this rehearsal by reducing the ability to concentrate.

Miller et al. (1972), using the Babcock Story Recall as the memory task, reported that intoxicated subjects introduced new material having an emotional tone with no specific source in the original story, along with arbitrary unrelated emotional material that radically altered the story. It seems as if these subjects are distracted by internal stimuli, rather than external stimuli such as the objects in the room that were so important to Weil and Zinberg's subjects. Tinklenberg et al. (1970) noted similar intermittent attention lapses that often interrupted speech patterns and seemed to be associated with the intrusion of extraneous perceptions and thoughts. The latter authors also pointed out that the impairments resulting from marijuana intoxication do not follow a smooth time function, but are episodic, brief, and not always voluntary.

Other investigators, using different tasks, also have usually found that marijuana causes memory decrements. Clark et al. (1970) found that reading comprehension was significantly impaired, and Zeidenberg et al. (1973) found a significant decrement in the ability to distinguish old from new trigrams. Halpern (1944) found impairment of both visual and object memory. Abel (1971b), using a task measuring delayed recognition memory, found a significant difference in terms of "hits," but not in terms of "false alarms." However, neither Hollister (1971) nor Waskow et al. (1970) found any significant effect for counting backward or saying the alphabet. Evidently these latter tasks are too simple or represent material that is too well-learned. These tasks have become automatized; they require minimal attention for successful performance.

The task of recalling digits also involves short-term memory, and thus is particularly vulnerable to lapses of concentration. Most investigators have found a significant impairment in digit recall (Melges et al., 1970; Tinklenberg et al., 1970; Dornbush et al., 1971; Rossi, 1973; Butler, 1973; Weingartner et al., 1972). Weingartner et al. (1972) note that there is a consistent drop in digit recall of 15 to 20%, and Butler (1973) reports a significant decrement when intoxicated, using 60 chronic users. Halpern (1944) found only digits backward impaired, and Waskow et al. (1970) and Hollister (1971) report no effect of marijuana on digit recall.

The study of Tinklenberg et al. (1970) is particularly interesting, since subjects were allowed to start over whenever their attention waned, thus presumably eliminating at least some of the effect of distraction. They still found an overall significant difference between the placebo and THC groups, but there was no significant dosage effect. The difference between the groups seemed to be due to a more general loss of information. According to Shiffrin and Atkinson (1969), information in the short-term memory store, if not attended to by the subject, will decay and be lost in a period of 30 seconds or less.

There is only one study that seems to show a failure of the retrieval process, as distinguished from difficulties in storage. Klonoff et al. (1973) found a deficiency in output, which they believe was due to a disturbance of central integrative processes. They studied visual-motor tasks under four experimental conditions: marijuana–marijuana, marijuana–placebo, placebo–marijuana, and placebo–placebo. Each of four groups of subjects was tested twice. Results indicated that the administration of marijuana compared to placebo during the first session did not result in a differential decrement in performance levels during the second. In other words, the effect of the drug state on learning during the second session was consistently unrelated to prior experience during the initial session. Thus, there was a difficulty in output, perhaps due to general disorganization or specifically to retrieval difficulties.

A word about state-dependent learning seems relevant here. It means that positive transfer of learning occurs when drug states are the same both during response acquisition and later testing, while negative transfer is found when drug state is changed. State-dependent learning is a special example of how storage affects retrieval. Shiffrin and Atkinson (1969) assume that storage and retrieval in the long-term memory store are parallel processes and seem to be basically correct, except insofar as state-dependent learning is not an all-or-none phenomenon. Chute and Wright (1973), studying rats in a passive-avoidance task, found that state-dependent learning occurred when a drug (sodium pentobarbital) was given immediately *after* acquisition of the task. It seems to be the storage process, rather than the stimulus sampling during immediate acquisition, that is crucial for memory.

The often-observed difficulty with time estimation is complex and may involve both distraction and shifting, rather than just shifting as previously hypothesized (DeLong and Levy, 1973). Most studies find an overestimation or underproduction of time intervals (Jones and Stone, 1970; Weil et al., 1968; Meyer et al., 1971; Rossi, 1973).* Tinklenberg et al. (1972) asked subjects to count silently during the Time Production Test and found an underproduction. It therefore seems possible, though not certain, that time estimation involves some kind of counting, either conscious or unconscious. What may be happening is that subjects count faster† than when they are not intoxicated. They do not lose count, as if distracted by a stimulus, but rather show a more subtle form of distraction. They are unable to hold the focus of attention long enough and involuntarily let it go too soon. According to Sack and Rice's model, it is not necessary to be distracted by a given identifiable stimulus. Rather, distraction is defined as an involuntary change in attentional focus, for whatever reason, internal or external, identifiable or unknown. It should be noted, however, that the actual tests they used in their study do have identifiable, visual characteristics which seem likely to produce distraction.

It seems also possible to say that the ability to shift the focus of attention voluntarily has been disturbed. It is not really perseveration, though, because the subjects are speeded up, not slowed down. It is a kind of perseveration in reverse. Further research should clarify this point.

Williams et al. (1946) found a misjudgment of time in the other direction; however, 4 subjects found time went much faster (as opposed to the usual subjective effect of slower) and 2 subjects found it went slightly slower.‡ Tart (1971) notes that this is an infrequent effect of the middle levels of marijuana intoxication, according to subjective reports. Souief (1967) reported that a majority of one group of users said time slowed, while a majority of another group said it speeded up. Of course, it is possible that some of the subjects confused subjective and objective time. If the effect of underestimation and overproduction of time is genuine, this may represent a true perseveration.

3. SHIFTING

Shifting, the third process, the ability to voluntarily shift from one task to another, is operationally defined by an anagrams test. So far only two

* Dornbush et al. (1971) found negative results.
† Not slower (DeLong and Levy, 1973).
‡ Dosage here was "good weed," according to the 6 subjects.

studies have used an anagrams test, and they found negative results—intoxicated subjects did not perform significantly poorer than controls (Abel, 1971a; Pearl, 1972). Miller and Drew (1972) have defined mental set-shifting in terms of Trail-Making B minus Trail-Making A.* In these studies, intoxicated subjects performed significantly worse than placebo controls (Miller and Drew, 1972; Drew et al., 1972). Klonoff et al. (1973) also found significantly poorer performance on the Trail-Making test when subjects were intoxicated. L. Rafaelsen et al. (1973) found that marijuana increased both time and errors on the finger labyrinth.

The pursuit meter, a dual-beam oscilloscope in which the subject uses a steering wheel to superimpose one beam on another, and the pursuit rotor, in which the subject tries to keep a stylus in contact with a spot on a moving turntable, involve similar types of performance. Perseveration, among other things, will affect performance on these tasks. Kiplinger et al. (1971), using the pursuit meter, found a significant performance decrement in intoxicated subjects, as did Manno et al. (1970). Evans et al. (1973), using low doses, some of which were lower than the amount of THC in the average street joint, also found a significant decrement in performance. Clark and Nakashima (1968), using the pursuit rotor, a cruder instrument, found no decrement except at the highest dose in a few subjects. Weil et al. (1968), also using the pursuit rotor, found a decrement for naive users, but not for chronics who improved slightly, while Meyer et al. (1971) found impairment more evident in casual than heavy users.

There are also several studies that have been done in the area of perception that show that marijuana causes a significant decrement in functioning. (There are also some in the expected direction, but not significant, which will not be discussed here.) These studies are not cognitive in the usual sense and do not fit well in the model of attention. Perceptual changes include significant decrements in judging the auditory intensity of tones (Myers and Caldwell, 1969; Caldwell et al., 1969), an increase in the autokinetic effect (Moskowitz et al., 1972) and glare recovery time (National Institute of Mental Health, 1972), decreased vigilance performance (Sharma and Moskowitz, 1973), and decreased stability of stance (Evans et al., 1973). While it is possible that perseveration is occurring in some of the above instances, one cannot be sure that the peripheral nervous system is not affected.

---

* These tests come from the Halstead-Reitan test battery, originally developed to measure organic brain damage.

B. Experimental Studies of Chronic Effects

Applying the attention model to the chronic effect findings should be done carefully because there is very little data available. Research has tended to focus on global constructs such as intelligence or organic brain damage rather than on the more specific cognitive constructs used in the acute research. No longitudinal studies are available; all the studies are cross-sectional.

So far all studies of this kind report no significant differences between users and nonusers. Jamaican users and nonusers were equated using an intelligence measure that did not correlate highly with measures of organicity (Rubin and Comitas, 1972; Bowman and Pihl, 1973). Reid (*Marihuana: A Signal of Misunderstanding*, 1972), using tests sensitive to organic brain functioning (Halstead-Reitan), found no overall impairment; but he did find that 2 out of 10 casual users and 2 out of 10 heavy users performed less well than would have been expected on the basis of IQ and education. Furthermore, Barratt *et al.* (1972) reported that in a sample of high school students the marijuana-only users showed poorer performance on the cognitive tasks than would have been expected considering their academic achievement. Halpern (1944), however, found no difference between prisoners who were long-term users and prisoners who were nonusers, although it is not clear how long they had been drug-free and what effect this would have.

1. DEGREE OF SELECTIVITY OR FIELD ARTICULATION

So far as the first factor, *degree of selectivity*, is concerned, three studies have now been done and they report no significant difference between users and nonusers. Barratt *et al.* (1972), using an embedded figures test, found no consistent relationship between users and nonusers. Neither did Cohen (1972), who used Witkin's Group Embedded Figures Test. Weckowitz and Janssen (1973), using 11 chronic users (marijuana or hashish three times a week) and 11 controls, also found no significant differences, but they found a trend toward better performance for the users on the Rod and Frame Test ($p < 0.10$).* This effect is the opposite of the acute effect. If it is not an artifact, it may represent the

---

* The users also did better on Witkin's Embedded Figures Test and the Stroop Color Word Test. These researchers also found that the users were better on the Guilford Induction Test, which included letter sets ($p < 0.05$) and figure classification ($p < 0.10$). It is hard to know for sure what Guilford's test measures, but in this sample results are consistent with selectivity.

result of learning to compensate for the drug's acute effect, or may be an indication that only relatively field-independent people become chronic users of marijuana.

2. RESISTANCE TO DISTRACTION

In the Weckowitz and Janssen study, users performed more poorly on Guilford's Number Facility Test, which measures short-term memory and thus distraction, although the difference between users and nonusers was not significant. It is hard to draw conclusions from this study—it is weak because the sample is so small and the study is *ex post facto*.

Three studies, however, have documented a significant decrement in what is probably resistance to distraction. One used the complicated calculating task of Melges *et al.* (1970) to measure temporal disintegration (W. G. Drew, personal communication). Another used the learning and free recall of paired-associates—a short-term memory task—and showed significant impairment for users as compared with nonusers (Entin and Goldzung, 1973). A third found a significant decrement for users on tests of speed and accuracy of psychomotor performance and memory span for digits and designs (Soueif, 1971). Bowman and Pihl (1973) studying Jamaican users, however, found no significant differences, using paired associates, reaction time, or digit span. Rubin and Comitas (1972), also studying Jamaicans, found users were significantly *better* at digit span, a short-term memory task; but they consider these results to be artifactual. Entin and Goldzung (1973) did not find scores on arithmetic problems to be significantly different and suggest as a reason the fact that the storage interval was a few seconds rather than a few minutes.

3. SHIFTING

The only study comparing heavy users and casual users (10 each) found that the heavy users underestimated or overproduced time intervals, although the difference was not significant (Rossi, 1973). It was found that the casual users were quite accurate, but after they had spent 21 days in the laboratory smoking marijuana every day their judgment closely resembled the predrug estimates of the heavy users. (After 21 days of smoking, the time estimates of the heavy users were slightly longer.) This effect is the opposite of the acute effect of underproducing and overestimating time and may come about as a compensation for the acute effect. It seems best understood as a kind of perseveration, a shifting difficulty. [Soueif (1971), though, found that chronic users were significantly *more accurate* in estimating time than the nonusers, both in the urban and rural samples.]

Other evidence of a difficulty with set-shifting has been reported by

Drew *et al.*, using Trail-Making B minus Trail-Making A as a measure. In a second sample, they failed to find a significant difference between light and heavy users, as opposed to users and nonusers, although they did find a difference on a slightly modified and more difficult form of the task when they included other independent variables in a regression analysis. Also, Barratt *et al.* (1972) found, using an item analysis of an embedded figures test, that chronic users performed more poorly on first exposure to a new level of problem difficulty, thus showing perhaps a difficulty in shifting set.

C. Clinical Studies of Chronic Effects

The other data existing on chronic users comes from studies using the psychiatric interview—studies that focused on the user without using a control group for purposes of comparison. There is a substantial weakness in this work since the subjects were psychiatric patients, whose pathology undoubtedly interacted with the effect of the drug. Further, the interview lacks some precision since it is not a source of quantitative data. But, such studies, while not useful for drawing firm conclusions, are good for suggesting hypotheses.

Kolansky and Moore (1972a,b) found that patients who used marijuana demonstrated various symptoms, including a slowed time sense, recent memory difficulty, poor concentration, and an inability to complete thoughts during verbal communication. These effects suggest a decreased resistance to distraction and difficulty with set-shifting. Scher (1970) found that his patients, who often held responsible positions, complained of cognitive inefficiency after several years of marijuana use. Kornhaber (1971, 1972) believed that one effect of marijuana on his adolescent patients was to impair the ability to concentrate and thus affect learning ability and judgment. Zinberg and Weil (1970) noted greater circumstantiality in daily users.

D. Studies of the Relationship of Marijuana Use to Motivation and Academic Achievement

The difficulties seen with concentration and set-shifting, if confirmed by further research, may explain the amotivational syndrome (McGlothlin and West, 1968). Middle-class students who used marijuana subtly became more introverted, more interested in the present than the future, and tended to drop out of college. They felt more creative, but actually became less productive. The creative feeling might actually be a tendency to be distracted by internal stimuli; the lessened productivity might be caused by general poor concentration. Never before have large numbers of intellectuals used marijuana. In India this practice has been viewed as a dissipation, and only laboring and religious groups used it (Kalant, 1972). The same thing seems to be true in Africa, the Middle East, and South America (Bouquet, 1951), in Egypt (Soueif, 1967), and Jamaica (Bowman and Pihl, 1973; Rubin and Comitas, 1972). Soueif (1971) found that the higher the level of education, the larger the discrepancy between users' and nonusers' test scores. Users usually performed more poorly.

Kupfer *et al.* (1973), in a study of the amotivational syndrome, found that the unmotivated light users had significantly higher depression and organicity scores as measured by a psychiatric interview questionnaire than the motivated light users. The heavy amotivational smokers were also higher on depression and organicity than the motivated heavy smokers. (There was also a greater percentage of unmotivated heavy smokers than unmotivated light smokers, but the difference was not significant.) These investigators interpret their results as demonstrating that impaired motivation may be a manifestation of depression rather than a consequence of frequent marijuana use.

It is not possible to tell from the above study whether the high organicity score (from poor concentration and memory) is a result of depression, drug use, premorbid personality, or some interaction of these variables. It does seem clear, however, that in the sample drawn by Kupfer *et al.* (1973) there are individual ways of reacting to the drug that overshadow the effects of frequency of use.

Academic achievement of marijuana users is also relevant to the issue of cognitive changes. Walters *et al.* (1972) reported no difference between users' and nonusers' college grades. They also found no significant change in grades following the beginning of use of marijuana, but they did find significantly more users were uncertain about career plans. [Hochman and Brill (1973) note that three times as many chronic users and nonusers quit jobs because they found them boring.] Finnell (1973) found that marijuana users had significantly higher aptitude tests, but no significant difference was found between users and nonusers on grades. However, those students who used only alcohol had the best grades, those using nothing had the next best grades, followed by students using marijuana. Those who used both marijuana and alcohol had the poorest grades. Grossman (1973) found that when aptitude was controlled (users had better scores) users performed more poorly than nonusers. There was great individual variation; however, some of the heaviest daily users got the best term grades in the sample. It was concluded that loss of motivation and poor performance may have caused drug use. Goode (1971) reports a curvilinear relationship between grades and marijuana use. Hochman and Brill (1973) report that duration and frequency of use is unrelated to college grades. Rodgers (1973), however, points out that in this study an A in one subject is treated as equivalent to an A in another, and some college majors have a higher percentage of users than others. This objection also can be raised for some of the other studies.

III. SUMMARY

It seems that a model of attention is most helpful in organizing the results of the studies of marijuana's cognitive effects. Without it, the literature seems scattered and unrelated. So far as the acute effects are concerned, there is evidence that all the factors of attention are affected, although the evidence is strongest for the second factor, resistance to distraction. There is too little experimental data to draw firm conclusions with regard to chronic effects, and it seems clear that more research needs to be done. Longitudinal studies including measures of attention are greatly needed, so that each individual can function as his own control. However, the results reported suggest that any cognitive deficit found in chronic users may well be a result of defects in attention.

REFERENCES

Abel, E. (1970). *Nature (London)* **227**, 1151–1152.
Abel, E. (1971a). *Nature (London)* **231**, 260–261.
Abel, E. (1971b). *Science* **173**, 1038–1040.
Barratt, E., Beaver, W., White, R., Blakeney, P., and Adams, P. (1972). *In* "Current Research in Marijuana" (M. F. Lewis, ed.), pp. 163–193. Academic Press, New York.
Bouquet, J. (1951). *Bull. Narcotics* **3**, 22–45.
Bowman, M., and Pihl, R. O. (1973). *Psychopharmacologia* **29**, 159–170.
Butler, J. L. (1973). *Dis. Abstr. 2B* **34**, 868–869.
Caldwell, D. F., Myers, S. A., Domino, E. F., and Merriam, P. E. (1969). *Percept. Mot. Skills* **29**, 755–759.
Chute, D. L., and Wright, D. C. (1973). *Science* **180**, 878–880.

Clark, L. D., and Nakashima, E. H. (1968). *Amer. J. Psychiat.* **125**, 379–383.
Clark, L. D., Hughes, R., and Nakashima, E. II. (1970). *Arch. Gen. Psychiat.* **23**, 193–198.
Cohen, G. H. (1972). *Diss. Abstr.* 5A **33**, 2162–2163.
Crancer, A., Dille, J. M., Delay, J. C., Wallace, J. E., and Haykin, M. D. (1969). *Science* **164**, 851–854.
Darley, C. F., Tinklenberg, J. R., Roth, W. T., Hollister, L. E., and Atkinson, R. C. (1973). *Memory & Cognition* **1**, 196–200.
DeLong, F. L., and Levy, B. I. (1973). *Psychol. Rep.* **33**, 907–916.
Dornbush, R. L., Fink, M., and Freedman, A. M. (1971). *Amer. J. Psychiat.* **128**, 194–197.
Dougherty, J. D. (1972). Section IV. Summary Progress Report.
Drew, W. G., Kiplinger, G. F., Miller, L. L., and Marx, M. (1972a). *Clin. Pharmacol. Ther.* **13**, 526–533.
Drew, W. G., Miller, L. L., Ables, B. M., Marx, D., and Marx, M. (1972b). Paper submitted to Committee on Problems of Drug Dependence.
Entin, E. E., and Goldzung, P. J. (1973). *Psychol. Rec.* **23**, 169–178.
Evans, M. A., Martz, R., Brown, D. J., Rodda, B. E., Kiplinger, G. F., Lemberger, L., and Forney, R. B. (1973). *Clin. Pharmacol. Ther.* **14**, 936–940.
Finnell, W. S. (1973). *Diss. Abstr.* 9A **33**, 4875–4876.
Gardner, R. W., and Moriarity, A. (1968). "Personality Structure at Pre-Adolescence." Univ. of Washington Press, Seattle.
Goode, E. (1971). *Nature (London)* **234**, 225–227.
Grossman, D. S. (1973). *Diss. Abstr.* 1B **34**, 392–393.
Halpern, F. (1944). In "The Marijuana Papers" (D. Solomon, ed.), pp. 290–314. Bobbs-Merrill, New York (reprinted, Signet Books, New York, 1966).
Hochman, J. S., and Brill, N. Q. (1973). *Amer. J. Psychiat.* **130**, 132–140.
Hollister, L. E. (1971). *Science* **172**, 21–29.
Hollister, L. E., and Gillespie, H. K. (1970). *Arch. Gen. Psychiat.* **23**, 199–203.
Jones, R. T., and Stone, G. (1970). *Psychopharmacologia* **18**, 108–117.
Kalant, A. (1969). *Science* **166**, 640.
Kalant, O. J. (1972). *Int. J. Addictions* **7**, 77–96.
Kiplinger, G. F., Manno, J. E., Rodda, B. E., and Forney, R. (1971). *Clin. Pharmacol. Ther.* **12**, 650–657.
Klonoff, H. K., Low, M., and Marcus, A. (1973). *Can. Med. Ass. J.* **108**, 150–156.
Kolansky, H., and Moore, W. T. (1972a). *Int. J. Psychiat.* **10**, 55–67.
Kolansky, H., and Moore, W. T. (1972b). *J. Amer. Med. Ass.* **222**, 35–41.
Kornhaber, A. (1971). *J. Amer. Med. Ass.* **215**, 1988.
Kornhaber, A. (1972). *Int. J. Psychiat.* **10**, 79–81.
Kupfer, D. J., Detre, T., Koral, J., and Fajans, P. (1973). *Amer. J. Psychiat.* **130**, 1319–1322.
Manno, J. E., Kiplinger, G. F., Haine, S. E., Bennett, I. F., and Forney, R. B. (1970). *Clin. Pharmacol. Ther.* **11**, 808–815.
"Marihuana: A Signal of Misunderstanding—The Technical Papers of the First Report of the National Commission on Marihuana and Drug Abuse." (1972). Appendix, Vol. 1, pp. 85–86. US Govt Printing Office, Washington, D.C.
McGlothlin, W. H., and West, L. J. (1968). *Amer. J. Psychiat.* **125**, 370–378.
Melges, F. T., Tinklenberg, J. P., Hollister, L. E., and Gillespie, H. K. (1970). *Science* **168**, 118–120.
Meyer, R. E., Pillard, R. C., Shapiro, L. M., and Mirin, S. M. (1971). *Amer. J. Psychiat.* **128**, 198–204.

Miller, L. L., and Drew, W. G. (1972). *Fed. Proc., Fed. Amer. Soc. Exp. Biol.* 31, 551.
Miller, L. L., Drew, W. G., and Kiplinger, G. F. (1972). *Nature (London)* 237, 172–173.
Moskowitz, M., Sharma, S., and Schapero, M. (1972). In "Current Research in Marijuana" (M. F. Lewis, ed.), pp. 129–150. Academic Press, New York.
Myers, S. A., and Caldwell, D. F. (1969). *New Physician* 18, 212–215.
National Institute of Mental Health. (1972). "Report on Marijuana and Health." US Govt. Printing Office, Washington, D.C.
Pearl, J. H. (1972). *Diss. Abstr. 5B* 33, 2329.
Rafaelsen, L., Christrup, H., Bech, P., and Rafaelsen, O. J. (1973). *Nature (London)* 242, 117–118.
Rafaelsen, O. J., Bech, P., Christiansen, J., Christrup, H., Nyboe, J., and Rafaelsen, L. (1973). *Science* 179, 920–923.
Rapaport, D., Gill, M. M., and Schafer, R. (1970). "Diagnostic Psychological Testing" (rev. ed.). Univ. of London Press, London.
Rodgers, T. C. (1973). *Amer. J. Psychiat.* 130, 140.
Rodin, E. A., Domino, E. F., and Porzak, J. P. (1970). *J. Amer. Med. Ass.* 213, 1300–1302.
Rossi, A. M. (1973). *Proc. 81st Annu. Conv. Amer. Psychol. Ass.* 8, 1029–1030.
Rubin, V., and Comitas, L. (1972). "A Report by the Research Institute for the Study of Man to the Center for Studies of Narcotic and Drug Abuse," Part II. Nat. Inst. Ment. Health, Washington, D.C.
Sack, S., and Rice, C. E. (1974). *Psychol. Rep.* 34, 1003–1012.
Scher, J. (1970). *J. Amer. Med. Ass.* 214, 1120.
Sharma, S., and Moskowitz, M. (1973). *Proc. 81st Annu. Conv. Amer. Psychol. Ass.* 8, 1035–1036.
Shiffrin, R. M., and Atkinson, R. C. (1969). *Psychol. Rev.* 76, 179–193.
Souief, M. I. (1967). *Bull. Narcotics* 19, 1–12.
Souief, M. I. (1971). *Bull. Narcotics* 23, 17–28.
Tart, C. T. (1971). "On Being Stoned: A Psychological Study of Marijuana Intoxication." Science and Behavior Books, Palo Alto, California.
Tennant, F. S., and Groesbeck, C. J. (1972). *Arch. Gen. Psychiat.* 27, 133–136.
Tinklenberg, J. R., Melges, F. T., Hollister, L. E., and Gillespie, H. K. (1970). *Nature (London)* 226, 1171–1172.
Tinklenberg, J. R., Kopell, B. S., Melges, F. T., and Hollister, L. E. (1972). *Arch. Gen. Psychiat.* 27, 812–815.
Walters, P. A., Jr., Goethals, G. W., and Pope, H. G. (1972). *Arch. Gen. Psychiat.* 26, 92–96.
Waskow, I. E., Olsson, J. E., Salzman, C., and Katz, M. (1970). *Arch. Gen. Psychiat.* 22, 97–107.
Weckowitz, T. E., and Janssen, D. V. (1973). *J. Abn. Psychol.* 81, 264–269.
Weil, A. T., and Zinberg, N. E. (1969). *Nature (London)* 222, 434–437.
Weil, A. T., Zinberg, N. E., and Nelsen, J. M. (1968). *Science* 162, 1234–1242.
Weingartner, H., Galanter, M., Lemberger, L., Roth, W. T., Stillman, R., Vaughn, T. B., and Wyatt, R. J. (1972). *Proc. 80th Ann. Conv. Amer. Psychol. Ass.* 7, 813–814.
Williams, E. G., Himmelsbach, C. K., and Wikler, A. (1946). *Pub. Health Rep.* 61, 1059–1083.
Witkin, H. A., Lewis, H. D., Hertzman, M., Machover, K., Meissner, P., Bretnoll, S., and Wapner, S. (1954). "Personality through Perception." Wiley, New York.

Witkin, H. A., Dyk, R. B., Faterson, H. F., Goodenough, D. R., and Karp, S. A. (1962). "Psychological Differentiation." Wiley, New York.
Zeidenberg, P., Clark, W. C., Jaffe, J., Anderson, S. W., Chin, S., and Malitz, S. (1973). *Comp. Psychiat.* 14, 549–556.
Zinberg, N. E., and Weil, A. T. (1970). *Nature (London)* 226, 119–123.

Chapter 6

PSYCHOLOGICAL AND NEUROPHYSIOLOGICAL EFFECTS OF MARIJUANA IN MAN: AN INTERACTION MODEL

HARRY KLONOFF AND MORTON D. LOW

I. Introduction 121
II. Methods 130
   A. Psychological Procedure 130
   B. Neurophysiological Procedure 132
III. Results 135
   A. Psychological Results 135
   B. Neurophysiological Results 141
IV. Discussion 145
   References 153

I. INTRODUCTION

Despite a large and growing number of published studies of the effects of cannabis derivatives in animals and man (The Le Dain Commission in 1972 listed 682 entries in its references and selected bibliography dealing with cannabis and its effects) there is still considerable controversy regarding the nature of the effects of marijuana on intellectual and cognitive functioning in man. Furthermore, the nature and degree of the physiological changes responsible for and associated with the subjective state of marijuana intoxication remain unclear.

If one seriously accepts methodological criteria (Klonoff, Chapter 1, this volume) in a critical review of the literature, the body of knowledge regarding marijuana and its effects shrinks exponentially. Turning first to the published studies that have dealt with the effects of marijuana on intellectual and cognitive functioning, the earliest culturally relevant experimental marijuana research is confined to three studies (Siler et al., 1933; Mayor's Committee on Marijuana, 1944; Williams and Oberst, 1946). The Mayor's study (1944) used 72 prisoners (48 were chronic users). Route of administration was oral as well as smoked, dose administered is not known exactly, nor is smoking procedure specified. The study concluded that: there was dose-related impairment with respect to static equilibrium, hand steadiness, and complex reaction time; there was a decrement in overall mental functioning and more particularly in memory, ability to handle numbers concepts, and problem solving ability; there were no significant changes in hand strength, auditory acuity, perception of length of lines, simple reaction time, or tapping speed.

The first published study that can withstand critical evaluation is that of Weil et al. (1968) who measured sustained attention, general alertness and muscular coordination, and attention of 17 subjects (9 naive and 8 experienced) under low dose (4.5 mg Δ^9-THC), high dose (18 mg Δ^9-THC), and placebo conditions, using a standardized smoking technique throughout. Sustained attention was not affected; general alertness and muscular coordination and attention decreased at both dose levels, but only for the naive subjects.

Subsequent to the study of Weil et al. (1968), a number of investigators between 1969 and 1973 have reported on the psychological effects of marijuana using a smoking route of administration and these are summarized below.

Caldwell et al. (1969) failed to find changes in either visual or auditory threshold following the smoking of 3.9 mg Δ^9-THC by 12 experienced subjects, using a semistandardized smoking procedure. In a second study by Caldwell et al. (1970), it was found that marijuana minimally affected sensory acuity in a group of 20 subjects who smoked a mean of 6.3 mg Δ^9-THC (subjective high procedure) in an unstandardized manner. Control groups were included in both studies.

Manno et al. (1970) measured motor performance and delayed auditory feedback in 12 experienced subjects. Subjects received placebo and two doses of marijuana (2.5 and 5 mg Δ^9-THC) in cigarette form administered in an unspecified manner, with no prior ingestion of alcohol and in combination with alcohol (0.05% alcohol in blood). Although marijuana impaired performance no dose-response phenomenon was demonstrated. The alcohol and marijuana exerted additive effects in motor performance.

Abel (1970, 1971a,b,c) has been concerned with measuring memory during marijuana and control conditions in experienced subjects (groups varied from 8 to 26 subjects), but with marijuana of unknown potency using unspecified smoking procedures. He reported that marijuana did not affect retrieval of information already present in memory, but did interfere with the initial learning (significantly affecting acquisition processes involved in the storage of information). The author suggested that an inability to concentrate may be the explanation for memory impairment after smoking marijuana; because of impaired concentration, rehearsal did not occur and information was not transferred to permanent memory.

Kiplinger and Manno (1971) and Kiplinger et al. (1971) measured motor performance, delayed auditory feedback, and stability of stance in 15 subjects (7 naive and 8 experienced). Cigarettes containing 5 mg Δ^9-THC, three much lesser dose levels, and a placebo were administered in an unspecified manner. Dose-dependent decrements were observed in almost all the measured variables.

Meyer et al. (1971) measured field dependence, attention, general alertness, time perception, task focusing, and muscular coordination in 12 subjects (6 heavy and 6 casual marijuana users). Experimental conditions were placebo, 2.3 mg Δ^9-THC, and self-selected amount of marijuana (average dose of casual users was 3.8 mg Δ^9-THC, of heavy users 3.4 mg Δ^9-THC). The smoking procedure was unspecified. Whereas no statistical analyses of data were made, the authors stated that most of the perceptual tests showed a mild degree of impairment, the impairment being more evident in the casual smokers.

Dornbush et al. (1971) and Dornbush and Freedman (1972) studied short-term memory, reaction time, and time estimation in 10 experienced subjects. Cigarettes contained two dose levels of THC, low (7.5 mg Δ^9-THC), high (22.5 mg Δ^9-THC), or placebo. The manner of smoking was unspecified. Short-term memory and reaction time were adversely affected only by the high dose of marijuana.

Le Dain (1972) measured short-term serial position memory and general alertness (digit symbol substitution) among other variables in subjects who smoked average doses of 0.7, 1.5, and 6.2 mg Δ^9-THC, using a standardized and closely controlled smoking technique. Impairment was found in the former but not the latter measure.

More recent investigators who used higher dose levels reported effects on new learning (Rickles et al., 1973, administered 14 mg Δ^9-THC and placebo) and attention (Galanter et al., 1973, administered 10 mg naturally occurring Δ^9-THC, 10 mg synthetic Δ^9-THC, and placebo).

A number of studies between 1968 and 1973 have reported the psychological effects of marijuana, using an oral route of administration, and these are summarized below. Clark and Nakashima (1968) and Clark et al. (1970) measured mirror tracing, depth perception, reaction time, time estimation, and learning in 18 and subsequently 12 naive subjects. The marijuana was administered by mouth as an alcohol extract. Learning, time estimation, and reaction time were most consistently affected by the drug.

Hollister and Gillespie (1970) measured muscular coordination and attention, general alertness, reaction time, muscular facility, flexibility of closure, and time estimation in 12 experienced subjects who had ingested median oral doses of 32 mg Δ^9-THC, ethanol, dextroamphetamine sulfate, and placebo. Only number facility was significantly affected by the marijuana.

Melges et al. (1970) and Tinklenberg et al. (1970) measured immediate or short-term memory in 8 subjects (prior drug history unspecified). Route of administration was oral; dose levels were 20, 40, and 60 mg Δ^9-THC; and a control (placebo) condition was included. Immediate memory was adversely affected, and the authors concluded that this impairment may hinder the individual's ability to compare current perceptions with memories. No consistent dose-response relationship was observed in their study.

Waskow et al. (1970) measured memory in 32 subjects (naive and experienced); route of administration was oral (20 mg Δ^9-THC). Little, if any, impairment of functioning was noted. Rafaelsen et al. (1971) measured memory and attention in 8 subjects who received oral doses of 8 to 16 mg Δ^9-THC. Decreased scores were observed only for the higher dose condition.

Darley et al. (1973) used a complex design which extended over 6 days with an initial administration of oral marijuana extract calibrated to 20 mg Δ^9-THC and subsequent doses of marijuana or placebo. The drug effect was explained as a change in the encoding processes of memory.

One study has used smoked and oral routes of administration. Jones and Stone (1970) measured muscular coordination and attention, time judgment, and general alertness in 10 heavy users of marijuana. Routes of administration were oral and smoked (4.5 mg Δ^9-THC), with the smoking procedure being unspecified. A placebo condition was also included. Only time estimation was adversely affected under marijuana by either route of administration.

6. Psychological and Neurophysiological Effects

The published studies that have dealt with the effects of marijuana on physiological functioning have shown few significant findings. The Le Dain report (1972) states in part: "The short-term physiological effects of a typical cannabis dose on normal persons are generally quite benign, and are apparently of little clinical significance." Presumably because of the absence of dramatic physiological changes, there have been no neurophysiological models, supported by experimental evidence, proposed to explain the brain mechanisms which must underlie the subjective experiential phenomena associated with cannabis intoxication. Typical of the summaries offered by various workers after analysis of their physiological data are the statements of Domino (1971) and Gale and Guenther (1971). Domino, speaking of cannabis and its natural or synthetic THC derivatives, states: "These agents are primary depressants of central nervous system function. However, they possess a unique spectrum of pharmacological actions with only superficial relation to various other psychoactive drugs. The chemistry and pharmacology of marijuana are distinct from other central nervous system depressants. . . ." Gale and Guenther state that: "The results of the present experiments support the concept that cannabis serves as an anti-anxiety agent and it is the reduction in anxiety that is desired by the long-term user."

The literature relevant to the neurophysiological changes induced by marijuana smoking presents conflicting data. Specifically, Wikler and Lloyd (1945) recorded a simple bipolar occipital electroencephalogram in each of 19 subjects before and after smoking 2 or 3 marijuana cigarettes of unspecified potency. They employed visual analysis only and found no change in the frequency of the Alpha rhythm in 13 of the 19 subjects, while the Alpha frequency increased slightly in 2 and decreased slightly in 3. The percent time Alpha was unchanged in 10 and decreased (average decrease of 19%) in 8 subjects.

Electroencephalographic studies during THC intoxication have also been reported by Hollister et al. (1970). In their study 16 subjects were given 32 mg of Δ^1-THC orally. Electroencephalograms (EEGs) were recorded during baseline testing and at 15 minute intervals for approximately 4 hours following administration of the drug. The EEG showed no changes attributable to drug effect on visual examination. The records did show some electrographic evidence of drowsiness, i.e., a slight increase in amplitude and slight slowing of posterior frequencies associated with a diminution in voltage activity in anterior distributions. Two of the 16 subjects showed some paroxysmal slowing of Alpha rhythm to 7 Hz. In this study simple analog frequency analysis of the EEG was employed. While it is not specified in their report from what scalp locations the samples were taken, the peak frequencies at 8.3 and 8.75 Hz for the drug and control subjects, respectively, suggest that the EEG was recorded from occipital or parietal derivations. Frequency analyzer outputs indicated significantly greater peaking of the EEG frequencies at 8.3 Hz while the subject was intoxicated with THC, a finding which was interpreted as suggesting "increased synchronization of posterior cerebral electrical activity."

Volavka et al. (1971) have performed both acute and chronic intoxication studies. They employed 10 paid volunteers (medical students) for the acute study, with a mean age of 22.5 years. Their marijuana contained 1.5% Δ^9-THC and they used both low- and high-dose levels (7.5 mg THC and 22.5 mg THC). Electroencephalograms were recorded over time, and computer analyses were done on activity from a single lead (vertex to occipital), using 20 second artifact-free epochs before and following smoking. They found an increase in percent time Alpha and an associated decrease in Theta and Beta activity. These effects were said to be most pronounced immediately after smoking. These authors also found dose-related increases in heart rate.

Two other groups of investigators have reported observations of scalp EEG activity during the acute marijuana intoxication state. Heath (1972) recorded from both scalp and implanted depth electrodes in one patient. Because of its contribution to the formation of a neurophysiological model of marijuana action in the brain, this chapter will be discussed in some detail later. A group of investigators in Detroit has reported a series of experiments evaluating the effects of marijuana smoking in healthy volunteers. Domino (1971), Johnson and Domino (1971), and Rodin et al. (1970) carried out three experiments with a total of 49 subjects. Their subjects smoked marijuana, supposed to contain 1.3% Δ^9-THC, to the point of refusal or to the state of the subject's usual "subjective high." Most subjects smoked 2 to 3 cigarettes. Pre- and post-smoking EEGs were done, and these were assessed visually as normal throughout the experiment, but showing a slight increase in Alpha amplitude post-smoking as compared to baseline. Power-density spectral analysis of a single parietal-occipital EEG lead showed a slight but significant shift from peak power at 11 Hz to a peak at 9–10 Hz. These authors also recorded visual, auditory, and somatosensory evoked responses (VER, AER, and SER) and found no significant changes in amplitude or latency measurements attributable to the drug. They did document a consistent and dose-related increase in heart rate, but could find no changes in visual brightness discrimination or in auditory frequency or intensity thresholds except for slightly poorer performance under drug conditions on auditory amplitude difference threshold measures.

Tinklenberg (1972) has reported findings contradictory to those of

Rodin et al. (1970) with respect to changes in auditory evoked potential measures. Tinklenberg studied 12 college age men, and each was given an oral dose of 0.35 mg/kg of Δ^1-THC. Tinklenberg reports an increase in amplitude and prolonged latency of the late (approximately 200 msec) negative and late positive components of the auditory evoked potential under THC as compared to placebo and alcohol. The author also reports a significant increase in contingent negative variation (CNV) amplitude after THC as compared to placebo and alcohol. To date this is the only report in the literature referring to the influence of cannabis derivatives on CNV parameters. The observation has significance in that the CNV is a slowly changing brain potential which may reflect the activity of brain mechanisms subserving processes of attention, motivation, and preparatory set (Tecce, 1972).

Lewis et al. (1973) have also reported findings which conflict with those of the Detroit group regarding the effects of THC on sensory evoked potentials. Lewis et al. recorded visual and somatosensory evoked potentials from 20 subjects after oral ingestion of placebo, 0.2, 0.4, or 0.6 mg/kg of Δ^9-THC extracted from raw marijuana. There were no statistically significant effects of THC on measured parameters (amplitude and latency of early and late components) of the SER, but there was a consistent dose-related increase in latency of all components of the VER. The investigators suggested that Δ^9-THC acts to increase the threshold of cortical and subcortical neurons involved in producing the VER.

Reports of the effects of chronic use of cannabis agents on the EEG are also contradictory. Williams et al. (1946) found what was described as "little significant EEG change" in their study of subchronic users of cannabis derivatives in high daily doses. The minor alterations seen in their subjects' EEGs in some cases disappeared after the drug was discontinued. Miras (1969) studied very heavy and chronic hashish users and found several isolated abnormal EEGs, but he had no systematic controls and had no follow-up examination to determine whether the abnormalities (chiefly some degree of slowing, continuous or episodic) would disappear after discontinuing drug use.

Worthy of special mention because it is an example of the misleading type of clinical "studies" of the effects of cannabis in man is a paper by Campbell (1971) reporting a comparison of the EEGs of 11 patients hospitalized for psychotic reactions occurring after using cannabis-containing agents and the EEGs of 3 other groups of patients, one of which included 11 persons with a history of cannabis use and no apparent psychiatric difficulty. This author reports an incredibly high incidence of EEG abnormality in both of the cannabis using groups, regardless of presence or absence of psychotic reaction (i.e., 90 and 73%, respectively).

To our knowledge there is no report anywhere in the world literature of such a high incidence of EEG abnormality associated with anything but the grossest of organic pathology. A clue to the reasons for the author's astonishing statistics may be the one illustration given as an example of "excessive Theta wave activity," apparently the most common "abnormality" encountered. The figure is not labeled with time or amplitude calibrations, and the montage is not clear. The head stamp indicates a basic 8-channel montage but only 6 channels are shown. Much of what the author describes as Theta activity appears to be artifact, and if the most obvious montage is in fact the one illustrated, this Theta activity is not really bitemporal as described but appears quite asymmetrically from the right ear and the entire left frontal area. For these reasons, and because his observations regarding the EEG patterns associated with cannabis use are so grossly at variance with other reports, we do not accept Campbell's claims as established or even valid.

Pivik et al. (1972) have recently assessed the effects of oral THC and Synhexyl on sleep patterns with 6 subjects. With doses ranging from 60–258 μg/kg, these investigators found that the drugs induced an increase in stage 4 and a decrease in REM sleep stages, both during normal sleep and sleep following REM deprivation.

Other investigators have looked for primarily autonomic or cardiovascular changes. Isbell and Jasinski (1969) and Jasinski et al. (1971) had their subjects smoke tobacco cigarettes injected with Δ^9-THC. Using two dose levels (75 and 225 μg/kg) and placebo, they found no significant effects on body temperature, systolic blood pressure, knee jerk threshold, or pupillary diameter. The smoked Δ^9-THC did produce a dose-related tachycardia.

Renault et al. (1971) administered marijuana to 10 male subjects ages 24 to 45. Their marijuana contained 1.5% Δ^9-THC and was administered in carefully measured doses of 62.5, 125, 250, and 435 mg of raw marijuana. The delivery of the smoke was precisely controlled using a spirometer, and the experimenters found a linear dose-effect curve for heart rate increase with replicable dose effects in individual subjects. The reported effects of Valsalva maneuvers during intoxication suggested that the heart rate changes were due to suppression of vagal tone.

Indications of altered autonomic tone have also been found by Gale and Guenther (1971) and Jones (1971). Gale and Guenther had 5 volunteer subjects bring their own marijuana to the laboratory where palmar galvanic skin response and finger plethysmograms were recorded before and after smoking. The marijuana was said to induce a significant reduction in basal skin conductance during tone-shock pairings, and the investigators attributed this decrease to a combination of lowered anxiety and peripheral or central anticholinergic effects of the drug.

Jones administered marijuana by smoking to 100 paid young volunteers. The raw material contained 0.9% Δ^9-THC, and each subject received approximately 9 mg of active ingredient. Jones found a significant increase in heart rate and a significant decrease in salivary flow, both observations consistent with an anticholinergic effect of the drug.

To summarize the literature, the reported neurophysiological changes induced by marijuana have included the following: (1) cardiovascular system: a significant and dose-related increase in heart rate; a minor decrease in systolic blood pressure; congestion and reddening of the conjunctiva of the eye; (2) central nervous system: minor changes in the power spectrum of the electroencephalogram; minor changes in sensory evoked potential parameters; an increase in the amplitude of the contingent negative variation (CNV); autonomic changes including decrease in salivation and decrease in basal skin resistance.

The electrophysiological experiments reported here were undertaken in an attempt to clarify some of the points of conflict in other published findings. Because of the previously suggested anticholinergic effects of cannabis derivatives in observations reported by others, respiration, heart rate, and galvanic skin response were recorded continuously throughout the experiments and were used as indicators both of anticholinergic effect and autonomic tone. The scalp EEG was also recorded continuously, primarily as an indicator of ongoing neocortical activity.

Because of the alterations in sensory perception very commonly reported during the marijuana experience and because of a conflict of reports in the literature, visual and auditory sensory evoked potentials were recorded. Parameters of such potentials are indicators both of the function of primary (classical) sensory pathways, including neocortical sensory receiving areas, and of central "processing" of incoming information and are affected by attention and subjective evaluation of the sensation.

Because of the emphasis in other literature on the learning–memory model in explaining the effects of marijuana and because most authors proposing such models claim that the functional defects associated with cannabis intoxication are chiefly the result of diminished attention or concentration on immediate tasks, CNVs were recorded in all our subjects. The CNV or contingent negative variation has been shown to be a very sensitive indicator of both attention and motivation (Tecce, 1972). It has also been shown that in auditory discrimination tasks, sequentially induced CNVs (before the discrimination and after the required response, in anticipation of a feedback signal containing information about the correctness of the response) can indicate not only the subject's immediate level of attention and interest in the task but also can reflect the effects of learning and certainty (Picton and Low, 1971). Such discrimination tasks with CNV recording were accordingly included in this study as indicators of learning, interest, and certainty of response correctness.

The specific goals of this study therefore were (1) to determine the effects of low- and high-doses of marijuana on neuropsychological functioning and learning; (2) to determine the effects of low- and high-doses of marijuana on neurophysiological functioning; and (3) to define more precisely, in neurophysiological terms, the mechanisms underlying the state of acute marijuana intoxication.

II. METHODS

Criteria for selection of volunteers and screening procedure, background characteristics of subjects, examination procedure, and marijuana and placebo were described by Klonoff (Chapter 1, this volume).

A. Psychological Procedure

1. EXPERIMENTAL DESIGN

The psychological phase of the study dealt with 81 non-naive subjects (38 men and 43 women) assigned to one of the following 7 counterbalanced conditions: marijuana/marijuana low-dose, 4 men and 5 women; marijuana low-dose/placebo, 5 men and 4 women; placebo/marijuana low-dose, 5 men and 3 women; marijuana/marijuana high-dose, 5 men and 8 women; marijuana high-dose/placebo, 5 men and 10 women; placebo/marijuana high-dose, 6 men and 8 women; and placebo/placebo, 8 men and 5 women.

The neurophysiological phase of the study dealt with 75 of these subjects assigned to one of the following conditions: low-dose marijuana (18), high-dose marijuana (29), and placebo (28).

2. MARIJUANA AND PLACEBO

Low dose was defined as standardized *Cannabis sativa* labeled as containing 0.69% Δ^9-THC, and high dose as containing 1.3% Δ^9-THC. Marijuana and placebo were administered in the form of cigarettes of standard size and weight (0.70 gm). For the neuropsychological examination the low-dose group smoked one 0.70 gm cigarette (4.8 mg Δ^9-THC) followed by one 0.35 gm cigarette 1 hour later (2.4 mg Δ^9-THC), and the high-dose group smoked one 0.70 gm cigarette (9.1 mg Δ^9-THC) followed by one 0.35 gm cigarette (4.5 mg Δ^9-THC) 1 hour later.

For the neurophysiological examination, the low-dose group smoked 4.8 mg Δ^9-THC and the high-dose group smoked 9.1 mg Δ^9-THC. Placebo was administered in an identical manner for the respective psychological and neurophysiological procedures and the smoking procedure was standardized throughout.

3. PSYCHOLOGICAL BATTERY

The screening battery consisted of the Wechsler Adult Intelligence Scale and the Minnesota Multiphasic Personality Inventory.

The neuropsychological test battery consisted of the following 13 tests and 32 variables (as multiple measures were obtained from some of the tests).

a. Halstead Category (1 Variable). A test of concept formation which requires postulation of hypotheses that appear reasonable with respect to recurring similarities and differences on the stimulus material, testing these hypotheses with respect to positive or negative reinforcement, and adapting hypotheses in accordance with the reinforcement accompanying each response.

b. Trail Making (3 Variables). A test of conceptual relations which requires immediate recognition of symbolic significance of numbers and letters; ability to scan, identify, and sequence; and flexibility in integrating numerical and alphabetical series under the pressure of time.

c. Halstead Tactual Performance (6 Variables). A test of tactile discrimination speed, incidental learning, and short-term memory which depends on tactile form discrimination, kinesthesis, manual dexterity, visualization of spatial configuration, and retention of spatial interrelationships.

d. Seashore Tonal Memory (1 Variable). A test of immediate memory which requires alertness and sustained attention, as well as the ability to perceive, retain, and compare different notes.

e. Benton Sentence Repetition (1 Variable). A test of immediate memory which requires a longer span of focused attention, involves progressive accumulation and recall of meaningful information.

f. Picture Recognition (1 Variable). A test of immediate memory which involves visual pattern discrimination and recognition of a stimulus within a serially presented series.

g. *Peterson Visual Memory (1 Variable)*. A test of immediate memory which involves retroactive interference (negative transfer) and measures the effect of an interpolated (intervening) activity on the retention and recall of a stimulus.

h. *Halstead Finger Tapping (2 Variables)*. A test of undirected motor speed for upper extremities which requires motor speed for brief intervals.

i. *Foot Tapping (2 Variables)*. A test of undirected motor speed for lower extremities which requires motor speed for brief intervals.

j. *Klove Grooved Steadiness (4 Variables)*. A test of directed motor steadiness which requires gross visual–motor coordination in one plane.

k. *Klove Maze Coordination (4 Variables)*. A test of dynamic motor coordination which requires gross visual–motor coordination in multiple planes.

l. *Klove Static Steadiness (4 Variables)*. A test of static fine visual–motor coordination which requires fine motor steadiness.

m. *Grooved Pegboard (2 Variables)*. A test of manipulative dexterity which requires speed, accuracy, and eye–hand coordination.

The duration of examination and re-examination 1 week later was approximately 1¾ hours. The order of presentation of the tests during both sessions was randomized from one subject to another in order to reduce bias that might result from examination (or reexamination) during maximal drug effect. The randomization obviated the need for time-response functions on the psychological data, permitting a statistical design of dose-response functions. Whereas curve of decay from maximal drug effect can be minimized by order of presentation, session-to-session practice effects were not susceptible to control and hence were included in the statistical analysis of data.

B. Neurophysiological Procedure

1. EXPERIMENTAL PROCEDURE

All neurophysiological experiments were done in the clinical investigation unit of a general hospital EEG laboratory. Throughout each experiment, continuous (except during smoking) recordings were made of scalp EEG, electrocardiogram (EKG), respiration (impedance pneumograph), galvanic skin response (GSR), and the electrooculogram (EOG). All physiological variables were recorded continuously on paper. Seven of these variables were simultaneously recorded on magnetic tape in FM mode for off-line computer analysis, including 5 EEG channels, the GSR, and the EOG.

Recording was done in a shielded, sound-deadened room with the subject seated in a comfortable lounge chair and facing the translucent screen of a visual stimulus-presentation module. The subject was asked to keep his eyes open throughout the experiment and to look at a target, except during 5 minutes of eyes-closed EEG. Auditory stimuli were tone bursts delivered binaurally through loud-speakers hung on one wall of the recording room. Motor responses, when required, were simple buttonpresses using a hand-held thumb switch.

The details and order of the experimental paradigms are given in Table I. Prior to paradigm 1, approximately 5 minutes of resting EEG was recorded with the subject's eyes closed. Immediately following paradigm 7 the subject was given one marijuana or placebo cigarette to smoke. As soon as smoking was finished the entire sequence was repeated. One complete sequence took approximately 40 to 45 minutes.

2. ANALYSIS OF NEUROPHYSIOLOGICAL DATA

Data analysis included visual assessment of the entire EEG record by one interpreter (MDL) according to traditional clinical EEG criteria; determination of heart rate from the Dynograph record measured during the first 20 seconds of paradigms 4, 5, 6, and 7 before and after smoking; determination of respiration rate at these same 4 points before and after smoking; determination of GSR reactivity as the ratio of visible changes in the GSR baseline to the number of trial sequences during paradigms 4, 5, 6, and 7; determination of the number of errors in response choice during discrimination tasks; and sensory evoked-potential averaging (measurements were made from the averaged C_z–A_1 lead in all cases).

Contingent negative variations were averaged off-line from the tape-recorded C_z–A_1 EEG channel using a PDP-12 computer; during discrimination-feedback trials, measurements were made of the S_1–$S_{2d\Delta}$-interval CNV area and of the post-$S_{2d\Delta}$ prefeedback area over the 1 second following the end of the $S_{2d\Delta}$-evoked response. The power spectrum of ongoing EEG was derived from four 4 second samples of artifact-free EEGs which were selected during paradigm 2 prior to smoking and from four similar samples during paradigm 2 after smoking (all samples were from the O_z–A_1 EEG lead).

TABLE I
Electrophysiological Experimental Procedures

Sequence	Paradigm	Description	# Trials	Purpose
1	S_1	Single stroboscopic light flash repeated every 4–5 seconds	64	Visual evoked response
2	S_2	Single 1 second tone burst, 1000 Hz, ~50 dB, repeated every 4–5 seconds	64	Auditory evoked response
3	$S_1 \ldots S_2$	Flash followed by tone. S_1–S_2 interval 1.4 seconds. Intertrial interval 2–3 seconds	32	Habituation
4	$S_1 \ldots S_2$-R	As in 3. Subject responds to S_2 by button-press R which terminates S_2. Intertrial interval 4–6 seconds	32	CNV measure of attention
5	$S_1 \ldots S_{2d\Delta}$-R $\ldots$ FB_{gb}	As in 4 but S_2 (randomly) d = 1000 Hz or Δ = 1200 Hz. Subject responds to Sd by pressing right button and to SΔ by pressing left button. Two seconds after R, a green light (good) or red light (bad) is lit. Intertrial interval 8–12 seconds	32	Auditory discrimination–feedback sequence. Measure of modality-specific memory, attention, and certainty
6	$S_1 \ldots S_{2d\Delta}$-R $\ldots$ FB_{gb}	As in 5, but $S_{2\Delta}$ = 1050 Hz	32	Discrimination more difficult
7	$S_1 \ldots S_{2d\Delta}$-R $\ldots$ FB_{gb}	As in 5, but $S_{2\Delta}$ = 1003 Hz	32	Discrimination very difficult

III. RESULTS

A. Psychological Results

1. SCREENING PSYCHOLOGICAL TESTS

a. Wechsler Adult Intelligence Scale. Mean Full-Scale IQ for the population of 81 volunteers was 122.60 (SD = 8.50), which is within the superior range of mental ability. Intellectual level was high, compared with the population in general, but consistent with the educational–occupational characteristics of the volunteers.

b. Minnesota Multiphasic Personality Inventory. Mean transformed scores for the validity and clinical scales for these 81 volunteers were as follows: L, 47.93; F, 55.69; K, 57.94; Hs, 50.32; D, 52.38; Hy, 56.94; Pd, 58.36; Mf, 56.52; Pa, 54.43; Pt, 57.22; Sc, 58.96; Ma, 61.09; Si, 50.17; Es, 60.79. The profile for the group is within normal limits, but the group measure would tend to obscure individual scale elevations.

2. SEX DIFFERENCES

Separate analyses for men and women were done for marijuana and placebo conditions for the initial and second sessions of the low- and high-dose groups. Of the 136 "t" test comparisons for the low-dose group, significantly different scores were obtained by men in five instances and by women in two instances. The same number of "t" test comparisons for the high-dose group revealed 8 significantly different values for the males and 11 for the females. The very small proportion of significant differences and the even distribution of these differences between the sexes obviates the need for considering sex as a variable in the data analysis.

3. GENERAL EFFECTS

Table II (columns 1–3) presents the results of the analysis of variance for the low-dose group and Table III (columns 1–3) for the high-dose group. There were distinct and numerous significant differences in performance between the subgroups of volunteers assigned to the various experimental conditions, more so for the high-dose group (11/13 tests and 20/32 variables) compared with the low-dose group (8/13 tests and 13/32 variables). Performance improved in the second session and in a comparable manner for both dose groups, i.e., learning occurred on 6/13 tests and 15/32 variables for the low-dose group and 5/13 tests and 12/32

TABLE II
Neuropsychological Results of F Tests for Low-Dose Group Analysis of Variance

Test no.	Variable no.	Test name	Between groups	Between trials	Groups × trials	Marijuana effect during initial session[a]	Marijuana effect during 2nd session (unrelated)[b]	Marijuana effect during 2nd session (related)[c]
1	1	Category Test (err.)	3.27[d]	47.77[e]	1.71	11.35[e]	0.17	1.48
2	2	Trail Making—A (time)	5.46[f]	7.59[f]	4.25[f]	9.28[f]	5.30[d]	1.12
	3	Trail Making—B (time)	10.37[e]	7.83[f]	4.12[f]	28.39[e]	5.25[d]	0.26
	4	Trail Making—Total (time)	9.96[e]	9.71[f]	4.06[f]	28.52[e]	6.57[o]	0.02
3	5	T.P.T.—Dom. (time)	0.45	20.37[e]	1.05	2.21	2.71	0.30
	6	T.P.T.—Non-Dom. (time)	1.00	8.94[f]	0.42	2.33	5.96[o]	0.23
	7	T.P.T.—Both (time)	1.19	6.00[o]	0.55	5.73[o]	3.41	0.38
	8	T.P.T.—Total (time)	1.05	16.92[e]	0.80	4.19[d]	5.72[o]	0.36
	9	T.P.T.—Memory (corr.)	1.47	5.95[o]	0.81	3.58	0.00	2.17
	10	T.P.T.—Location (corr.)	0.81	5.72[o]	0.38	0.31	0.01	0.44
4	11	Seashore Tonal Memory (err.)	2.62[d]	0.21	0.54	0.93	1.30	2.14
5	12	Sentence Repetition (corr.)	10.69[e]	0.07	4.04[f]	7.17[f]	14.17[e]	2.89
6	13	Picture Recognition—Total (err.)	0.71	2.95	0.28	2.94	0.01	0.04
7	14	Visual Memory (err.)	9.45[e]	7.09[f]	3.25[d]	20.89[e]	6.95[f]	0.08
8	15	Finger Tapping—Dom. (corr.)	1.09	0.10	1.25	3.52	0.13	0.23
	16	Finger Tapping—Non-Dom. (corr.)	1.01	0.85	0.08	1.72	0.04	0.32
9	17	Foot Tapping—Dom. (corr.)	1.00	0.31	0.18	0.24	0.65	2.91
	18	Foot Tapping—Non-Dom. (corr.)	1.15	0.07	0.06	0.94	0.28	0.03

6. Psychological and Neurophysiological Effects

10	19	Grooved Steadiness—Dom. (time)	2.09	6.52^a	1.41	12.50^e	0.37	1.08
	20	Grooved Steadiness—Dom. (corr.)	5.22^f	4.00^d	2.86^d	15.06^e	0.31	0.20
	21	Grooved Steadiness—Non-Dom. (time)	0.31	2.66	0.20	1.39	1.82	1.06
	22	Grooved Steadiness—Non-Dom. (corr.)	0.11	2.45	0.05	0.13	0.45	2.45
11	23	Maze Coordination—Dom. (time)	0.64	3.28	0.36	1.98	3.78^d	0.01
	24	Maze Coordination—Dom. (corr.)	0.57	2.80	0.37	1.77	3.01	0.02
	25	Maze Coordination—Non-Dom. (time)	1.14	4.45^d	0.76	1.02	0.05	0.01
	26	Maze Coordination—Non-Dom. (corr.)	0.73	8.69^f	0.38	0.69	0.24	0.27
12	27	Static Steadiness—Dom. (time)	10.43^e	1.30	4.21^f	12.97^e	14.64^e	1.32
	28	Static Steadiness—Dom. (corr.)	5.20^f	0.67	1.72	3.57	10.16^f	1.25
	29	Static Steadiness—Non-Dom. (time)	6.77^e	0.15	3.17^d	4.47^d	8.62^f	0.98
	30	Static Steadiness—Non-Dom. (corr.)	3.50^a	0.02	2.44	1.76	8.98^f	1.18
13	31	Grooved Pegboard—Dom. (time)	2.70^d	2.07	1.13	1.87	8.11^f	0.02
	32	Grooved Pegboard—Non-Dom. (time)	2.49	0.41	0.33	0.00	1.27	0.13

^{a} $(\underline{M_1M_2} + M_1P_2) - (\underline{P_1M_2} + P_1P_2)$.

^{b} Marijuana effect during second session unrelated to experimental condition in initial session $(M_1M_2 + P_1M_2) - (M_1P_2 + P_1P_2)$.

^{c} Marijuana effect during second session related to experimental condition in initial session $(M_1\underline{M_2} - M_1\underline{P_2}) - (P_1\underline{M_2} - P_1\underline{P_2})$.

^{d} $p < 0.05$.

^{e} $p < 0.001$.

^{f} $p < 0.01$.

^{g} $p < 0.02$.

TABLE III
Neuropsychological Results of F Tests for High-Dose Group Analysis of Variance

Test no.	Variable no.	Test name	Between groups	Between trials	Groups × trials	Marijuana effect during initial session[a]	Marijuana effect during 2nd session (unrelated)[b]	Marijuana effect during 2nd session (related)[c]
1	1	Category Test (err.)	5.61[d]	60.06[d]	2.17	26.40[d]	4.30[e]	0.01
2	2	Trail Making—A (time)	2.22	0.01	1.77	5.79[f]	8.42[g]	0.09
	3	Trail Making—B (time)	7.99[d]	4.16[e]	6.21[d]	18.95[d]	17.03[d]	0.04
	4	Trail Making—Total (time)	7.63[d]	2.86	5.65[d]	18.48[d]	18.23[d]	0.09
3	5	T.P.T.—Dom. (time)	0.75	44.32[d]	7.16[d]	16.77[d]	7.70[g]	0.14
	6	T.P.T.—Non-Dom. (time)	1.23	14.35[d]	3.91[g]	11.57[d]	4.19[e]	1.43
	7	T.P.T.—Both (time)	1.76	15.47[d]	1.85	5.09[e]	3.08	0.49
	8	T.P.T.—Total (time)	3.71[f]	34.72[d]	6.27[d]	16.28[d]	7.28[g]	0.78
	9	T.P.T.—Memory (corr.)	2.50	6.25[f]	1.19	3.83[e]	0.80	0.13
	10	T.P.T.—Location (corr.)	1.27	12.73[d]	0.75	0.48	0.37	0.95
4	11	Seashore Tonal Memory (err.)	2.03	1.25	0.42	0.09	0.98	0.01
5	12	Sentence Repetition (corr.)	17.38[d]	3.63	5.58[d]	21.97[d]	3.25	1.43
6	13	Picture Recognition—Total (err.)	5.73[d]	2.26	3.10[e]	6.13[f]	7.58[g]	0.48
7	14	Visual Memory (err.)	9.33[d]	2.98	3.87[g]	15.19[d]	15.47[d]	0.15
8	15	Finger Tapping—Dom. (corr.)	5.59[d]	0.63	0.82	4.78[e]	6.58[f]	0.54
	16	Finger Tapping—Non-Dom. (corr.)	3.02[e]	0.51	1.32	6.79[g]	5.85[f]	0.62
9	17	Foot Tapping—Dom. (corr.)	0.90	2.15	0.36	0.94	0.00	0.32
	18	Foot Tapping—Non-Dom. (corr.)	0.99	0.98	0.40	2.12	1.64	0.07

6. Psychological and Neurophysiological Effects

10	19	Grooved Steadiness—Dom. (time)	2.94[e]	1.50	2.14	7.93[a]	5.45[f]	2.55
	20	Grooved Steadiness—Dom. (corr.)	2.68[e]	1.63	1.83	8.30[a]	5.00[e]	1.49
	21	Grooved Steadiness—Non-Dom. (time)	1.58	1.08	0.66	8.34[a]	4.62[e]	0.30
	22	Grooved Steadiness—Non-Dom. (corr.)	1.78	0.55	0.71	5.64[f]	9.21[a]	1.02
11	23	Maze Coordination—Dom. (time)	3.29[f]	1.39	2.30	10.87[a]	2.39	0.90
	24	Maze Coordination—Dom. (corr.)	4.14[a]	6.83[a]	2.72[e]	12.88[a]	2.06	1.60
	25	Maze Coordination—Non-Dom. (time)	2.92[e]	5.83[f]	2.11	4.46[a]	2.66	0.09
	26	Maze Coordination—Non-Dom. (corr.)	4.71[a]	4.58[e]	2.94[e]	4.67[e]	4.27[e]	0.11
12	27	Static Steadiness—Dom. (time)	2.85[e]	0.31	3.78[f]	19.57[d]	8.78[a]	1.56
	28	Static Steadiness—Dom. (corr.)	4.53[a]	0.10	4.31[a]	15.09[d]	11.78[d]	1.41
	29	Static Steadiness—Non-Dom. (time)	1.61	0.29	6.20[d]	13.20[d]	18.49[d]	0.00
	30	Static Steadiness—Non-Dom. (corr.)	4.70[a]	0.00	3.98[a]	10.16[a]	12.68[d]	0.06
13	31	Grooved Pegboard—Dom. (time)	25.39[d]	7.53[a]	7.64[d]	25.24[d]	2.50	0.29
	32	Grooved Pegboard—Non-Dom. (time)	16.28[d]	2.12	3.64[f]	18.47[d]	2.69	0.06

[a] $(M_1M_2 + M_1P_2) - (P_1M_2 + P_1P_2)$.

[b] Marijuana effect during second session unrelated to experimental condition in initial session $(M_1M_2 + M_1P_2) - (M_1P_2 + P_1M_2)$.

[c] Marijuana effect during second session related to experimental condition in initial session $(M_1M_2 - M_1P_2) - (P_1M_2 - P_1P_2)$.

[d] $p < 0.001$.

[e] $p < 0.05$.

[f] $p < 0.02$.

[g] $p < 0.01$.

variables for the high-dose group. The high-dose group, however, showed a greater incidence of differential change within experimental conditions between sessions, i.e., significant improvement occurred on 8/13 tests and 16/32 variables for the high-dose group compared with 5/13 tests and 8/32 variables for the low-dose group.

4. DRUG EFFECTS ON PERFORMANCE AND LEARNING

The data for the low- and high-dose groups were now analyzed to provide information about (1) drug-effect, i.e., marijuana compared with placebo conditions in the first session (column 4 of Tables II and III); (2) effect of drug-state on learning, i.e., marijuana compared with placebo conditions in the second session (the same tests were administered during the initial and second sessions), regardless of experimental condition (marijuana or placebo) in the first session (column 5 of Tables II and III); and (3) effect of drug-state on learning in the second session when prior experience (the experimental condition of the first session) is taken into account (column 6 of Tables II and III).

Drug-effect, i.e., adverse effect on performance during the first session, was noted frequently for the low-dose group, i.e., for 7/13 tests and 12/32 variables (Table II, column 4). The drug effect on performance was, however, much more striking and generalized for the high-dose group, i.e., for 11/13 tests and 28/32 variables (Table III, column 4).

For the low-dose group, the drug-state (marijuana compared with placebo conditions) did affect learning during the second session, but the extent of impairment of performance remained unchanged from that noted during the initial session, i.e., marijuana resulted in significantly different scores in 7/13 tests and 13/32 during the second session. For the high-dose group, there was also a drug-effect on learning during the second session; although the extent of impairment on performance was less striking than in the first session, the impairment was still generalized and still significantly higher when compared with the low-dose group, i.e., marijuana affected 9/13 tests and 20/32 variables (column 5 of Tables II and III).

But the effect of drug-state on learning during the second session was consistently unrelated to prior experience during the initial session, for both the low- and high-dose groups. Specifically, we were unable to demonstrate that the administration of marijuana compared to placebo during the first session resulted in a differential decrement in performance levels during the second session (column 6 of Tables II and III).

5. DOSE-EFFECT RELATIONSHIPS

Of the tests and variables adversely affected by the drug in the first session, a dose-related decrement in performance levels was demonstrated for 4/13 of these tests and 16/32 of these variables. Of the tests and variables adversely affected by the drug in the second session, a dose-related decrease in performance was shown for 5/13 of these tests and 13/32 of these variables.

A number of the tests in the neuropsychological battery were more sensitive to impairment during the drug-state regardless of dose and repeated administration of these tests. It can be noted from column 4 of Tables II and III that during the initial session, scores on the same 7/13 tests and 12/32 variables were significantly different for both low- and high-dose groups. The significant differences noted in the first session decreased to the same 4/13 tests and 10/32 variables for both dose groups during the second session (column 5 of Tables II and III). The most sensitive to impairment regardless of dose or session reduced to 4/13 tests and 7/32 variables (columns 4 and 5 of Tables II and III).

6. ACUTE EFFECTS AND CEREBRAL DYSFUNCTION

The presence of significant differences between marijuana and placebo conditions for various mental processes leads to one set of inferences and conclusions. But when these significant differences for the marijuana compared with the placebo group derive from scores which are usually associated with cerebral dysfunction, the inferences and conclusions may be more clinical in nature. The results of two tests of the Halstead Battery —Category (a measure of concept formation visually mediated) and Tactual Performance Total (a measure of form discrimination and spacial configuration kinesthetically mediated)—illustrate this phenomenon (Table IV). As has already been pointed out, neither of these tests was found to be dose related during the initial session, and only the Category test was dose related during the second session. In comparing the findings of these two tests during the initial session with ascertained cutoff points (Table IV), it is evident that the result of the Category test is beyond normal limits for both marijuana dose groups while the score from the Tactual Performance test is outside normal limits for only the high-dose group.

B. Neurophysiological Results

1. VISUAL ASSESSMENT OF THE EEG

Of the 75 baseline records obtained, only 5 were abnormal by clinical criteria. The abnormal records included 3 with paroxysmal, generalized slow and sharp activity and 2 with focal slow activity. This represents an abnormality rate of 6.6%, which is well within the expected range for a

TABLE IV

Mean Scores of Category and Tactual Performance Tests for Low- and High-Dose Marijuana Groups

Test	Session	Placebo	Marijuana low-dose	Percent of change	Marijuana high-dose	Percent of change	Cut-off point
Category	First	−35.91	−53.28[a]	48	−56.71[a]	58	51 errors or more
	Second	−17.59	−18.65	6	−25.41[b]	25	—
Tactual performance total	First	−11.32	−13.82[b]	22	−16.70[a]	47	15.7 minutes or more
	Second	− 6.65	− 9.95[c]	49	−10.26[d]	54	—

[a] $p < 0.001$.
[b] $p < 0.05$.
[c] $p < 0.02$.
[d] $p < 0.01$.

normal population. The focal abnormalities were both occipital-temporal in location, one left- and one right-sided.

None of the records changed significantly after smoking, except one with a right occipital-temporal slow focus which showed a very slight increase in slowing after placebo, and one with paroxysmal slow and sharp activity which improved slightly after a high dose of active marijuana.

2. COMPUTER ANALYSIS OF EEG

The results of the computer-derived power density spectral analysis of occipital EEG activity are summarized in Table V. Peak power (mean)

TABLE V

EEG Power Spectral Analyses

Measured parameter	N	Baseline	N	Placebo	N	Drug low	N	Drug high
Mean of peak power (value)	75	309	28	308	18	310	29	181[a]
Mean of peak power (freq.)	75	10.0	28	10.0	18	10.0	29	10.2
Peak of mean spectra (value)	75	218	28	211	18	232	29	143[a]
Peak of mean spectra (freq.)	75	10.4	28	10.2	18	9.8	29	10.5

[a] Significant difference from baseline $p < 0.05$.

was very close to 10 Hz during baseline recording and this peak point was not changed significantly by administration of placebo or either dose of drug. There was a slight tendency, however, for the peak power point to shift to the left under low drug condition.

There was a significant decrease in power at the peak frequency (10.2 to 10.5 Hz) following the high dose of the drug and a tendency, though not significant, to an increase in power at the peak frequency (9.8 to 10.0 Hz) following the low-dose.

3. VISUAL AND AUDITORY EVOKED POTENTIALS

Measuring peak latency and peak-to-peak amplitude of the late negative deflection, VER parameters were unchanged following either drug dose. The AER latency was slightly but significantly ($p < 0.05$) prolonged following high drug dose (137 msec) as compared to placebo (119 msec).

4. RESPIRATION

Mean respiration rate was 16.3/minute during baseline trials, 15.7/minute during placebo trials, and tended to be slightly but not significantly higher during drug trials, with means of 16.4 and 16.6/minute after low and high drug doses respectively.

5. HEART RATE

Figure 1 illustrates the observed heart rate changes. Marijuana smoking induced a very rapid, significant dose-related increase in heart rate which began to diminish within 22 minutes after smoking was completed. The rate diminished progressively thereafter, but was still significantly higher than baseline levels near the end of the recording period (44 minutes after beginning smoking).

6. GSR REACTIVITY

The GSR reactivity ratio decreased significantly throughout both baseline (0.89) and placebo (0.76) trials, for both low- (0.55, $F = 25.63$) and high- (0.52, $F = 48.96$) dose groups, as compared to the baseline condition.

7. CNV

The only significant change was in the magnitude of the CNV after smoking marijuana containing 4.8 mg Δ^9-THC. Under low-dose conditions subjects developed significantly larger amplitude CNVs (22.3 μV) than during placebo trials (15.6 μV).

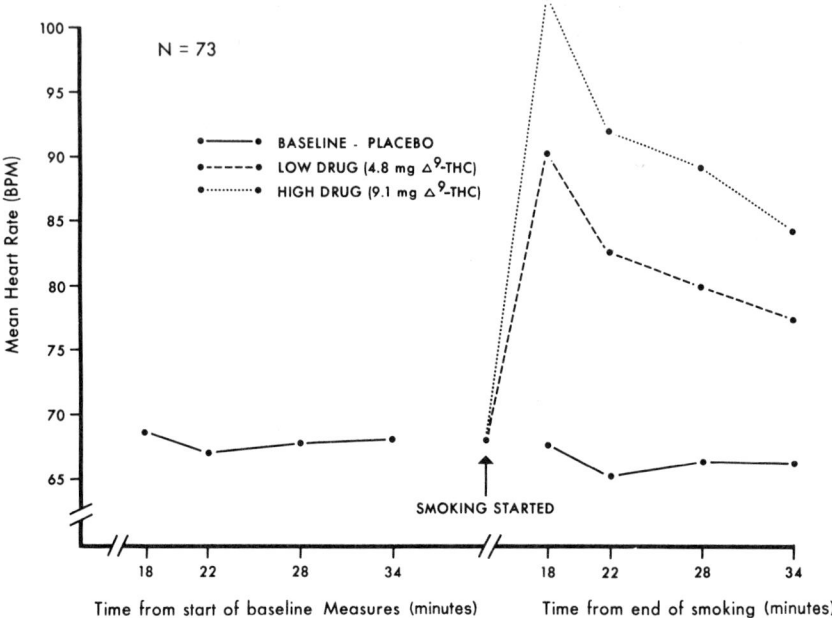

Fig. 1. Graph of observed heart rate vs. time through baseline and postsmoking recording. Each mean heart rate observation following either high or low dose of marijuana is significantly higher than the corresponding baseline and placebo value ($p < 0.05$ at least). Note that total (baseline) $N = 73$, placebo $N = 29$, low drug $N = 16$, and high drug $N = 28$. (From Low et al., 1973.)

8. DISCRIMINATION–FEEDBACK CNVS

There was a slight but insignificant tendency for the CNV area to decrease and for the postresponse area to increase as the discrimination task became more difficult during both baseline and placebo trials. The difficulty in discrimination was indicated by a significant increase in the average number of response errors from paradigm 5 to paradigm 7 (<2 to 6 per task set).

Following marijuana smoking there was a marked change in the relative magnitudes of the pre-$S_{2d\Delta}$ CNV and the post-R CNV, with the post-R area tending to become larger than the pre-$S_{2d\Delta}$ CNV. The mean number of response errors was significantly higher during all three discrimination trial sets after smoking either low (3.69, 5.56, and 8.94 per task set) or high (3.12, 6.20, and 10.28) doses of marijuana than during baseline (1.64, 2.24, and 6.17) or placebo (1.64, 2.82, and 5.93) trials. There was a slightly higher response–error rate during paradigms 6 and

7 after the high drug dose as compared to the low drug dose, but no clear-cut dose effect as in the heart rate changes.

IV. DISCUSSION

If one is to generalize from findings of a particular study, the dose level should be relevant to the sociocultural scene as well as to other laboratory studies that have employed marijuana in a standardized manner. The data regarding social usage of marijuana are sparse. Le Dain (1972), after reviewing the literature, reported that in North America most users smoke less than 10 mg Δ^9-THC to get "stoned." In Commission laboratory experiments, doses of about 6 mg Δ^9-THC were smoked to produce "high effects." Our low dose of 4.8 mg followed by an additional 2.4 mg 1 hour later is therefore comparable with Le Dain's definition of a socially relevant dose. Data are, however, available regarding the use of higher dose levels in studies. Some of the more credible investigators in the field, such as Weil et al. (1968) and Dornbush et al. (1971), used 18 and 22.5 mg Δ^9-THC, respectively (delivered by smoking). Our high dose of 9.1 mg followed by an additional 4.5 mg 1 hour later falls far short of doses defined as high by some laboratory investigators. Furthermore, questionnaires completed by the subjects included in this study regarding their use of marijuana in a social context indicate that our high dose is relevant to the social scene.

The even distribution of the very limited number of significant differences of men compared with women on the neuropsychological tests, for the low- and high-dose groups, leads us to conclude that there are no discernible sex differences with respect to the effect of marijuana on mental processes. The Mayor's Committee on Marijuana (1944) found test results for their female subjects that were not entirely similar to those obtained for the men, but only 5 women were included in the study and their performance showed great variability. Of more recent studies, only Abel (1971c) included female subjects, and Hollister and Gillespie (1970) included one female subject. There was no mention of sex differences in these articles.

The dose of marijuana defined as high (9.1 mg Δ^9-THC reinforced by an additional 4.5 mg 1 hour later) administered during the initial session resulted in significant impairment in all four mental processes and, furthermore, the effect was generalized to all modalities (visual, tactile, and auditory). It is noteworthy that the dose of marijuana defined as low (4.8 mg Δ^9-THC reinforced by 2.4 mg 1 hour later) also resulted in significant impairment in these four mental processes and all modalities. There were, however, some selective differences in the pattern of impairment between the low- and high-dose groups. Concept formation was as adversely affected by the low dose of marijuana as by the high dose. Memory, on the other hand, was selectively affected only by the low dose; specifically, tactile short-term memory and auditory immediate memory of notes were not affected, but auditory immediate memory of meaningful information was significantly impaired. Whereas visual immediate memory was unaffected, the more complex form of visual immediate recall was significantly impaired. Tactile form discrimination was also selectively impaired. But the most striking reduction in effect in the low- compared with the high-dose group was evident in the motor sphere. Specifically, of the five tests and 16 variables impaired in the high-dose group, only the two steadiness tests and four variables were impaired in the low-dose group.

The same trend was noted for the second compared with the first session, the second session having been purposefully included to measure learning or practice effect. For the high-dose group, concept formation remained significantly impaired. There was, however, sufficient learning with respect to auditory memory of meaningful information so that this variable did not discriminate between marijuana and placebo conditions. Both tests of visual memory remained impaired. Tactile form discrimination was somewhat less affected by learning. The improvement due to learning was proportional in the motor tasks. For the low-dose group there was a differential learning effect on concept formation, in that Trail Making but not Category remained significantly impaired. It should be noted that the Category test is the more pointed and powerful test of reasoning. With respect to memory, auditory immediate memory of meaningful information remained significantly impaired as did visual recall involving retroactive interference. Tactile discrimination also remained apparently unchanged in terms of impairment. The extent of impairment in the motor sphere increased during the second session. This could possibly be explained on the basis of order effect, in that these particular tests may have been readministered at a time of maximal drug effect. Another possible explanation is variability within data for these two tests.

How can one account for such disorganization, transient in nature, in terms of a brain-behavior model? Melges et al. (1970) referred to the effects of marijuana on cognitive operations as temporal disintegration, relating the disintegration of sequential thought to impaired immediate memory. The present study found the disintegrative effects to be more generalized. Whereas most problems in concept formation involve the

6. Psychological and Neurophysiological Effects

effective use of stored information, one could not account for the rather profound impairment in concept formation noted in this study for both the low- and high-dose groups during the initial session solely on the basis of memory impairment. The decrement in performance on motor tasks is unrelated to memory impairment. One would accordingly have to posit a drug-related effect on the individual's central integrative processes, the disturbance in brain function being transient in nature. A finding that merits further investigation is the extent of disorganization in concept formation, as reflected by the Category test, and the low threshold for disorganization in terms of dose of marijuana. Whereas the scores on the Category test were beyond the cut-off point and within the cerebral dysfunction range, further generalizations would be unwarranted at this point.

The effects of marijuana on learning as well as on memory might be explained by the same model. Learning refers to a change in behavior which is brought about through practice, and the second session in this study was designed to measure learning. Memory involves three stages: input (registration), storage (retention), and output (recall). One must then distinguish those drug effects on learning that are the result of effects on memory storage from other effects due to attentional, perceptual, and motivational influences. Regarding memory, output (recall) can fail because the subject cannot adopt the set that will enable him to make the appropriate response available to him. Inappropriate set can occur at time of input (registration) or at output (recall), independent of registration. In the present study, marijuana effects on mental processes were noted on reexamination (during the second session), but we were not able to demonstrate by statistical analysis that these drug effects were related to prior experimental conditions (marijuana or placebo administrations during the initial session). Whereas the drug has a demonstrable effect on learning, the influence on learning is unrelated to prior experience. Furthermore, the impairment noted during the initial session could not have been the result of faulty acquisition or a faulty set at time of input, as these would have precluded other stages of memory and subsequent learning. The impairment must therefore be in the storage or output processes, more probably the latter in view of lack of interference with learning regardless of prior experimental conditions.

How does one now reconcile generalized disintegrative effects during the initial session with transfer of sufficient information to ensure learning during the second session? One possible explanation is that the information was coded into storage during the initial session but the output was faulty, due to interference with central integrative processes. The interference was, however, transitory, and by the time the subject appeared for the second session the previously learned information was available, and to the same extent as for the group who received placebo during the initial session. The readministration of the drug still resulted in a generalized impairment of mental processes but to a lesser extent for the particular mental processes, owing to prior experience (with marijuana or placebo) and learning. The model of learning proposed in this chapter is different from the one suggested by Abel (1971c) who, in his studies of the effects of marijuana on memory, concluded that marijuana affects concentration and input of information and, as a result, storage and adequate recall are precluded.

Our heart rate data are consistent with those of many other investigators (Rodin et al., 1970; Jasinski et al., 1971; Renault et al., 1971). It is clear that marijuana smoking produces an almost immediate tachycardia, that this tachycardia is dose-related, and that the initial rate increase is sustained for only a relatively short period of time. However, marked subjective and objective effects of the drug may persist while the heart rate returns toward resting levels.

There is no clear parallel between heart rate and GSR reactivity changes, although they both show a suggestively bimodal pattern, with initial short-lived changes which could be attributed to marked anticholinergic activity, either central or peripheral. That these initial effects give way to qualitatively different effects within approximately 30 to 35 minutes after starting to smoke is suggested by the rapidly decreasing heart rate near the end of this time period and by the change in GSR reactivity pattern to follow more closely the pattern obtained with placebo.

The EEG spectral analysis during low drug dose conditions shows trends (statistically not significant) similar to those described by Hollister et al. (1970), Volavka et al. (1971), and Rodin et al. (1970), i.e., a very slight shift downward in the peak frequency and a slight increase in the power of the peak frequency of the occipital EEG. These trends are reversed, however, under high drug dose conditions, in which we found a significant decrease in the power of the peak frequency. This decrease indicates "desynchronization" of alpha activity and suggests a greater or qualitatively different effect of high doses of THC on this measure of corticodiencephalic tone than is induced by low doses.

These differences are paralleled by differences in AER latencies and CNV magnitude and emphasize the crucial importance of specifying dose when discussing the effects of drugs like the cannabis derivatives. Under low drug dose conditions, we observed a significant increase in CNV magnitude as compared to placebo during the simple reaction-time paradigm. No significant changes in this CNV measure were induced by high drug doses, however. These data confirm the report of Tinklenberg (1972) and lend support to the idea that during the initial phase of the marijuana experience the brain mechanisms subserving attention are enhanced rather than diminished.

We have observed a slight increase in AER latency under high drug dose conditions, but no significant changes in AER amplitude or in VER parameters. These findings support partially the conclusions of Tinklenberg (1972) and, together with the CNV data, suggest that while attention mechanisms are undisturbed, high doses of THC may alter perception by interfering with cognitive read-out functions. The observed change in AER latency was in the relatively late negative component, the amplitude of which has been shown to be diminished during inattention (Haider et al., 1964) and whose latency is presumably related in part to the efficiency of cognitive processes occurring after the arrival of the sensation in the primary auditory cortex.

That attention mechanisms per se are not necessarily disturbed by marijuana is also suggested by the results of the discrimination–feedback experiments. During the first discrimination task set the pre-$S_{2d\Delta}$ CNV tended to be higher under low drug dose than placebo conditions, although this difference was not statistically significant; only under high-dose conditions relatively late in the recording session was there a significant diminution in the magnitude of the prediscrimination CNV compared to placebo.

This significant diminution in the pre-$S_{2d\Delta}$ CNV area under high drug dose during discrimination tasks 2 and 3 must be interpreted in the light of the subject's involvement in the whole task and of the changes occurring after the response. The difference between the pre-$S_{2d\Delta}$ CNV and the prefeedback CNV is interpreted as an indication of the subject's certainty of correctness of response choice, since the post-R prefeedback CNV directly reflects interest in the information conveyed by the feedback signal. If one subtracts post-R area from CNV area, the result is positive in some relation to the subject's degree of certainty of the correctness of his choice of response to $S_{2d\Delta}$. That this is a reasonable interpretation is supported by previous evidence (Picton and Low, 1971).

The absolute measure of correctness of response choice is the number of response errors, fewer errors indicating better discrimination. The large number of errors made during drug trials, even while the subjects were interested and attentive and were receiving specific feedback information about correctness of response, clearly indicates a performance deficit induced by the drug.

In context with the results of our neuropsychological experiments and with other reported findings, these observations can form the basis of a reasoned hypothesis of the neural mechanisms responsible for the marijuana experience.

First, it is clear that smoked marijuana has at least a qualitative bimodal effect over time, with an initial relatively brief "rush" lasting approximately 30 to 35 minutes and a subsequent longer period of "quieter" action. This sequence fits almost exactly with the known time frame of biotransformation of Δ^9-THC to 11-OH THC (Lemberger et al., 1971) and with the subjective reports of many users. It is possible that Δ^9-THC is itself in general terms an "activator" or stimulant, while its metabolites such as 11-OH THC are predominantly "depressant" to the CNS.

Second, dose is critically important in determining not only the duration of effects as has been claimed by some, but also the qualitative nature of the effects themselves, perhaps in a successive-threshold fashion.

Third, marijuana induces changes in brain function which can be profound but which are associated with only relatively minor measurable changes using standard electrophysiological recording techniques such as the EEG. This fact alone strongly implicates subcortical, medial, or basal brain structures as being primarily responsible for the experiential and performance changes induced.

We have demonstrated in these experiments that marijuana interferes with performance in a manner which cannot be explained on the basis of decreased attention or altered retention of learned information. The results of the neuropsychological experiments in particular indicate that the functional change produced is one which results in altered concept formation or appraisal. The neurophysiological data support this conclusion in demonstrating changes in AER latency and marked disturbances in sensory discrimination task performance.

Appropriate action in response to any sensory input depends on a complex neural pathway serving sensation, perception, appraisal, evaluation or concept formation, and motor response. According to Arnold (1970) and MacLean (1970), the appraisal or evaluation function is likely mediated by relays from cortical sensory receiving areas to the adjoining limbic system.

Shute and Lewis (1961) have shown that the main afferent pathways to the hippocampus are cholinergic in type. Our experiments and others have demonstrated that marijuana exerts an anticholinergic effect.

Clinical evidence has shown that abnormal discharges in or near the limbic cortex may produce feelings of depersonalization, distortions of perception, alterations in time sense, and feelings of fear or paranoia (Penfield and Jasper, 1954). All these subjective states may occur, and some are very common as part of the marijuana experience. Pleasant feelings, euphoria, happiness, and placidity are also very common ele-

6. Psychological and Neurophysiological Effects 151

ments of the marijuana experience, and it is notable that the septal region, which appears to function as a major coordinating center for the entire limbic system, is by far the most effective target for self-stimulation experiments with a variety of mammals, including man. Delgado (1970) has demonstrated that electrical stimulation of limbic structures, especially the hippocampus, often produces pleasant sensations, elation, deep thoughtful concentration, relaxation, and colored visions in human subjects with chronically implanted depth electrodes.

Finally, the paper previously referred to by Heath (1972) and one by McIsaac et al. (1971) provide objective evidence that the primary physiological and chemical changes induced by marijuana do occur in limbic-diencephalic structures. Heath recorded electrical activity from multiple subcortical brain regions and from scalp electrodes in one psychiatric patient. Recordings were made repeatedly over several weeks during all states of consciousness and during intoxication with marijuana, alcohol, and amphetamines and while smoking tobacco. Only during marijuana intoxication and only associated with "rushes" of euphoria, Heath recorded marked changes in electrical activity patterns from the septal region. There were no significant changes in the activity in any other area including the scalp-recorded EEG.

McIsaac et al. injected squirrel monkeys with radioactive Δ^9-THC and, using radioautographic techniques, showed that very high concentrations appeared in the limbic system, diencephalon (excluding hypothalamus) midbrain, and frontal and cerebellar cortex within 15 minutes and remained in these regions at higher concentrations than in other brain areas for up to 4 hours. They also noted a differential effect of dose on the behavior of the monkeys, with low doses producing apparently diminished anxiety, moderate doses inducing stimulation, and high doses producing incapacitation.

This may be the most inclusive neural model of the physiological basis of the marijuana experience: Δ^9-THC and its metabolites act primarily to alter the normal functional relationship between paleocortical limbic system structures and the neocortex. This alteration may vary from stimulation of limbic activity to depression (or disinhibition to increasing inhibition) depending on dose, time, prior set, and current setting. The major elements of the marijuana experience, including altered perception, mood, and performance, may all be explained on this basis. The most striking objective change, i.e., a general cognitive performance decrement, may be the result of the loss of an accurate concept formation, appraisal, or evaluation stage in the stimulus cue performance sequence, normally subserved by neocortical–limbic circuits. The occasional "bad trip," which occurred with 3 of our subjects only and which from our observations appears to occur only if the individual is already feeling badly or is apprehensive about the experimental situation, emphasizes the importance of set and setting in determining the quality of the emotional aspects of the experience.

The model would explain not only the major elements of the acute marijuana experience itself but also the occasionally reported "flashback" phenomenon and possibly some of the cannabis-mobilized psychoses. It is well known to neurophysiologists that the limbic system, and the hippocampus in particular, has a very low threshold for activation by mechanical, chemical, or electrical stimulation. Once activated, neuronal discharges tend to spread throughout all limbic circuits without very readily involving other brain areas. These phylogenetically old neural structures also have a marked tendency to persist in an altered functional state for long periods after the initial stimulus has been withdrawn. In this regard, it is perhaps significant that Heath (1972) has recorded bursts of high voltage spike and slow activity from limbic areas as the only consistent electrographic abnormality in a large number of patients during periods of psychotic behavior.

Because of the intense current interest of society in the subject of drugs and their effects on people, it is inevitable that investigators with research data will be asked for interpretations of those data in philosophical–sociological terms. While such interpretations can mislead the unwary if it is not made clear where the evidence stops and speculation begins, if carefully made they can provide a valuable perspective for laymen and may stimulate other scientists in different disciplines to seek new directions for future investigation.

With the disclaimer, then, that what follows here is a speculative interpretation on a social level, we believe that the neurophysiological model proposed might also explain the devotion to the marijuana experience of millions of young and not-so-young individuals in present-day society. In terms of the relationships among the three brain levels suggested by MacLean (1970), cannabis may allow the individual to exist at a phylogenetically old mammalian level, literally within the emotional brain itself, free from the conflict which is constant between the old sensory and feeling-oriented system and the newly imposed "civilization brain."

Such "regression in service of the ego" is not new in our society, nor is it unique to the marijuana experience. It is practiced regularly with at least some cultural approval and even encouragement in the form of tobacco smoking, alcohol consumption, some forms of psychotherapy, the use of tranquillizers, "back to earth" activities, and even in the rituals, ceremonies, and ordinances of many lodges, fraternal organizations, and religions. In this regard, the crucial questions regarding the marijuana experience have to do with the degree of certainty about the transient or temporary nature of the regression measured against the survival value to the individual of that particular form of experience!

ACKNOWLEDGMENTS

This research was supported by Grant 610-25-1, National Health Grants, Ottawa, Canada. The authors wish to express their appreciation to: A. M. Marcus, M.D., Associate Professor, Department of Psychiatry, Head, Division of Forensic Psychiatry, U.B.C.; H. Sanders, Ph.D., Associate Professor, Department of Pharmacology, U.B.C.; C. Fibiger, Ph.D., J. C. Yuille, Ph.D., I. Gillespie, M.D., I. Heller, M.D., B. Simpson, R.N., H. Hoodless, B.Sc., S. Svitorka, B.A., R.E.T., S. Y. Th'ng, R.E.T., E. Holmes, B.Sc., M. Gregg, Ph.D., K. Low, the Health Sciences Centre Hospital, U.B.C. and the Vancouver General Hospital for their cooperation and for providing the necessary research facilities, and to the Digital Equipment Corporation, Vancouver office, for providing the PDP-12 computer used in some of the data analysis.

REFERENCES

Abel, E. L. (1970). *Nature (London)* 227, 1151–1152.
Abel, E. L. (1971a). *Nature (London)* 231, 58.
Abel, E. L. (1971b). *Nature (London)* 231, 260–261.
Abel, E. L. (1971c). *Science* 173, 1038–1040.
Arnold, M. B. (1970). *In* "Physiological Correlates of Emotion" (P. Black, ed.), p. 261. Academic Press, New York.
Caldwell, D. F., Myers, S. A., Domino, E. F., and Merriam, P. E. (1969). *Percept. Mot. Skills* 29, 755–759.
Caldwell, D. F., Myers, S. A., and Domino, E. F. (1970). *In* "Psychotomimetic Drugs" (D. H. Efron, ed), p. 299. Raven Press, New York.
Campbell, D. R. (1971). *Can. Psychiat. Ass. J.* 16, 161–165.
Clark, L. D., and Nakashima, E. N. (1968). *Amer. J. Psychiat.* 125, 379–384.
Clark, L. D., Hughes, R., and Nakashima, E. N. (1970). *Arch. Gen. Psychiat.* 23, 193–198.
Darley, C. F., Tinklenberg, J. R., Hollister, T. E., and Atkinson, R. C. (1973). *Psychopharmacologia* 29, 231–238.
Delgado, J. M. R. (1970). *In* "Physiological Correlates of Emotion" (P. Black, ed.), p. 189. Academic Press, New York.
Domino, E. F. (1971). *Ann. N.Y. Acad. Sci.* 191, 181–191.
Dornbush, R. L., and Freedman, A. M. (1972). *Psychopharmacol. Bull.* 8, 19–20.
Dornbush, R. L., Fink, M., and Freedman, A. M. (1971). *Amer. J. Psychiat.* 128, 194–197.
Galanter, M., Weingartner, H., Vaughan, T. B., Roth, W. T., and Wyatt, R. J. (1973). *Arch. Gen. Psychiat.* 28, 278–281.
Gale, E. N., and Guenther, G. (1971). *Brit. J. Addict.* 66, 188–194.

Haider, M., Spong, P., and Lindsley, D. B. (1964). *Science* **145**, 180–182.
Heath, R. G. (1972). *Arch. Gen. Psychiat.* **26**, 577–584.
Hollister, L. E., and Gillespie, H. (1970). *Arch. Gen. Psychiat.* **23**, 199–203.
Hollister, L. E., Sherwood, S. L., and Cavasino, A. (1970). *Pharmacol. Res. Commun.* **2**, 305–308.
Isbell, H., and Jasinski, D. R. (1969). *Psychopharmacologia* **14**, 115–123.
Jasinski, D. R., Haertzen, C. A., and Isbell, H. (1971). *Ann. N.Y. Acad. Sci.* **191**, 196–205.
Johnson, S., and Domino, E. F. (1971). *Clin. Pharmacol. Ther.* **12**, 762–768.
Jones, R. T., and Stone, G. (1970). *Psychopharmacologia* **18**, 108–117.
Jones, R. T. (1971). *Pharmacol. Rev.* **23**, 359–369.
Kiplinger, G. F., and Manno, J. E. (1971). *Pharmacol. Rev.* **23**, 339–347.
Kiplinger, G. F., Manno, J. E., Rodda, B. E., and Forney, R. B. (1971). *Clin. Pharmacol. Ther.* **12**, 650–657.
Le Dain Commission. (1972). "A Report of the Commission of Inquiry into the Non-Medical Use of Drugs." Information Canada, Ottawa.
Lemberger, L., Axelrod, J., and Kopin, I. J. (1971). *Pharmacol. Rev.* **23**, 371–380.
Lewis, E. G., Dustman, R. E., Peters, B. A., Straight, R. C., and Beck, E. C. (1973). *Electroencephalogr. Clin. Neurophysiol.* **35**, 347–354.
McIsaac, W. M., Fritchie, G. E., Idanpaan-Heikkila, J. E., Ho, B. T., and Englert, L. F. (1971). *Nature (London)* **230**, 593–594.
MacLean, P. D. (1970). *In* "The Neurosciences: Second Study Program" (F. O. Schmitt, ed.), p. 336. Rockefeller Univ. Press, New York.
Manno, J. E., Kiplinger, G. F., Haine, S. C., Bennett, I., and Forney, R. (1970). *Clin. Pharmacol. Ther.* **11**, 808–815.
Mayor's Committee on Marijuana. (1944). "The Marijuana Problem in the City of New York" (G. B. Wallace, chairman). Jacques Cattell Press, New York.
Melges, F. T., Tinklenberg, J. R., Hollister, L. E., and Gillespie, H. K. (1970). *Science* **168**, 1118–1120.
Meyer, R. E., Pillard, R. C., Shapiro, L. M., and Mirin, S. M. (1971). *Amer. J. Psychiat.* **128**, 198–204.
Miras, C. H. (1969). *In* "Drugs and Youth" (J. R. Wittenborn et al., eds.), p. 191. Thomas, Springfield, Illinois.
Penfield, W., and Jasper, H. H. (1954). "Epilepsy and the Functional Anatomy of the Human Brain." Little, Brown, Boston, Massachusetts.
Picton, T. W., and Low, M. D. (1971). *Electroencephalogr. Clin. Neurophysiol.* **31**, 451–456.
Pivik, R. T., Zarcone, V., Dement, W. C., and Hollister, L. E. (1972). *Clin. Pharmacol. Ther.* **13**, 426–435.
Rafaelsen, L., Bech, P., Christrup, H., and Rafaelsen, O. J. (1971). Rigshospitalet Psychochemistry Institute, Copenhagen (unpublished manuscript).
Renault, P. F., Schuster, C. R., Heinrich, R., and Freeman, D. X. (1971). *Science* **174**, 589–591.
Rickles, W. H., Cohen, M. J., Whitaker, C. A., and McIntyre, K. E. (1973). *Psychopharmacologia* **30**, 349–354.
Rodin, E. A., Domino, E. F., and Porzak, J. P. (1970). *J. Amer Med. Ass.* **213**, 1300–1302.
Shute, C. C. D., and Lewis, P. R. (1961). *Bibl. Anat.* **2**, 34–49.
Siler, J. F., Sheep, W. L., Bates, L. B., Clark, G. F., Cook, G. W., and Smith, W. A. (1933). *Mil. Surg.* **73**, 269–280.

Tecce, J. J. (1972). *Psychol. Bull.* **77,** 73–108.
Tinklenberg, J. R. (1972). *Psychopharmacol. Bull.* **8,** 9–10.
Tinklenberg, J. R., Melges, F. T., Hollister, L. E., and Gillespie, H. K. (1970). *Nature (London)* **226,** 1171–1172.
Volavka, J., Dornbush, R. L., Feldstein, S., Clare, G., Zaks, A., Fink, M., and Freedman, A. M. (1971). *Ann. N.Y. Acad. Sci.* **191,** 206–215.
Waskow, I. E., Olsson, J. E., Salzman, C., and Katz, M. (1970). *Arch. Gen. Psychiat.* **22,** 97–107.
Weil, A. T., Zinberg, N., and Nelsen, J. (1968). *Science* **162,** 1234–1242.
Wikler, A., and Lloyd, B. (1945). *Fed. Proc., Fed. Amer. Soc. Exp. Biol.* **4,** 141–142.
Williams, E., and Oberst, F. W. (1946). *Pub. Health Rep.* **61,** 1.
Williams, E., Himmelsbach, C. K., Wikler, A., Ruble, D., and Lloyd, B. (1946). *Pub. Health Rep.* **61,** 1059–1083.

Chapter 7

CANNABIS: NEURAL MECHANISMS AND BEHAVIOR

LOREN L. MILLER AND WILLIAM G. DREW

I.	Introduction	158
II.	Cognitive Effects of Cannabis in Man	158
III.	Hippocampus and Memory	160
IV.	Hippocampus and Internal Inhibition	163
V.	Cholinergic System, Memory, and Inhibition	164
VI.	Comparison of Cannabinoids, Anticholinergics, and Hippocampectomy	165
	A. Maze Learning and Performance	165
	B. Sequential Behavior	166
	C. Memory	166
	D. Attention	167
	E. Conditioned Fear	167
	F. Avoidance Learning and Performance	168
	G. Resistance to Extinction	169
	H. State Dependence	169
	I. DRL Schedules	170
	J. Passive Avoidance	170
	K. Habituation	170
VII.	Evidence That Cannabinoids Exert Actions within the Limbic System	171
VIII.	Evidence That Cannabinoids Exert Actions on Cholinergic Mechanisms	173
IX.	Data Inconsistent with the Cholinergic Hypothesis	175
X.	Effects of THC on Neuroendocrine Systems	177
XI.	Comparison of THC, the Extraadrenal Actions of ACTH, and Hippocampectomy	178
	A. Behavioral	178
	B. Pharmacological	179
XII.	Summary	181
	References	182

I. INTRODUCTION

Although the actions of cannabinoids on human cognition are now beginning to be defined, there exists a paucity of data or, for that matter, speculation as to possible neural and chemical mechanisms which may mediate the behavioral effects of this class of compounds. The purpose of this chapter is to develop a working model which incorporates a number of existing findings pertaining to the behavioral actions of cannabis in man. Animal data pertinent to the hypothesis are also entertained in an effort to be sufficiently assiduous.

Attempting to relate much of the animal literature to the human findings is difficult. However, research in our laboratory as well as an examination of the literature suggests that it is possible to incorporate within a single theoretical framework numerous findings at both the behavioral and pharmacological level.

II. COGNITIVE EFFECTS OF CANNABIS IN MAN

Habitual smokers of marijuana describe the effects of the drug in terms of a "high"; reporting feelings of relaxation, contentment, happiness, and increased clarity of sensing and thinking (Ames, 1958; Bromberg, 1934; Tart, 1970). An examination of these descriptions reveals that subjective estimates of increased clarity of sensing and thinking and clinical observations rarely coincide. Beringer (1932, as related by Ames, 1958) spoke of cannabis-induced "fragmentation of thought processes," "disturbances of memory," and "interruptions in the stream of thought." Bromberg (1934) in his description of the "complete acute marijuana intoxication syndrome," stated that anxiety occurred within 10 to 30 minutes after smoking and was often accompanied by panic states and even fear of death. Later, calmness, euphoria, talkativeness, and exhilaration became pronounced along with paresthesia. As a result, there was "an astounding feeling of lightness to the limbs and body . . . Elation continues: He laughs uncontrollably and explosively for brief periods of time without, at times, the slightest provocation; if there is a reason, it quickly fades, the point of the joke is lost immediately. Speech is rapid, flighty . . . ideas flow quickly . . . these flighty ideas are not deep enough to form an engram that can be recollected—hence, the confusion that appears on trying to remember what was thought" (Bromberg, 1934). Objective substantiation of some of these observations has been gained in recent studies employing known doses of Δ^9-THC in marijuana or Δ^9-THC administered orally (Hollister, 1971).

While some of the extreme reactions seen with marijuana (i.e., panic states, hallucinations, and delusions) are most likely the result of the employment of abnormally large doses of THC, consistent cognitive alterations are found at low and moderate dose levels. For example, time sense disturbances have been observed within such a number of diverse techniques (Clark et al., 1970; Jones and Stone, 1970; Tinklenberg et al., 1972; Weil et al., 1968; Williams et al., 1946) that it is generally held that marijuana (at low dose levels) subjectively slows the perception of time. In other words, subjects tend to overestimate the passage of time.

Concomitant with, or perhaps incidental to, time sense disturbances are disruptions in various aspects of memory functioning. It has been reasoned by Melges et al. (1970, 1971) that impaired performance on a goal-directed serial alternation task (a task which requires a subject to add and subtract numbers mentally until some specified number is reached) and disrupted speech patterns which are often found following marijuana intoxication (Weil and Zinberg, 1969) may be related to the "temporal incoordination of recent memories with intentions." According to one experimental subject, "I can't remember what I just said or what I want to say . . . because there are just so many thoughts that are broken in time, one chunk there and one chunk here." Thus, performance on the goal-directed serial alternation task is characterized by a "difficulty in retaining, coordinating and serially indexing those memories, perceptions and expectations that are relevant to the attainment of some goal." This phenomenon has been termed "temporal disintegration."

Recent observations in our laboratory lend support to the idea that memory loss during the intoxicated state and disrupted time sense may somehow be related. In one study, subjects were required to learn and recall a short narrative while under the influence of marijuana or placebo. A low dose of Δ^9-THC contained in the marijuana cigarette (25 μg/kg) significantly impaired recall measured in terms of number of story units remembered. Two dimensions which characterized forgetting were (1) the introduction of material not originally included in the narrative—subjects tended to introduce arbitrary and unrelated material often having a strong emotional tone during story recall; and (2) distortions of temporal context—facts were recalled out of their proper chronological order (Drew et al., 1972a; Miller et al., 1972). The former results offer support for the observations of Tinklenberg et al. (1972) that marijuana, through its capacity to speed up an internal biological clock, induces disorganization along a temporal continuum of memory storage. The introduction of new material during recall might be an attempt by an intoxicated subject to compensate for a memory deficit.

It was felt that the insufficiency in timing behavior, as well as the apparent incidence of confabulations, was strongly reminiscent of the memory deterioration found in Korsakoff patients (Drew et al., 1972a). This disorder, while often associated with chronic alcoholism, has been attributed to central nervous system damage to the limbic system. More accurately, lesions specific to the fornices (Hassler and Riechert, 1957), mammillary bodies, and hippocampus (Barbizet, 1963; Brion, 1969; Kahn and Crosby, 1972) and dorsal medial nucleus of the thalamus (Meissner, 1968) characterize the syndrome. Brion (1969) stated that lesions characterizing this syndrome are bilateral, involving the hippocampo–mammillo–thalamo–cingular limbic circuit, while Adams (1969) describes the defect in terms of a bilateral infarction of the medial aspects of the temporal lobes, particularly the hippocampus and parahippocampal convolutions and fornices.

In a number of human investigations, attempts have been made to ascertain whether memory storage or retrieval processes were affected by cannabis. Based on the results of a number of studies it has been concluded that the major action of marijuana is that of attenuating the passage of information from short-term to long-term memory, thereby affecting storage processes. That is, material acquired prior to intoxication is retained while material learned during the intoxication period tends not to be fully consolidated (Abel, 1971; Darley et al., 1973). It is striking that the acquisition of new information and/or the passage of information from short- to long-term memory under cannabinoids is similar to the primary memory deficits found in temporal lobe and Korsakoff patients (DeJong, 1973; Meissner, 1968).

These findings, as well as those mentioned previously, have led us to speculate that the effects of marijuana on cognition may be mediated by certain limbic structures, especially the hippocampus. We have further reasoned that the biochemical substrate for the effect of cannabis on numerous types of behaviors in human subjects and animals is cholinergic in nature. The rest of this chapter is devoted to exploring this hypothesis.

III. HIPPOCAMPUS AND MEMORY

Experimental interest in the various limbic system structures as possible neural loci crucial to memory and learning developed largely from human clinical data. Although a number of structures such as the amygdala, cingulate gyrus, mammillary bodies, and septum have all, at one time or another, been implicated as possible sites of memory formation and learning, the hippocampus has been most prominently mentioned. Klüver and Bucy (1939) initially noted severe behavioral changes in monkeys following bilateral resection of the temporal lobe. An important part of the overall behavioral anomaly was "psychic blindness." Monkeys presented with objects repeatedly would examine each as if viewing them for the first time. Scoville and Milner (1957) and Penfield and Milner (1958) reported severe recent memory loss in patients with surgical resections of the temporal lobes including the hippocampus. These patients exhibited severe anterograde amnesia which extended to the span of immediate memory. Although some retrograde amnesia was also present, I.Q., reasoning, perception, and other aspects of general intelligence remained intact. According to Milner (1958) the memory deficit in temporal lobe patients appeared twofold: (1) Patients could recall a stimulus several minutes after exposure unless distracted (the trace effects of a stimulus were left intact only as long as interference was eliminated); and (2) regardless of whether interference did or did not occur, information was not consolidated into long-term memory (i.e., the acquisition and utilization of cues was not possible).

Many similarities exist between the cognitive deterioration found in Korsakoff patients and the cognitive deficits of temporal lobe patients. In fact, it has been suggested that ablation of the temporal lobe and hippocampus produces a Korsakoff-like syndrome (Magoun, 1963). Earlier investigations showed that although some simple memories were retained, overall retention in these patients was greatly impaired (Nyssen, 1957). Talland (1965) found them not only inferior in recalling stories, but apt to substitute erroneous data and introduce extraneous material during recall. Meissner (1968) has suggested that memory impairments found in these patients may reflect an inability to habituate or to ignore trivial stimuli in addition to a deficit in consolidating recently acquired information.

Interestingly, earlier investigations of this syndrome suggested that fundamental to the amnesic syndrome was the inability to temporally order experience; memories might be retained but could not be evoked in sequential order (Van der Horst, 1956). Bernard (1951) suggested that the Korsakoff patient had difficulty in comparing present information with preceding and subsequent experiences. This was a result of disorganization in thinking along a temporal dimension. In fact, Williams and Zangwill (1952) already had described the sequential disturbances of memory in Korsakoff patients as that of an "agnosia of succession."

One of the more controversial issues in the specification of memory deficits found in amnesic patients is whether memory over brief intervals (short term) is affected by insult to the hippocampus and related limbic structures. A good deal of support exists for the view that the passage of information from short-term to long-term memory is blocked by hippocampal damage (DeJong, 1973; Kesner, 1973), but findings pertaining to short-term memory disruption per se are discordant. Widely divergent findings on this issue have surfaced in both the human and animal literature.

Drachman and Arbit (1966) found that hippocampal patients have a normal immediate memory span for subspan digits, but are impaired on superspan digits even after multiple repetitions. Wickelgren (1968) has found a normal decay function for a temporal lobe patient on a short-term recognition memory test. Baddeley and Warrington (1970) reported that amnesics are not impaired on the Peterson-Peterson short-term memory test. Similar results have been found by Sidman *et al.* (1968) on a delayed matching-to-sample task. On the other hand, Korsakoff patients not only evidence deficiencies in their ability to consolidate information, but also display poor short-term memory (Cermak *et al.*, 1971; Cermak and Butters, 1972). Both proactive interference (interference with memory due to previously presented information) and failure to verbally encode new information are responsible for this dual memory dysfunction.

It is feasible that some of the divergent results in the Korsakoff literature may be attributable to the influence of interference. For example, Cermak and Butters (1972) found such patients more sensitive than controls to the effects of proactive inhibition on a short-term memory task. Moreover, Korsakoff patients were more deficient under a massed practice condition than when practice was distributed. This strongly suggests that inhibition accrues during massed practice at a faster rate for Korsakoff patients relative to controls. When inhibition is allowed to dissipate with spaced trials, the recall of Korsakoff patients approaches normality. A similar interpretation has been offered by Correll and Scoville (1970) for the finding that monkeys with bilateral rhinencephalic lesions show poorer learning at short than at long intertrial intervals.

The animal literature appears to be at least as disparate as the human data with regard to the above issue. Both Correll and Scoville (1965) and Drachman and Ommaya (1964) found no deficiencies on delayed matching-to-sample tasks in hippocampal monkeys. Orbach *et al.* (1960) found no deficits in delayed alternation in hippocampectomized monkeys. However, severe reductions in delayed alternation have been found in rats with hippocampal lesions (Racine and Kimble, 1965). Stepien *et al.* (1960) found that two monkeys with amygdala-hippocampal lesions were impaired on a delayed comparison task (opening a door resulted in reinforcement if two stimuli presented successively were the same, but were not reinforced if the two stimuli were different). Adequate performance on this task requires inhibition of a response. This latter point is of great importance in at least one widely held theory of hippocampal functioning.

Although damage to the hippocampus does appear to result in some kind of memory disruption, a number of investigators have generally discounted all memory interpretations of hippocampal functioning (Douglas, 1967; Kimble, 1968; Isaacson, 1972). Isaacson (1972) has indicated that the correlation between memory loss and hippocampal damage is less than perfect. The major difficulty with the memory loss idea is that bilateral hippocampal damage in nonhuman organisms does not produce significant memory loss. For example, hippocampally lesioned rats acquire an avoidance response faster than controls and display retention 24 hours later (Isaacson *et al.*, 1961). Other studies have shown that hippocampal animals are normal in the learning of many types of discrimination problems (Kimble, 1963; Kimble and Kimble, 1965; Truax and Thompson, 1969). Superior learning ability at long rather than short intertrial intervals would also discount a recent memory interpretation (Correll and Scoville, 1970). It would appear that the memory hypothesis may not be encompassing enough to describe many of the behavioral effects of hippocampal lesions.

IV. HIPPOCAMPUS AND INTERNAL INHIBITION

A more encompassing hypothesis of hippocampal functioning has been proposed by Kimble (1968) and Douglas (1967). Since the recent memory hypothesis has come under attack mainly because of inconsistencies in the animal literature, an hypothesis which explained much of the animal data and at the same time incorporated the human data was needed.

According to Douglas (1967), the major function of the hippocampus is to "exclude stimulus patterns from attention through a process of efferent control of sensory reception known as gating." There are two types of gating:

1. *Nonspecific.* This type of gating is responsible for the exclusion of extraneous stimuli during concentration of attention, protecting memory traces from interference during consolidation. Recent memory loss is theoretically caused by a lack of nonspecific gating and, consequently, interference with selective consolidation occurs. Kimble (1968) states

that the hippocampus may be the organ of internal inhibition. Internal inhibition may protect consolidation processes from further modification serving as a strengthening factor in the process of memory storage. Via this mechanism, an observed deficit in recent memory could occur in an organism with an intact ability to store and recall information if that organism lacked a neural mechanism for the reduction and prevention of interference.

2. *Specific.* This type of gating acts to inhibit the perception of specific stimuli which have been associated with nonreinforcement. This would be important to such processes as error reduction, habituation, reversal learning, and extinction. Indeed, hippocampal animals display profound deficits on tasks in which some inhibition of behavior is required (Kimble, 1968). For example, hippocampal rats display greater resistance to extinction (Niki, 1962) and continued approach responding in a passive avoidance situation (Kimble, 1963; Kimura, 1958; Liss, 1968; McCleary, 1961). Thus, the hippocampus appears to be responsible for the normal behavioral braking which is provided for by the development of internal inhibition. The organism with hippocampal damage would be less apt to inhibit or alter its responses to initially prepotent environmental stimuli and consequently would display less flexible and hence less adaptive behavior.

V. CHOLINERGIC SYSTEM, MEMORY, AND INHIBITION

The search for biochemical, physiological, and pharmacological correlates or learning, memory, and inhibition have centered around cholinergic mechanisms involved in the mediation of behavior. Douglas suggested that cholinergic neurons within the hippocampal systems may be involved in gating. Should this be the case, anticholinergic drugs should severely disrupt hippocampal gating functions. In fact, all sensory input to the hippocampus could be blocked at the periphery by anticholinergic drugs. If the gating hypothesis is valid the effects of hippocampectomy and treatment with anticholinergic drugs should produce strikingly similar results. Such similarities do exist and will be dealt with in Section VI of this chapter.

That various aspects of memory formation are mediated by changes at cholinergic synapses, especially within the hippocampus, has been demonstrated in a number of studies (Adams *et al.*, 1969; Deutsch, 1971; Wiener and Messer, 1973). Deutsch (1971) has shown that anticholinesterases may increase conduction and consolidation. Scopolamine produces opposite effects and interferes with retention. Erickson and Patel (1969) found that post-trial stimulation of the hippocampus facilitated avoidance learning, an effect which was blocked by atropine.

Carlton (1969) has tried to explain the action of anticholinergic drugs on numerous aspects of behavior by hypothesizing that these agents interfere with an inhibitory process that is common to a variety of situations. Anticholinergics appear to attenuate inhibition which normally accrues to stimuli associated with nonreward. This interpretation is very similar to Kimble's internal inhibition hypothesis of hippocampal functioning and certainly corresponds to the specific gating mechanism proposed by Douglas. More direct evidence that a cholinergic inhibitory system exists within the hippocampus has been provided by Warburton (1969). He showed that a successive go, no-go discrimination was disrupted because of increased responding on nonreinforced trials following the injection of atropine into the ventral hippocampus.

VI. COMPARISON OF CANNABINOIDS, ANTICHOLINERGICS, AND HIPPOCAMPECTOMY

The behavioral effects of treatment with cannabis and its derivatives, anticholinergics, and damage to the hippocampus are strikingly similar. To our knowledge only a few studies have directly compared cannabinoids and anticholinergics while no studies have compared all three. A great majority of works have assessed individually the effect of each treatment. In this section, we shall attempt to make appropriate comparisons across investigations and treatments.

A. Maze Learning and Performance

The acquisition and performance of maze behaviors are disrupted by treatment with cannabinoids, anticholinergics, and following hippocampectomy. Although Carlini and Kramer (1965) showed that rats treated with cannabis extract display superior maze acquisition, later investigations have not replicated these findings. Rather, severe disruption of maze behavior has been noted (Carlini et al., 1970; Orsingher and Fulginiti, 1970). Both hippocampectomy (Jarrard and Lewis, 1967; Kaada et al., 1961; Stein and Kimble, 1966) and anticholinergics (Domer and Schueler, 1960; Whitehouse, 1964; Whitehouse et al., 1964) impair the acquisition and performance of maze behavior, presumably by retarding the development and/or display of inhibition so that error tendencies are increased or less readily eliminated. The mechanisms by which cannabinoids impair learning and performance in the maze are unknown. However, interference with inhibition is a tenable, although unexplored, possibility.

B. Sequential Behavior

Cannabinoids, hippocampectomy, and anticholinergics impair performance in human beings and animals on a number of tasks, the performance of which is dependent on the sequential integration of responses. In man, goal-directed serial alternation is one such task and is reportedly disrupted by Δ^9-THC (Melges et al., 1970, 1971). Nonspatial single alternation has been found to be disrupted by Δ^9-THC (Miller et al., 1973a), atropine (Warburton, 1969), and hippocampal lesions (Franchina and Brown, 1970). Hippocampectomy disrupts behavioral chaining on a sequential bar pressing task by producing perseverative responding (Kimble and Pribram, 1963). Hippocampectomy, anticholinergic drugs, and low doses of Δ^9-THC impair spontaneous alternation (Drew et al., 1973; Kirkby et al., 1967; Meyers and Domino, 1964; Roberts et al., 1962). Although a number of these authors interpret impaired sequential behavior as being reflective of short-term memory disruption, an inhibition notion is probably a more parsimonious alternative if other data are considered.

C. Memory

Although treatment with anticholinergics and cannabinoids as well as hippocampectomy has considerable influence on memory formation, it is still debatable as to the manner in which memory is affected. The primary deficit following hippocampectomy is an inability to consolidate new information, or an impairment in long-term memory (DeJong, 1973; Drachman and Arbit, 1966; Kesner, 1973). Whether hippocampal damage affects short-term memory per se has been a polemic question with little resolution (see Section III). However, recent evidence indicates that the hippocampus may participate in both short-term and long-term memory (Glick and Greenstein, 1973). On the other hand, marijuana has been implicated in memory loss over a few seconds or minutes as well as reducing the passage of labile information from the short-term store to long-term memory. Two studies have presented strong evidence for the latter (Abel, 1971; Darley et al., 1973). Other studies have shown that marijuana impairs short-term memory as measured by delayed matching-to-sample tasks in monkeys (Ferraro and Grilly, 1973; Zimmerberg et al., 1971) and on the Peterson-Peterson short-term recognition task in man (Dornbush et al., 1971).

There appears to be a dearth of objective experimentation pertinent to the cognitive effects of scopolamine in man. However, it seems clear that both short-term memory and consolidation are impaired by anticholinergics (Ketchum et al., 1973; Safer and Allen, 1971). On the other hand, data bearing on animal memory and cholinolytics are very broad (see Carlton, 1969). Short-term memory, as measured by delayed matching-to-sample, is impaired by anticholinergics (Glick and Jarvik, 1970; Robustelli et al., 1969). Other evidence exists which indicates that scopolamine influences the registration and storage of information (Glick and Zimmerberg, 1972).

None of the above treatments interfere with the recall of information from long-term storage in man, although there has been some suggestion that marijuana may in some cases affect retrieval processes (Klonoff et al., 1973).

D. Attention

Grastyan et al. (1959) have postulated that the hippocampus may function to prevent the diversion of attention during learning. Indeed, hippocampal lesions produce inattentiveness in animals (Altman et al., 1973) and human beings (Meissner, 1967). Both cannabis and scopolamine interfere with different aspects of attention in man. Marijuana has been shown to interfere with concentration so that verbal information is not consolidated (Abel, 1971), while both scopolamine and marijuana impair vigilance (Casswell and Marks, 1973; Safer and Allen, 1971). All three treatments nullify latent learning which is thought to be a measure of the ability of an organism to attend to relevant environmental stimuli (Kimble and Greene, 1968; Miller and Drew, 1973; Whitehouse, 1964).

E. Conditioned Fear

When a neutral stimulus is paired with a punishing stimulus such as shock, the neutral stimulus acquires the ability to elicit conditioned fear. This once neutral stimulus can therefore suppress some ongoing behavior independent of further pairings with shock. The behavioral suppression obtained has been termed the conditioned emotional response (CER).

Under all three conditions, the acquisition and/or retention of the CER is impaired. Lesions specific to the ventral hippocampus (McGowan, 1972) impair the acquisition of the CER as does post-trial stimulation of the hippocampus (Shinkman and Kaufman, 1972). Reduced emotionality and impaired memory appear to be responsible for deficits in CER acquisition. On the other hand, impaired CER performance under anticholinergics has been attributed to a lack of inhibitory control or to drug state change effects (Carlton, 1969; Carlton and Markiewicz, 1971). It has been suggested that lack of suppression under cannabinoids may be related to their ability to reduce fear or anxiety rather than to an interference with consolidation (Abel, 1969; Gonzalez, et al., 1972). However, cannabinoids probably do not reduce fear or alleviate anxiety since some experiments suggest that emotionality is increased under this class of drugs (Jaffe and Baum, 1971; Potvin and Fried, 1972).

F. Avoidance Learning and Performance

Even though impaired shuttle box acquisition has been reported following treatment with THC (Henriksson and Jarbe, 1971), most reports indicate that chronic treatment with different cannabinoids facilitates acquisition in both the shuttle box and operant chamber (Barry and Kubena, 1971; Goldberg et al., 1973; Walters and Abel, 1970). Divergent results may be attributable to the finding that animals displaying poor acquisition or low baseline levels of responding improve under THC and marijuana, while the opposite is found for animals showing superior acquisition or high levels of baseline avoidance (Park and Tilton, 1970; Pirch et al., 1972a). Contrary to the acquisition findings, cannabinoids consistently depress a highly trained avoidance response (Barry and Kubena, 1970; Grunfeld and Edery, 1969; Newman et al., 1972; Orsingher and Fulginiti, 1970; Webster et al., 1971).

The facilitation of avoidance by cannabinoids may be due to a reduction in behavioral freezing (Barry and Kubena, 1971). A similar argument has been made for the facilitation seen with scopolamine. However, anticholinergics may disrupt a highly trained avoidance response through the introduction of competing behaviors previously eliminated during training (Carlton and Markiewicz, 1971). Scopolamine, like cannabinoids, has also been found to reduce the avoidance responding of good performers in the shuttle box and to increase the number of avoidance responses given by poor performers (Rech, 1968).

Two-way active avoidance responding in the shuttle box is facilitated following hippocampal lesions (Liss, 1968; Olton and Isaacson, 1968), but one-way avoidance acquisition is depressed (Isaacson et al., 1961). Scopolamine produces corresponding effects (Suits and Isaacson, 1968). A comparison of one-way and two-way avoidance learning following treatment with cannabinoids has not been made.

G. Resistance to Extinction

Increased resistance to extinction has been reported under all three conditions, but this finding appears to be task related. Hippocampectomy and scopolamine produce increased resistance to extinction on appetitive tasks (Hearst, 1959; Jarrard and Isaacson, 1965; McCoy, 1972; Niki, 1962). However, rats display decreased resistance to extinction on a maze habit under cannabis extract (Gonzalez and Carlini, 1971). Decreased resistance to extinction may be due to an alteration of appetitive motivation especially with higher doses of THC (Elsmore and Fletcher, 1972).

Both lesions of the hippocampus (Isaacson et al., 1961) and treatment with hashish resin (Jaffe and Baum, 1971) increase resistance to extinction of an avoidance response.

H. State Dependence

State-dependent learning or dissociation refers to the finding that better retention is found if an organism is trained and tested in the same drug state than if trained in one state and tested in another (Overton, 1968). Cannabinoids produce dissociation in both active (Barry and Kubena, 1971; Goldberg et al., 1973; Henriksson and Jarbe, 1971) and passive avoidance situations (Glick and Milloy, 1972). Scopolamine produces similar actions for passive avoidance learning (Meyers, 1965), conditioned suppression (Berger and Stein, 1969), and in numerous appetitively motivated tasks (Overton, 1968). It has been shown that dissociation may be more pronounced in the asymmetrical (D-ND) than symmetrical (ND-D) direction for both scopolamine and THC (Berger and Stein, 1969; Goldberg et al., 1973). Dissociation on verbal and visual memory tasks in man has also been reported (Hill et al., 1973; Overton, 1968; Rickles et al., 1973).

Both cannabinoids and anticholinergics have been employed as discriminative stimuli for various learned responses (Henriksson and Jarbe, 1972; Kubena and Barry, 1972; Overton, 1968). That is, different drug states can control separate sets of responses.

I. drl Schedules

The most reliable comparison that can be made among the three treatments is the effect each has on a differential reinforcement of low rate (drl) schedule. On this schedule, an organism must space its responses for some period of time in order to receive a reinforcement. Treatment with cannabinoids and anticholinergics or hippocampal lesions results in an increase in response rate and reduction in the number of reinforcements (Carlton, 1961; Clark and Isaacson, 1965; Ellen and Powell, 1962; Ferraro et al., 1971, 1972; Jarrard, 1965; Pradhan et al., 1972; Pradhan and Roth, 1968). Though somewhat questionable, the drl schedule has typically been considered a measure of an organism's ability to efficiently time its responding. A recent study by Cappell et al. (1972) with human subjects has shown that marijuana produces a dose-related disruption of drl performance. Alcohol did not disrupt timing behavior. Both hippocampectomy (Meissner, 1968) and treatment with marijuana (Melges et al., 1970, 1971) have been associated with a disruption of time sense in man. Under both conditions, time is thought to pass more slowly. Therefore, subjects tend to overestimate the passage of time.

J. Passive Avoidance

Both the acquisition and retention of passive avoidance have been found to be affected by hippocampectomy and anticholinergics (Blanchard and Fial, 1968; Calhoun and Smith, 1968; Kimble et al., 1966; McCleary, 1961; Meyers, 1965). Cannabinoids apparently have little effect on passive avoidance (Goldberg et al., 1973; Miller et al., 1973b; Padina and Musty, 1973). One exception is a study by Glick and Milloy (1972) which indicated that THC could disrupt retention of passive avoidance through a process of dissociation.

K. Habituation

Habituation most simply defined is a decrease in responsivity to a stimulus which has been repeatedly presented. Dishabituation refers to an increase in responsivity to the originally presented stimulus on presentation of some novel stimulus. Hippocampectomy, cannabinoids, and anticholinergics have been reported to retard habituation of the exploration of some novel environment (Brown, 1971; Carlton, 1966; Leaton, 1965, 1968). Tetrahydrocannabinol increases the spontaneous wheel activity of rats previously habituated to the wheels (Drew and Miller, 1973). Other investigators have alluded to the possible attenuating actions of cannabis on habituation (Masur et al., 1971; Miller and Drew, 1973).

VII. EVIDENCE THAT CANNABINOIDS EXERT ACTIONS WITHIN THE LIMBIC SYSTEM

A number of polygraph studies indicate that marijuana and THC alter electrographic activity within certain limbic system structures. Like anticholinergics, Δ^8- and Δ^9-THC attenuate and/or abolish theta activity recorded from the hippocampus while greatly reducing cortical electrogenesis (Lipparini et al., 1969). Spindling and high-voltage slow activity have been observed in recordings of activity in the hippocampus, ventromedial hypothalamus, and amygdala of the chronically implanted cat by Hockman et al. (1971) and in our laboratory (unpublished observations). During exposure to marijuana smoke, Heath (1973) found that marijuana induced changes in monkey limbic areas which were similar to those produced in a human subject (Heath, 1972). In monkeys, septal activity was slowed with some sharp waves occurring around a 20–30 second period. The recorded activity of the septum in the human subject was similar to that previously obtained in pleasureful and euphoric states (Heath, 1964; Heath et al., 1968). Additional information recorded from the intoxicated monkeys indicated that spindling activity was also present in the septum, cerebellar nuclei, and the hippocampus as well as from the temporal and occipital neocortices (Heath, 1973). Martinez et al. (1972), in a study on the effects of intravenously infused THC in the awake rhesus monkey, reported similar findings. All recording sites including the dorsal hippocampus evidenced "epileptiform activity" across a 1.6 to 12.8 mg/kg dose range.

A number of reports indicate that cannabinoids possess antiepileptic activity. Dimethylheptylpyran has antiepileptic activity in rats (Loewe and Goodman, 1947) and epileptic children (Davis and Ramsey, 1949) while Δ^9-THC also blocks seizure activity following electroconvulsive shock (Sofia et al., 1971) and following more discrete stimulation of subcortical structures (Wada et al., 1973). That these antiepileptic effects might reflect an action on the hippocampus seems supported by the observations that THC had no effect on the hippocampal after discharge produced by reticular formation stimulation in the rabbit (Lipparini et al., 1969). Moreover, Izquierdo et al. (1973) have recently reported that cannabidiol, cannabinol, and the two THCs decreased rat dorsal hippocampal seizure discharges induced by electrical stimulation. These workers found that cannabidiol effectively blocked K^+ efflux from afferently stimulated hippocampus, suggesting that an interference with hippocampal K^+ release may reflect one mechanism of action of the cannabinoids.

Izquierdo and Nasello (1973) found that cannabidiol depressed the hippocampal facilitation of evoked responses in the rat as well as their post-tetanic potentiation. In comparison with diphenylhydantoin (80 mg/kg i.p.), cannabidiol (3.5 mg/kg) blocked the normal increase in hippocampal RNA levels pursuant to afferent stimulation. The same dose level of cannabidiol given as a pretrial injection significantly reduced the number of conditioned avoidance responses in a shuttle box avoidance task, but did not affect (post-trial) retention. Izquierdo and Nasello (1973) related these findings to the cannabidiol-induced impairment of K^+ efflux from the hippocampus.

McIsaac et al. (1971) studied the distribution of labeled Δ^9-THC within the squirrel monkey brain. Though labeled THC was observed in all brain sites, these investigators called attention to the high concentration that appeared within the amygdala and hippocampus. It was suggested that an interaction between the frontal cortex and hippocampus could underlie the temporal dysfunction in the sequential storage of memories.

Recently, Drew and Slagel (1973) have shown that Δ^9-THC can block the uptake of labeled corticosterone in the hippocampus and septum of adrenalectomized rats. This blockade was selective in regard to a variety of other central structures. In view of the findings of other investigators that the hippocampus is a major central target tissue for corticosterone uptake (McEwen et al., 1972; Stevens et al., 1971; Gerlach and McEwen, 1972), these results demonstrate conclusively that cannabinoids exert actions within the hippocampus. The implications of these findings will be discussed in a later section of this chapter.

The data presented above offer support for the hypothesis that cannabinoids produce marked effects within the limbic system. Although cannabinoids may affect many limbic structures, the data support the hypothesis that one prime target site for cannabinoid action is the hippocampus.

VIII. EVIDENCE THAT CANNABINOIDS EXERT ACTIONS ON CHOLINERGIC MECHANISMS

A number of reports indicate that cannabinoids affect cholinergic mechanisms. At first glance it might be concluded that THC produces classic anticholinergic-like effects at muscarinic receptors since both THC and scopolamine produce "dry mouth" (Johnson and Domino, 1971) and attenuate the bradycardia induced by vagal stimulation in anesthetized dogs (Cavero et al., 1972; Gill et al., 1970; Kubena et al., 1971a). However, it is doubtful that THC exerts major actions on muscarinic receptors in view of other findings. Cavero et al. (1972) have shown that even though THC greatly reduces salivation produced by electrical stimulation of the chorda tympani, this effect apparently is not the result of an action on the receptor element since muscarine still induces marked sialorrhea. Stellate ganglion transmission also is not blocked by THC. Hence, Cavero et al. concluded that THC may affect the release of acetylcholine (ACh). This hypothesis is supported by the work of Gascon and Pérès (1973) who reported that Δ^8- or Δ^9-THC do not possess ACh agonistic activity in the guinea pig vas deferens, rat phrenic nerve-diaphragm preparation, or in the isolated guinea pig ileum. In fact, Δ^8-THC was found to interfere with the release of ACh in the guinea pig gut. These data strongly suggest that THC *does* interfere with *in vitro* ACh release in peripheral tissue preparations. However, the data available on central cholinergic effects of cannabinoids presents a somewhat different picture.

Tetrahydrocannabinol produces a dose-dependent increase in measurable brain levels of ACh in mice (Domino, 1971). Scopolamine, likewise, increases the neocortical release of ACh in the rat (Bartolini and Pepeu, 1967). Since anticholinergics increase measurable ACh levels by either increasing ACh release or by blocking cholinergic receptors (Abood, 1968), it is not clear which mechanism is operating for THC. Though this similarity suggests a scopolamine-like mechanism of action for THC, such a conclusion might not be warranted in view of the findings that other drugs (e.g., *d*-amphetamine) without scopolamine-like effects also induce neocortical ACh release (see Nistri et al., 1972). Both Δ^9-THC and intraventricularly applied hemicholinium (HC-3) will induce ACh release from the young rat brain (Domino, 1971). Yet when administered together, THC at larger dose levels (i.e., 10 and 32 mg/kg) blocked the HC-3-induced release of ACh. This latter finding may parallel to some extent the capacity of THC to inhibit angiotensin-induced ACh release from the guinea pig gut (Gascon and Pérès, 1973), but whether similar mechanisms are at play remains unknown.

In considering the effects of THC on the metabolism of ACh, an equally disparate set of results presents itself. The centrally active anticholinesterase, physostigmine, will shorten barbiturate sleeping time (White, 1966), but cannabinoids potentiate this effect (Dagirmanjian and Boyd, 1962; Garriott et al., 1967; Kubena and Barry, 1970) as will atropine and scopolamine (Giarman and Pepeu, 1962; White et al., 1961). In addition, there are several reports which indicate that cannabinoids may potentiate the overt behavioral hyperactivity induced by amphetamines (Dagirmanjian and Boyd, 1962; Garriott et al., 1967). It is well known that anticholinergics will produce the same effect (Carlton and Didamo, 1961; White, 1963). These similarities regarding pharmacological interactions make it difficult to conceptualize THC as having anticholinesterase-like actions. In fact, these effects are more like those of an anticholinergic. However, the simultaneous administration of physostigmine and THC, both at dose levels far below their respective, LD_{50}'s, results in very high mortality owing possibly to an extreme cholinergic crisis (Rosenblatt et al., 1972). The implication of these results is that THC acts synergistically with physostigmine. Contrary to this view, Gascon and Pérès (1973) found no anticholinesterase activity of THC in the rat phrenic nerve-diaphragm preparation. However, THC did modify the effects of physostigmine in this preparation, and the suggestion was advanced that THC may facilitate physostigmine-induced ACh release.

Based on the foregoing it is a gross understatement to say that the actions of cannabinoids on cholinergic mechanisms are complex and not fully understood. Although no study has reported a direct action on cholinergic mechanisms within the hippocampus or septum, the likelihood that the cholinergic systems within these structures would be spared seems very remote. Indeed, some evidence rather strongly suggests that THC may act on cholinergic drinking centers within the hypothalamus. Kilbey et al. (1973) found in rats that parenterally administered THC in conjunction with carbachol injections to the anterior hypothalamus blocked the increase in water consumption normally produced by carbachol. In a second experiment, THC and atropine were administered to the lateral hypothalamus. Both drugs blocked deprivation-induced drinking. These results appear at first glance to suggest an atropine-like effect of THC. It should be noted however, that carbachol (carbamylcholine) is an unusual, long-acting cholinergic agonist. Its peculiarity derives from the fact that it will elicit emotional behavior if applied to the hypothalamus (Baxter, 1967) and that this effect of carbachol cannot be mimicked with ACh or a combination of ACh and physostigmine (Baxter, 1967, 1969). Thus, carbachol would also appear to have properties other than those normally associated with cholinergic receptor occupation and as such cautions against drawing too hastily the conclusion that THC is like scopolamine.

While little direct information exists regarding THC-induced impairment of ACh uptake mechanisms, there are a number of studies available which suggest a rather speculative, but intriguing, possibility. Domino *et al.* (1968) have reported that HC-3 administered to dogs via the intraventricular route produced marked electrographic changes within the limbic system. At 40 minutes postinjection, marked spiking was observed in a variety of limbic structures, but especially in certain amygdalar nuclei. Though cortical desynchrony was evident, hippocampal theta activity was abolished. This pattern changed over time such that by 4 hours postinjection both the neocortex and limbic system evidenced a rather diffuse synchrony with spiking. It is interesting that THC produces in rabbits a strikingly similar electrographic profile. Lipparini *et al.* (1969) reported that within 30 minutes of the intravenous administration of 2 mg/kg THC, the rabbit cortex exhibited desynchronized activity concomitant with the absence of hippocampal theta rhythm. Spike and wave patterns were also much in evidence at this time. At 5 to 6 hours postinjection however the cortex exhibited marked synchrony. In view of other reports of spiking within the basolateral amygdala mentioned above, it would appear that some overlap exists between the pharmacological profiles offered the THC and HC-3. Thus, as witnessed by certain electrographic indices, THC and HC-3 produce somewhat similar effects at the cortical and limbic levels, suggesting the speculative possibility that "THC may be exerting an HC-3-like action on the uptake of ACh" (Drew and Miller, 1974). Indeed, Gascon and Pérès (1973) have presented data strongly suggestive of the possibility that not only may THC inhibit or interfere with ACh release but that it may also affect ACh uptake mechanisms as well.

IX. DATA INCONSISTENT WITH THE CHOLINERGIC HYPOTHESIS

From the above there appears to be a large number of instances in which the behavioral and pharmacological changes induced by cannabinoids are strikingly similar to those produced by anticholinergics and following hippocampal lesions. Cannabinoid-induced changes in behavior seem, for the present, to be explainable by assuming that cannabinoids affect internal inhibition mechanisms currently thought to be dependent on hippocampal integrity and especially on the cholinergic systems therein. However, this hypothesis, while accounting for a number of behavioral effects of cannabinoids, must be considered tentative at this point. Certain dissimilarities in the behavioral and pharmacological effects of cannabinoids, anticholinergics, and the hippocampectomized state exist which are difficult to explain by the anticholinergic hypothesis.

One rather obvious difference which exists between the three outlined treatment states is the effect of each on passive avoidance learning. Passive avoidance situations are greatly affected by hippocampal damage and by treatment with the belladonna alkaloids, but apparently are not influenced to any great extent by cannabinoids (e.g., THC) except through a process of dissociation (Glick and Milloy, 1972). This may be attributable to the fact that both hippocampectomy and anticholinergics produce a more highly aroused, active organism while cannabinoids predominantly induce motor inactivity. Since poor performance in passive avoidance situations is strongly correlated with high activity levels under anticholinergics (Calhoun and Smith, 1968), it may be understandable, in view of the biphasic locomotor actions of cannabinoids, why no detrimental effects of THC can be demonstrated. In other words, this represents a situation in which the locomotor depressant actions of cannabinoids favor superior performance. However, on most other types of tasks, poor performance is generally attributable to the locomotor depressant actions of cannabinoids. For example, cannabinoids produce decreases in responding on a variety of schedules of reinforcement. An obvious exception is that of drl responding where increased responding is observed, albeit less efficient.

On the pharmacological level, one of the more consistently noted effects of cannabinoid administration is hypothermia. While this is discussed fully later in this chapter, it is mentioned here since there is no counterpart response observable after administration of the belladonna alkaloids; in fact, just the opposite occurs (Goodman and Gilman, 1965). Hippocampectomized laboratory animals show little change in body temperature.

Another difficulty with the anticholinergic hypothesis is that euphoria and other cognitivelike states are not observed after treatment with anticholinergics unless toxic levels are administered, but there the disturbed state of mind might more aptly be termed delusional. While there may be a tendency toward euphoria in hippocampectomized subjects, this trend is at best only mild.

These findings, as are certain others, are inconsistent with the anticholinergic hypothesis of cannabinoid action. Some of the inconsistencies may be accounted for within another hypothetical framework—the neuroendocrine system.

X. EFFECTS OF THC ON NEUROENDOCRINE SYSTEMS

Since the hippocampus had been shown to be a primary CNS target organ for the uptake of corticosterone (McEwen et al., 1969), Drew and Slagel (1973) examined the uptake of corticosterone in the presence of THC. The presence of THC exerted a marked influence on the selective uptake of the labeled corticosterone by the rat hippocampus and septum compared with cortical uptakes. At 3 mg/kg, THC produced a slight but nonsignificant increase in hormone uptake, while at 9 mg/kg, hormone uptake was significantly antagonized.

This finding is important for a variety of reasons. The hippocampus and septum have been thought to exert a feedback regulation on the hypothalamo–pituitary–adrenal axis (Knigge and Hays, 1963; Mangili et al., 1966; Dallman and Yates, 1967). Accordingly, the finding that Δ^9-THC impairs the uptake of corticosterone by the hippocampus is in line with the findings of Kubena et al. (1971b) who showed that Δ^9-THC activates the pituitary–adrenal axis in the rat. Their suggestion that a central stimulation probably accounts for increased corticosterone secretion seen following Δ^9-THC is supported by the results of Ling et al. (1973) who found no effect of Δ^9-THC on the *in vitro* corticosteroid output from the rat adrenal gland either in the presence or absence of ACTH. Accordingly then, THC treatment may result in a dysfunctioning within inhibitory feedback loops which, according to Yates et al. (1971), may be rate sensitive or level sensitive. As a result, the lack of inhibitory feedback in the presence of THC may increase the release of ACTH by the pituitary and thereby increase the production of corticosteroids. As a consequence, some of the actions of THC might then be explainable on the basis of secondary effects which could be dependent on the increased release of ACTH.

In postulating that THC exerts part of its actions via the feedback-inhibition release of ACTH, it is necessary that ACTH be capable of inducing a variety of extraadrenal actions. Such extraadrenal actions of ACTH are well known and these effects and their similarity to those induced by THC represent the final section of this chapter.

XI. COMPARISON OF THC, THE EXTRAADRENAL ACTIONS OF ACTH, AND HIPPOCAMPECTOMY

A. Behavioral

ACTH and related peptides exert certain behavioral effects which are very similar to those seen with Δ^9-THC. ACTH and other peptides (e.g., α-MSH) (Sandman et al., 1973) inhibit the extinction of avoidance responding in rats (Murphy and Miller, 1955; Miller and Ogawa, 1962; De Wied, 1966). Moreover, these peptides will likewise inhibit the extinction of appetitively motivated behaviors (Gray, 1971). These effects apparently occur as extraadrenal actions of ACTH since De Wied (1969) has determined their independence from any action on the adrenal cortex. As mentioned earlier, both hippocampally lesioned rats (Isaacson et al., 1961) and hashish resin treated rats (Jaffe and Baum, 1971) exhibit an increased resistance to extinction of avoidance responses. Since drugs which block extinction also will produce dishabituation (see Carlton, 1969; Thompson and Spencer, 1966) it is relevant to indicate that our laboratory has recently demonstrated that low doses of Δ^9-THC will induce dishabituated responding in rats who were at the time of testing habituated to running wheels (Drew and Miller, 1973).

Fear-motivated behaviors are markedly affected by ACTH and ACTH-like peptide hormones (De Wied, 1969). Similarly, there are indications that behavioral changes seen with Δ^9-THC and other cannabinoids may be the result of enhanced fear. A number of investigators report marked increases in squealing in rats treated with THC (Drew et al., 1972b; Ling et al., 1973). Behavioral freezing is also noted (Drew et al., 1972b).

Not only will circulating ACTH produce extraadrenal actions, but, obviously, "adrenal" effects as well. Both the adrenal and extraadrenal actions of ACTH influence avoidance learning, and by understanding these influences certain avoidance learning problems may be resolved. Corticosterone, whose production is dependent on ACTH, is the predominant cortical hormone in the rat. Its actions on avoidance learning have been extensively investigated and a rather interesting pattern of results has emerged. As summarized by Endröczi (1972), "an excess increase of tonic internal inhibition as the result of corticosteroid treatment may lead to suppression of learning in active avoidance situations" . . . [but would have] . . . "just the opposite effect . . . in passive avoidance conditions." In other words, corticosterone enhances learning of passive avoidance responses. In fact, Dupont et al. (1970) have shown a positive correlation between elavated plasma corticosterone levels and passive avoidance learning while showing a negative or inverse correlation between corticosterone levels and active avoidance learning. Δ^9-THC does not appear to impair passive avoidance in the rat (Miller et al., 1973b) or in the mouse (Goldberg et al., 1973). Hippocampectomy however does disrupt passive avoidance, and as Antelman and Brown (1972) have suggested, this may be related to chronically elevated ACTH levels. Hippocampectomy results in chronically elevated ACTH levels in rats (Fendler et al., 1961). However, as Endröczi (1972) has pointed out it is not always possible to compare the actions of corticosteroids with those of ACTH in behavioral situations since the actions of ACTH are more "species-dependent" than are those of the corticosteroids and are often opposite in magnitude. This may unfortunately hinder a more specific or definitive evaluation of the actions of THC on avoidance learning behaviors in experimental situations based on the neuroendocrine hypothesis of THC action.

As reviewed by De Wied (1969, 1971), ACTH will facilitate the acquisition of avoidance tasks. Δ^9-THC can likewise facilitate the acquisition of avoidance tasks especially following repeated high dose level administrations in rats (Barry and Kubena, 1971). However, lower doses given acutely or chronically do not seem to depress acquisition (Henriksson and Jarbe, 1971). This issue obviously needs further resolution.

It is interesting to note some additional extraadrenal actions of ACTH as they compare to the actions of THC on other behaviors. For example, ACTH 1–10 markedly impairs latent learning in the rat (Dupont et al., 1970). We have shown that Δ^9-THC abolishes latent learning in rats at a time when interference with appetitive motivation is highly unlikely (Miller and Drew, 1973). In another vein, cannabinoids, inclusive of THC, typically induce marked euphoric states in man. Both ACTH 1–24 and ACTH 1–10 produce a long-lasting "euphoria" in man (Endröczi, 1972). Moreover, restlessness is also induced.

B. Pharmacological

A variety of neuropharmacological observations support the possibility that cannabinoids and especially Δ^9-THC exert actions which may be related to or dependent on the release of ACTH. Lipparini et al. (1969), as discussed earlier, found that Δ^9-THC reduced EEG amplitude and abolished hippocampal theta waves. Later in the intoxication, spike and wave complexes appeared and with higher doses became relatively continuous. Similar effects have been reported by other laboratories (Masur and Khazan, 1970; Pirch et al., 1972b) for the rat. The electrographic effects of ACTH are similar to the effects of THC. Kawakami et al. (1967) reported changes in hippocampal activity following 0.5 unit of ACTH. ACTH reduced both the amplitude and frequency of the theta waves. ACTH also reportedly generates sporadic spindlelike bursts in the amygdala.

The well-known hypothermic effects of cannabinoids, while being difficult to account for solely by assuming responsibility by an anticholinergic mechanism, might be explained by the action of THC on the release of ACTH. Douglas and Paton (1952) found ACTH to reduce body temperature in the rabbit following intravenous injection. The temperature drop was in excess of $1°C$ within an hour of injection and remained depressed for another hour. In all, the effect persisted for about 3 hours. In addition, pyrogen-induced fever was found to be blocked by ACTH. These effects are thought to reflect the actions of corticosteroids (Atkins et al., 1955; Petersdorf et al., 1957; Chowers et al., 1968). Hypothermia is observed in a variety of laboratory animals following the administration of a number of cannabis preparations: for example, marijuana extract (Miras, 1965; Garattini, 1965; Gill et al., 1970), Δ^9-THC (Holtzman et al., 1969; Lomax, 1971; Kaymakcalan and Deneau, 1972; Haavik and Hardman, 1973), and DMHP (Hardman et al., 1971). The hypothermic actions of cannabinoids in man are less clear. Hypothermia has been observed in man following DMHP (Sim and Tucker, 1963). However Δ^9-THC may not reduce body temperature in man (Hollister and Richards, 1968; Hosko et al., 1973). In animals at least, and perhaps also in man, the hypothermia observed is partially dependent on the ambient temperature (Hardman et al., 1971; Gill et al., 1970; Lomax, 1971; Haavik and Hardman, 1973).

Paton et al. (1972) have recently reported that both cannabis extract and Δ^9-THC can abolish the pyrogenic response to International standard pyrogen in rabbits. Since ACTH, probably via an action on the adrenal cortex, can reduce body temperature and counteract pyrogen-induced fever in rabbits, it is suggested that the hypothermic actions of cannabinoids may be due to their secondary effects on the pituitary–adrenal axis.

As mentioned earlier, cannabinoids possess antiepileptic activity. Very recently, Izquierdo et al. (1973) have demonstrated that "cannabidiol, cannabinol, Δ^9- and Δ^8-tetrahydrocannabinol, in that order or potency, decreased the susceptibility of rat dorsal hippocampus to seizure discharges caused by afferent stimulation." Izquierdo et al. found that cannabidiol blocked K^+ efflux from the rat hippocampus and suggested that this mechanism accounted for the antiepileptic activity. It is tempting to suggest that cannabinoids exert such actions because of their secondary actions on the pituitary–adrenal axis. ACTH and the adrenal cortical hormones exert marked influences on brain tissue excitability (Woodbury, 1954; Woodbury et al., 1957; Valkana et al., 1967; Valkana and Timiras, 1968). This regulatory influence on CNS excitability becomes "operative only when changes in excitability occur; the adrenocortical hormones then act to restore normal brain excitability, regardless of the direction in which the deviation tends" (Woodbury et al., 1957). In fact this system may account not only for the antiepileptic activity of the cannabinoids but may underlie the reported biphasic locomotor and cognitive actions of the cannabinoids. It is feasible that the initial locomotor-stimulating actions of THC may reflect increased CNS excitability effected by ACTH since ACTH seems to increase brain excitability (Pincus et al., 1951; Woodbury and Vernadakis, 1967). The later appearance of locomotor depression may reflect the actions of a number of cortical hormones. For example, deoxycorticosterone and progesterone exhibit anestheticlike effects in animals (Selye, 1941) while progesterone has been known for some time to possess soporific activity (Merryman et al., 1954). On the other hand, the utility of ACTH and adrenal hormones have clinical efficacy only in certain seizure disorders (see Schmidt and Wilder, 1968, for review).

Thus, as postulated by Drew and Slagel (1973) the possibility exists that many of the behavioral, electrographic, and pharmacological actions of THC may be secondary effects which could be dependent on the increased release of ACTH.

XII. SUMMARY

We have attempted to show the feasibility of the hypothesis that cannabinoids exert a number of actions on the limbic system and especially within the hippocampus. The many behavioral similarities between anticholinergics, cannabinoids, and hippocampectomized animals make it difficult to discount the hypothesis that cannabinoids affect hippocampal neural functioning. It is suggested than many of the cognitive and behavioral alterations produced by cannabinoids may be attributable to disturbances with those mechanisms responsible for the phenomenon of internal inhibition. Specifically, cannabinoids seem to affect cholinergic mechanisms through some interference with the release of ACh and secondarily may influence behavior through their complex actions on limbic–neuroendocrine feedback loops which regulate the hypothalamo-pituitary–adrenal axis.

REFERENCES

Abel, E. L. (1969). *Psychon. Sci.* 16, 44.
Abel, E. L. (1971). *Science* 173, 1038–1040.
Abood, L. G. (1968). *U.S., Pub. Health Serv., Publ.* 1836, 683–692.
Adams, H. E., Hoblit, P. R., and Sutker, P. B. (1969). *Physiol. & Behav.* 4, 113–116.
Adams, R. D. (1969). In "The Pathology of Memory" (G. A. Talland and N. C. Waugh, eds.), pp. 91–106. Academic Press, New York.
Altman, J., Brunner, R. C., and Bayer, S. A. (1973). *Behav. Biol.* 8, 557–596.
Ames, F. (1958). *J. Ment. Sci.* 104, 972–999.
Antelman, S. M., and Brown, T. S. (1972). *Physiol & Behav.* 9, 15–20.
Atkins, E., Allison, F., Smith, M. R., and Wood, W. B. (1955). *J. Exp. Med.* 101, 353–366.
Baddeley, A. D., and Warrington, E. K. (1970). *J. Verb. Learn. Verb. Behav.* 9, 176–189.
Barbizet, J. (1963). [N.S.] 26, 127–155.
Barry, H., III, and Kubena, R. K. (1970). *Proc. 78th Annu. Conv. Amer. Psychol. Ass.* 5, 805–806.
Barry, H., III, and Kubena, R. K. (1971). *Proc. 79th Annu. Conv. Amer. Psychol. Ass.* 6, 747–748.
Bartolini, A., and Pepeu, G. (1967). *Brit. J. Pharmacol. Chemother.* 31, 66–73.
Baxter, B. L. (1967). *Exp. Neurol.* 19, 412–432.
Baxter, B. L. (1969). *Exp. Neurol.* 23, 220–229.
Berger, B. D., and Stein, L. (1969). *Psychopharmacologia* 14, 351–358.
Bernard, P. (1951). *La Raison* 2, 93–101.
Blanchard, R. J., and Fial, R. A. (1968). *J. Comp. Physiol. Psychol.* 66, 606–612.
Brion, S. (1969). In "The Pathology of Memory" (G. A. Talland and N. C. Waugh, eds.), pp. 29–39. Academic Press, New York.
Bromberg, W. (1934). *Amer. J. Psychiat.* 91, 303–330.
Brown, H. (1971). *Psychopharmacologia* 21, 294–301.
Calhoun, W. H., and Smith, A. A. (1968). *Psychopharmacologia* 13, 201–209.
Cappell, H., Webster, C. D., Herring, B. S., and Ginsberg, R. (1972). *J. Pharmacol. Exp. Ther.* 182, 195–203.
Carlini, E. A., and Kramer, C. (1965). *Psychopharmacologia* 7, 175–181.
Carlini, E. A., Hamaoui, A., Bieniek, D., and Korte, F. (1970). *Pharmacology* 4, 359–368.
Carlton, P. L. (1961). *Pharmacologist* 3, 60.
Carlton, P. L. (1966). *Psychon. Sci.* 5, 347–348.
Carlton, P. L. (1969). In "Reinforcement and Behavior" (J. T. Tapp, ed.), pp. 286–327. Academic Press, New York.
Carlton, P. L., and Didamo, P. (1961). *J. Pharmacol. Exp. Ther.* 132, 91–96.
Carlton, P. L., and Markiewicz, B. (1971). In "Pharmacological and Biophysical Agents and Behavior" (E. Furchgott, ed.), pp. 345–373. Academic Press, New York.
Casswell, S., and Marks, D. (1973). *Nature (London)* 241, 60–61.

Cavero, I., Buckley, J. P., and Jandhyala, B. S. (1972). *Eur. J. Pharmacol.* **19**, 301–304.
Cermak, L. S., and Butters, N. (1972). *Neuropsychologia* **10**, 89–95.
Cermak, L. S., Butters, N., and Goodglass, H. (1971). *Neuropsychologia* **9**, 307–315.
Chowers, I., Conforti, N., and Feldman, S. (1968). *Amer. J. Physiol.* **213**, 538–542.
Clark, L. D., Hughes, R., and Nakashima, E. N. (1970). *Arch. Gen. Psychiat.* **23**, 193–198.
Clark, L. V. H., and Isaacson, R. L. (1965). *J. Comp. Physiol. Psychol.* **59**, 137–140.
Correll, R. E., and Scoville, W. B. (1970). *J. Comp. Physiol. Psychol.* **70**, 464–469.
Dagirmanjian, R., and Boyd, E. S. (1962). *J. Pharmacol. Exp. Ther.* **135**, 25–33.
Dallman, M. F., and Yates, F. E. (1967). *Proc. Roy. Soc. Med.* **60**, 904–905.
Darley, C. F., Tinklenberg, J. R., Roth, W. T., Hollister, L. E., and Atkinson, R. C. (1973). *Memory & Cognition* **1**, 196–200.
Davis, J. P., and Ramsey, H. (1949). *Fed. Proc., Fed. Amer. Soc. Exp. Biol.* **8**, 284–285.
DeJong, R. N. (1973). *J. Neurol. Sci.* **19**, 73–83.
Deutsch, J. A. (1971). *Science* **174**, 788–794.
De Wied, D. (1966). *Proc. Soc. Exp. Biol. Med.* **122**, 28–32.
De Wied, D. (1969). In "Frontiers in Neuroendocrinology" (W. F. Ganong and L. Martini, eds.), pp. 97–140. Oxford Univ. Press, London and New York.
De Wied, D. (1971). In "The Hypothalamus" (L. Martini, M. Motta, and F. Fraschini, eds.), pp. 1–8. Academic Press, New York.
Domer, F. R., and Schueler, F. W. (1960). *Arch. Int. Pharmacodyn. Ther.* **127**, 449–458.
Domino, E. F. (1971). *Ann. N.Y. Acad. Sci.* **191**, 166–191.
Domino, E. F., Yamamoto, K., and Dren, A. T. (1968). *Prog. Brain Res.* **28**, 113–133.
Dornbush, R. L., Fink, M., and Freedman, A. M. (1971). *Amer. J. Psychiat.* **128**, 194–197.
Douglas, R. J. (1967). *Psychol. Bull.* **67**, 416–442.
Douglas, W. W., and Paton, W. O. M. (1952). *Lancet* **1**, 342.
Drachman, D. A., and Arbit, J. (1966). *Arch. Neurol. (Chicago)* **15**, 52–61.
Drachman, D. A., and Ommaya, A. K. (1964). *Arch. Neurol. (Chicago)* **10**, 411–425.
Drew, W. G., and Miller, L. L. (1973). *Pharmacology* **9**, 41–51.
Drew, W. G., and Miller, L. L. (1974). *Pharmacology* **11**, 12–32.
Drew, W. G., and Slagel, D. E. (1973). *Neuropharmacology* **12**, 909–914.
Drew, W. G., Kiplinger, G. F., Miller, L. L., and Marx, M. (1972a). *Clin. Pharmacol. Ther.* **13**, 526–533.
Drew, W. G., Miller, L. L., and Wikler, A. (1972b). *Psychopharmacologia* **23**, 289–299.
Drew, W. G., Miller, L. L., and Baugh, E. L. (1973). *Psychopharmacologia* **32**, 171–182.
Dupont, A., Endröczi, E., and Fortier, C. (1970). In "The Influence of Hormones on the Central Nervous System" (D. H. Ford, ed.), pp. 451–462. Karger, Basel.
Ellen, P., and Powell, E. W. (1962). *Exp. Neurol.* **6**, 538–547.
Elsmore, T. F., and Fletcher, W. V. (1972). *Science* **175**, 911–912.
Endröczi, E. (1972). In "Hormones and Behavior" (S. Levine, ed.), pp. 173–207. Academic Press, New York.
Erickson, C. A., and Patel, J. B. (1969). *J. Comp. Physiol. Psychol.* **68**, 400–406.
Fendler, K., Karmos, G., and Telegdy, G. (1961). *Acta Physiol.* **20**, 293–297.
Ferraro, D. P., and Grilly, D. M. (1973). *Science* **179**, 490–492.

Ferraro, D. P., Grilly, D. M., and Lynch, W. C. (1971). *Psychopharmacologia* **22**, 333–351.
Ferraro, D. P., Lynch, W. C., and Grilly, D. M. (1972). *Pharmacology* **7**, 273–282.
Franchina, J. J., and Brown, T. S. (1970). *J. Comp. Physiol. Psychol.* **70**, 66–72.
Garattini, S. (1965). *Ciba Found. Study Group* **21**, 70–82.
Garriott, J. C., King, L. J., Forney, R. B., and Hughes, F. W. (1967). *Life Sci.* **6**, 2119–2128.
Gascon, A. L., and Pérès, M. T. (1973). *Can. J. Physiol. Pharmacol.* **51**, 12–21.
Gerlach, J. L., and McEwen, B. S. (1972). *Science* **175**, 1133–1136.
Giarman, H. J., and Pepeu, G. (1962). *Brit. J. Pharmacol. Chemother.* **19**, 226–234.
Gill, E. W., Paton, W. D. M., and Pertwee, R. G. (1970). *Nature (London)* **228**, 134–36.
Glick, S. D., and Greenstein, S. (1973). *J. Comp. Physiol. Psychol.* **82**, 188–194.
Glick, S. D., and Jarvik, M. E. (1970). *J. Comp. Physiol. Psychol.* **73**, 307–313.
Glick, S. D., and Milloy, S. (1972). *In* "Current Research in Marijuana" (M. F. Lewis, ed.), pp. 1–24. Academic Press, New York.
Glick, S. D., and Zimmerberg, B. (1972). *Behav. Biol.* **7**, 245–254.
Goldberg, M. E., Hefner, M. A., Robichaud, R. C., and Dubinsky, B. (1973). *Psychopharmacologia* **30**, 173–184.
Gonzalez, S. C., and Carlini, E. A. (1971). *Psychon. Sci.* **24**, 203–204.
Gonzalez, S. C., Karniol, I. G., and Carlini, E. A. (1972). *Behav. Biol.* **7**, 83–94.
Goodman, L. S., and Gilman, A., eds. (1965). "The Pharmacological Basis of Therapeutics," 3rd ed. Macmillan, New York.
Grastyan, E., Lissak, K., Madaraoz, I., and Donhoffer, H. (1959). *Electroencephalogr. Clin. Neurophysiol.* **11**, 409–430.
Gray, J. A. (1971). *Nature (London)* **229**, 52–54.
Grunfeld, Y., and Edery, H. (1969). *Psychopharmacologia* **14**, 200–210.
Haavik, C. O., and Hardman, H. F. (1973). *J. Pharmacol. Exp. Ther.* **187**, 568–574.
Hardman, H. F., Domino, E. F., and Seevers, M. H. (1971). *Pharmacol. Rev.* **23**, 295–315.
Hassler, R., and Riechert, T. (1957). *Acta Neurochir.* **5**, 330–340.
Hearst, E. (1959). *J, Pharmacol. Exp. Ther.* **126**, 349–358.
Heath, R. G. (1964). *In* "The Role of Pleasure in Behavior" (R. G. Heath, ed.), pp. 219–243. Harper (Hoeber), New York.
Heath, R. G. (1972). *Arch. Gen. Psychiat.* **26**, 577-584.
Heath, R. G. (1973). *Neuropharmacology* **12**, 1–14.
Health, R. G., John, S. B., and Fontana C. J. (1968). *In* "Computers and Electronic Devices in Psychiatry" (N. Kline and E. Laska, eds.), pp. 178–189. Grune & Stratton, New York.
Henriksson, B. G., and Jarbe, T. (1971). *Psychopharmacologia* **22**, 23–30.
Henriksson, B. G., and Jarbe, T. (1972). *Psychon. Sci.* **27**, 25–26.
Hill, S. Y., Schwin, R., Powell, B., and Goodwin, D. W. (1973). *Nature (London)* **243**, 241–242.
Hockman, C. H., Perrin, R. G., and Kalant, H. (1971). *Science* **172**, 968–970.
Hollister, L. E. (1971). *Science* **172**, 21–29.
Hollister, L. E., and Richards, R. K. (1968). *Clin. Pharmacol. Ther.* **9**, 783–791.
Holtzman, D., Lovell, R. A., Jaffe, J. H., and Freedman, D. X. (1969). *Science* **163**, 1464–1467.
Hosko, M. H., Kochar, M. S., and Wang, R. I. H. (1973). *Clin. Pharmacol. Ther.* **14**, 344–352.

Isaacson, R. L. (1972). *Neuropsychologia* 10, 47–64.
Isaacson, R. L., Douglas, R. J., and Moore, R. Y. (1961). *J. Comp. Physiol. Psychol.* 54, 625–628.
Izquierdo, I., and Nasello, A. G. (1973). *Psychopharmacologia* 31, 167–176.
Izquierdo, I., Orsingher, O. A., and Berardi, A. C. (1973). *Psychopharmacologia* 38, 95–102.
Jaffe, P. B., and Baum, M. (1971). *Psychopharmacologia* 20, 97–102.
Jarrard, L. E. (1965). *Psychon. Sci.* 2, 115–116.
Jarrard, L. E., and Isaacson, R. L. (1965). *Nature (London)* 207, 109–110.
Jarrard, L. E., and Lewis, T. C. (1967). *Amer. J. Psychol.* 80, 66–72.
Johnson, S., and Domino, E. F. (1971). *Clin. Pharmacol. Ther.* 12, 762–768.
Jones, R. T., and Stone, G. C. (1970). *Psychopharmacologia* 18, 108–117.
Kaada, B. R., Rasmussen, E. W., and Kvein, O. (1961). *Exp. Neurol.* 3, 333–335.
Kahn, E. A., and Crosby, E. C. (1972). *Neurology* 22, 117–125.
Kawakami, M., Seto, K., Terasawa, E., and Yoshida, K. (1967). *Progr. Brain Res.* 27, 69–102.
Kaymakcalan, S., and Deneau, G. A. (1972). *Acta Med. Turc., Suppl.* 1, 1–27.
Kesner, R. (1973). *Psychol. Bull.* 80, 177–203.
Ketchum, J. S., Sidell, F. R., Crowell, E. B., Aghajanian, G. K., and Hayes, A. H. (1973). *Psychopharmacologia* 28, 121–145.
Kilbey, M. M., Forbes, W. B., and Olivetti, C. C. (1973). *Behav. Biol.* 8, 679–685.
Kimble, D. P. (1963). *J. Comp. Physiol. Psychol.* 56, 273–283.
Kimble, D. P. (1968). *Psychol. Bull.* 70, 285–295.
Kimble, D. P., and Greene, E. G. (1968). *Psychon. Sci.* 11, 99–100.
Kimble, D. P., and Kimble, R. J. (1965). *J. Comp. Physiol. Psychol.* 60, 474–476.
Kimble, D. P., and Pribram, K. H. (1963). *Science* 139, 824–825.
Kimble, D. P., Kirkby, R. J., and Stein, D. G. (1966). *J. Comp. Physiol. Psychol.* 61, 141–143.
Kimura, D. (1958). *Can. J. Psychol.* 12, 213–218.
Kirkby, R. J., Stein, D. G., Kimble, R. J., and Kimble, D. P. (1967). *J. Comp. Physiol. Psychol.* 64, 342–345.
Klonoff, H. K., Low, M., and Marcus, A. (1973). *Can. Med. Ass. J.* 108, 150–156.
Klüver, H., and Bucy, P. C. (1939). *Arch. Neurol. Psychiat.* 42, 979–1000.
Knigge, K. M., and Hays, M. (1963). *Proc. Soc. Exp. Biol. Med.* 114, 67–69.
Kubena, R. K., and Barry, H., III. (1970). *J. Pharmacol. Exp. Ther.* 173, 94–100.
Kubena, R. K., and Barry, H., III. (1972). *Nature (London)* 235, 397–398.
Kubena, R. K., Cavero, I., Jandhyala, B. S., and Buckley, J. P. (1971a). *Pharmacologist* 13, 311.
Kubena R. K., Perhatch, J. L., Jr., and Barry, H., III. (1971b). *Eur. J. Pharmacol.* 14, 89–92.
Leaton, R. H. (1965). *J. Comp. Physiol. Psychol.* 59, 325–330.
Leaton, R. N. (1968). *J. Comp. Physiol. Psychol.* 66, 524–527.
Ling, G. M., Thomas, J. A., Usher, D. R., and Singhal, R. L. (1973). *Int. J. Clin. Pharmacol.* 7, 1–5.
Lipparini, F., DeCarolis, A. S., and Longo, V. G. (1969). *Physiol. & Behav.* 4, 527–532.
Liss, P. (1968). *J. Comp. Physiol. Psychol.* 66, 193–197.
Loewe, S., and Goodman, L. S. (1947). *Fed. Proc., Fed. Amer. Soc. Exp. Biol.* 6, 352.
Lomax, P. (1971). *Res. Commun. Chem. Pathol. Pharmacol.* 2, 159–167.
McCleary, R. A. (1961). *J. Comp. Physiol. Psychol.* 54, 605–613.

McCoy, D. F. (1972). *Psychol. Rep.* 30, 867–873.
McEwen, B. S., Weiss, J. M., and Schwartz, L. S. (1969). *Brain Res.* 16, 227–241.
McEwen, B. S., Magnus, C., and Wallach, G. (1972). *Endocrinology* 90, 217–226.
McGowan, B. K. (1972). *Behav. Biol.* 7, 841–852.
McIsaac, W. M., Fritchie, G. E., Indanpan-Heikkila, J. E. H., Ho, B. T., and Englert, L. E. (1971). *Nature (London)* 230, 1118–1120.
Magoun, H. W. (1963). "The Waking Brain." Thomas, Springfield, Illinois.
Mangili, G., Motta, M., and Martini, L. (1966). *In* Neuroendocrinology" (L. Martini and W. F. Ganong, eds.), Vol. 1, pp. 297–370. Academic Press, New York.
Martinez, J. L., Stadnick, S. W., and Schaeppi, U. H. (1972). *Life Sci.* 11, 643–651.
Masur, J., and Khazan, N. (1970). *Life Sci.* 9, 1275–1280.
Masur, J., Martz, R. M. W., and Carlini, E. A. (1971). *Psychopharmacologia* 19, 388–397.
Meissner, S. J. (1967). *Int. J. Neuropsychiat.* 3, 298–310.
Meissner, S. J. (1968). *J. Neuropsychiat.* 4, 6–20.
Melges, F. T., Tinklenberg, J. R., Hollister, L. E., and Gillespie, H. K. (1970). *Science* 168, 1118–1120.
Melges, F. T., Tinklenberg, J. R., Hollister, L. E., and Gillespie, H. K. (1971). *Arch. Gen. Psychiat.* 21, 564–567.
Merryman, W., Boiman, R., Barnes, L., and Rothchild, I. (1954). *J. Clin. Endocrinol. Metab.* 14, 1567–1569.
Meyers, B. (1965). *Psychopharmacologia* 8, 111–119.
Meyers, B., and Domino, E. F. (1964). *Arch. Int. Pharmacodyn. Ther.* 150, 525–529.
Miller, L. L., and Drew, W. G. (1973). *Nature (London)* 243, 473–474.
Miller, L. L., Drew, W. G., and Kiplinger, G. F. (1972). *Nature (London)* 237, 172–173.
Miller, L. L., Drew, W. G., and Wikler, A. (1973a). *Psychopharmacologia* 28, 1–11.
Miller, L. L., Drew, W. G., and Joyce, P. (1973b). *Behav. Biol.* 8, 421–426.
Miller, R. E., and Ogawa, N. (1962). *J. Comp. Physiol. Psychol.* 55, 211–213.
Milner, B. (1958). *Res. Publ., Ass. Res. Nerv. Ment. Dis.* 36, 244–257.
Miras, C. J. (1965). *Ciba Found. Study Group* 21, 37–53.
Murphy, J. V., and Miller, R. E. (1955). *J. Comp. Physiol. Psychol.* 48, 47–49.
Newman, L. M., Lutz, M. P., Gould, M. H., and Domino, E. F. (1972). *Science* 175, 1022–1023.
Niki, H. (1962). *Jap. Psychol. Res.* 4, 139–153.
Nistri, A., Bartolini, A., Deffenu, G., and Pepeu, G. (1972). *Neuropharmacology* 11, 665–674.
Nyssen, R. (1957). *Acta Neurol. Psychiat. Belg.* 57, 639–666.
Olton, D. S., and Isaacson, R. L. (1968). *Physiol. & Behav.* 3, 719–724.
Orbach, J., Milner, B., and Rasmussen, T. (1960). *Arch. Neurol. (Chicago)* 3, 230–251.
Orsingher, O. A., and Fulginiti, S. (1970). *Pharmacology* 3, 337–344.
Overton, D. A. (1968). *U.S., Pub. Health Serv., Publ.* 1836, 918–930.
Padina, R. J., and Musty, R. E. (1973). *Proc. 81st Annu. Conv. Amer. Psychol. Ass.* 8, 993–994.
Park, Y. Y., and Tilton, B. E. (1970). *Proc. West. Pharmacol. Soc.* 13, 151–155.
Paton, W. D. M., Pertwee, R. G., and Temple, D. (1972). *In* "Cannabis and its Derivatives" (W. D. M. Paton and J. Crown, eds.), pp. 50–75. Oxford Univ. Press, London and New York.
Penfield, W., and Milner, B. (1958). *Arch. Neurol. Psychiat.* 79, 475–497.

Petersdorf, R. G., Keene, W. R., and Bennett, I. L. (1957). *J. Exp. Med.* **106**, 787–809.
Pincus, J. B., Natelson, S., and Lugovoy, J. K. (1951). *Proc. Soc. Exp. Biol. Med.* **78**, 24–27.
Pirch, J. H., Osterhalm, K. C., Barratt, E. S., and Cohn, R. A. (1972a). *Proc. Soc. Exp. Biol. Med.* **141**, 590–592.
Pirch, J. H., Cohn, R. A., Barnes, P. R., and Barratt, E. S. (1972b). *Neuropharmacology* **11**, 231–240.
Potvin, R. J., and Fried, P. A. (1972). *Psychopharmacologia* **26**, 369–378.
Pradhan, S. N., and Roth, T. (1968). *Psychopharmacologia* **12**, 358–366.
Pradhan, S. N., Bailey, P. T., and Ghosh, P. (1972). *Psychon. Sci.* **27**, 179–181.
Racine, R. J., and Kimble, D. P. (1965). *Psychon. Sci.* **3**, 285–286.
Rech, R. H. (1968). *Psychopharmacologia* **12**, 371–383.
Rickles, W. H., Jr., Cohen, M. J., Whitaker, C. A., and McIntyre, K. E. (1973). *Psychopharmacologia* **30**, 349–354.
Roberts, W. W., Dember, W. N., and Brodwick, M. (1962). *J. Comp. Physiol. Psychol.* **55**, 695–700.
Robustelli, F., Glick, S. D., Goldfarb, T. L., Geller, A., and Jarvik, M. E. (1969). *Commun. Behav. Biol.* **3**, 101–109.
Rosenblatt, J. E., Janowsky, D. S., Davis, J. M., and El-Yousef, M. K. (1972). *Res. Commun. Chem. Pathol. Pharmacol.* **3**, 474–482.
Safer, D. J., and Allen, R. P. (1971). *Biol. Psychiat.* **3**, 347–355.
Sandman, C. A., Kastin, A. J., Schally, A. V., Kendall, J. W., and Miller, L. H. (1973). *J. Comp. Physiol. Psychol.* **84**, 386–390.
Schmidt, R. P., and Wilder, J. B. (1968). "Epilepsy," pp. 163–164. Davis, Philadelphia, Pennsylvania.
Scoville, W. B., and Milner, B. (1957). *J. Neurol., Neurosurg. Psychiat.* [N.S.] **20**, 11–21.
Selye, H. (1941). *J. Pharmacol. Exp. Ther.* **73**, 172–141.
Shinkman, P. G., and Kaufman, K. P. (1972). *J. Comp. Physiol. Psychol.* **80**, 283–292.
Sidman, M., Stoddard, L. T., and Mohr, J. P. (1968). *Neuropsychologia* **6**, 245–254.
Sim, V. M., and Tucker, L. M. (1963). "Summary Report on EA 1496 and EA 2233 (U)." AD342 332, pp. 1–65. Defense Documentation Center for Scientific and Technical Information, Cameron Station, Alexandria, Virginia.
Sofia, R. D., Kubena, R. K., and Barry, H. (1971). *Pharmacologist* **13**, 246.
Stein, D. G., and Kimble, D. P. (1966). *J. Comp. Physiol. Psychol.* **62**, 243–249.
Stepien, L. S., Cordau, J. P., and Rasmussen, T. (1960). *Brain* **83**, 470–489.
Stevens, W., Grosser, B. I., and Reed, D. J. (1971). *Brain Res.* **35**, 602–607.
Suits, E., and Isaacson, R. L. (1968). *Int. J. Neuropharmacol.* **7**, 441–446.
Talland, G. A. (1965). "Deranged Memory." Academic Press, New York.
Tart, C. T. (1970). *Nature (London)* **226**, 701–704.
Thompson, R. F., and Spencer, W. A. (1966). *Psychol. Rev.* **73**, 16–43.
Tinklenberg, J. R., Kopell, B. S., Melges, F. T., and Hollister, L. E. (1972). *Arch. Gen. Psychiat.* **27**, 812–815.
Truax, T., and Thompson, R. (1969). *J. Comp. Physiol. Psychol.* **67**, 228–234.
Valkana, T., and Timiras, P. S. (1968). *Fed. Proc., Fed. Amer. Soc. Exp. Biol.* **27**, 470.
Valkana, T., Vernadakis, A., and Timiras, P. S. (1967). *Neuroendocrinology* **2**, 326–329.
Van der Horst, L. (1956). *Evol. Psychiat.* **1**, 189–205.
Wada, J. A., Sato, M., and Corcoran, M. E. (1973). *Exp. Neurol.* **39**, 157–165.

Walters, G. D., and Abel, E. L. (1970). *J. Pharm. Pharmacol.* **22**, 310–312.
Warburton, D. M. (1969). *Physiol. & Behav.* **4**, 641–644.
Webster, C. D., Willinsky, M. D., Herring, B., and Walters, G. (1971). *Nature (London)* **232**, 498–501.
Weil, A. T., and Zinberg, N. E. (1969). *Nature (London)* **222**, 434–437.
Weil, A. T., Zinberg, N. E., and Nelson, J. M. (1968). *Science* **162**, 1234–1242.
White, R. P. (1963). *Arch. Int. Pharmacodyn. Ther.* **145**, 1–17.
White, R. P. (1966). *Recent Advan. Biol. Psychiat.* **8**, 127–139.
White, R. P., Nash, C. B., Westerbeke, E. J., and Possanza, G. J. (1961). *Arch. Int. Pharmacodyn. Ther.* **132**, 349–363.
Whitehouse, J. M. (1964). *J. Comp. Physiol. Psychol.* **57**, 13–15.
Whitehouse, J. M., Lloyd, A. J., and Fifer, S. A. (1964). *J. Comp. Physiol. Psychol.* **58**, 475–476.
Wickelgren, W. A. (1968). *Neuropsychologia* **6**, 235–244.
Wiener, N. I., and Messer, J. (1973). *Behav. Biol.* **9**, 227–234.
Williams, E. G., Himmelsbach, C. K., Wikler, A., Ruble, D. C., and Lloyd, B. J. (1946). *Pub. Health Rep.* **61**, 1059–1083.
Williams, M., and Zangwill, O. L. (1952). *J. Neurol., Neurosurg. Psychiat.* [N.S.] **15**, 54–58.
Woodbury, D. M. (1954). *Recent Progr. Horm. Res.* **10**, 107.
Woodbury, D. M., and Vernadakis, A. (1967). In "Neuroendocrinology" (L. Martini and W. F. Ganong, eds.), Vol. 2, pp. 335–375. Academic Press, New York.
Woodbury, D. M., Timiras, P. S., and Vernadakis, A. (1957). In "Hormones, Brain Function, and Behavior" (H. Hoagland, ed.), pp. 27–54. Academic Press, New York.
Yates, F. E., Russell, S. M., and Maran, J. W. (1971). *Annu. Rev. Physiol.* **33**, 393–444.
Zimmerberg, G., Glick, S. D., and Jarvik, M. E. (1971). *Nature (London)* **233**, 343–345.

Chapter 8

MARIJUANA AND BEHAVIOR: HUMAN AND INFRAHUMAN COMPARISONS

LOREN L. MILLER

I. Introduction	189
II. Memory and Acquisition	191
III. Timing Behavior	202
IV. State-Dependent Learning	206
V. Attention and Habituation	212
VI. Summary and Discussion	216
References	217

I. INTRODUCTION

Any attempt at an overall evaluation of the effects of a pharmacological agent on human behavior would be seriously deficient in scope if it failed to take into account findings obtained from infrahuman organisms. This is especially true of cannabinoids and other so called "drugs of abuse" since these drugs are used illegally and little quantifiable data exist concerning their effects on behavior. Unfortunately, there is a paucity of specific, comparative, behavioral pharmacological data relating to the effects of cannabinoids. However, if one were willing to admit conditionally certain classes of infrahuman data that do exist as evidence pertaining to the reported actions of cannabinoids in man, then a number of deficiencies and disparaties in the human research area could be substantially diminished.

In compiling the evidence to be presented in this chapter, it can be maintained that it is scientifically proprietous to assume that if a behavior is altered in a similar manner across species by a given agent, that agent is producing a general effect. By correlating a wide variety of behavioral similarities and dissimilarities produced by a drug or different classes of drugs, subsequent behavioral changes might be understood in terms of a single mechanism. The key to a successful science of behavioral pharmacology lies in experimentally producing similar behavior patterns not only within species but across species, so that drug effects can be legitimately evaluated.

That is not to say that such a course can be taken without reservations, for it has been argued that the generality of laws of behavior across species is limited. Ethologists hold that all learning and conditioning must be evaluated in terms of previous experience and evolutionary development. Forming generalizations about behavior across species must proceed with caution (Burghardt, 1973). Furthermore, pharmacodynamic differences exist between species so that factors such as absorbtion, metabolism, and distribution of various agents must be considered. Finally, genetic differences in reaction to drugs are found so that drug-behavior interactions can vary within strains within a species (Weiss and Laties, 1967). However, the latter authors suggest that "a continuity in biological systems does exist and transcends different species so that behavioral similarities across species are more profound than dissimilarities. Arguments which assert a sharp discontinuity between man and other living creatures in the fundamental mechanisms of behavior are asserting one of biology's least likely possibilities." Much evidence suggests that behavioral control can be exerted over man just as it can in lower organisms. For example, behavior modification techniques so popular in psychotherapy today have their basis in animal laboratory demonstrations of behavioral control.

The generality of behavioral processes and the methods used to study or influence these processes can be assessed by establishing functional relationships (Sidman, 1960). For example, a behavioral pharmacologist would attempt to determine the effects of a wide range of doses on a given behavior, or establish a functional relationship between the dosage of a drug and the class of responses it is affecting.

The generality of the observed functional relationship can be investigated by replicating the function under novel conditions and with different species. When similar functions are established for different species, a true science of comparative behavioral pharmacology must emerge.

A comparative behavioral pharmacology of cannabis as well as other drugs of abuse has proceeded in rather a diametrical fashion in comparison to other agents (i.e., medical drugs). Traditionally, drugs are screened in animals where behavioral and physiological effects are noted; the drugs are then modified so that adverse effects in man are minimal. The agents are then distributed for use. Illegal drugs such as cannabis enjoy no such luxury. Although used for centuries, the illegal status of cannabis has afforded it a rather dubious reputation so that any systematic research with humans or animals has only recently occurred. Since numerous behavioral effects in man have been noted under cannabis, investigators have tried to specify and quantify these actions in animals.

The purpose of this chapter is to compare the behavioral actions of cannabinoids in humans with those found in infrahumans, with special reference to acquisition and retention processes, timing behavior, state-dependent learning, and attention. The discovery of similarities and differences in the action of cannabinoids in humans and infrahumans has theoretical relevance for the determination of the mechanism(s) by which cannabinoids influence these behavioral processes.

II. MEMORY AND ACQUISITION

Early investigations of the acute marijuana intoxication syndrome are replete with descriptions of thought disturbance and memory loss (Bromberg, 1934; Ames, 1958). Recent work employing the smoking method or using oral forms of cannabinoids has objectively confirmed these earlier observations (Abel, 1970, 1971; Melges *et al.*, 1970; Hollister, 1971; Miller *et al.*, 1972). However, while many investigators have shown that marijuana has some gross effect on memory, many of these studies have been *demonstration* oriented rather than *hypothesis* oriented. That is, they have failed to specify what aspects of memory are particularly affected by marijuana.

For a number of years psychologists have debated the question of whether there is a single mechanism involved in memory or whether there are two mechanisms which differ in their capacity for storing information. The issue of whether a "unitary" or "dualistic" theory of memory is most appropriate has never been resolved. In the last decade, however, research of both a psychological and neurophysiological nature has supported the validity of dividing memory into short-term and long-term components (Shiffrin and Atkinson, 1969; Kesner, 1973). A model of memory similar to that proposed by Shiffrin and Atkinson is presented in Fig. 1. The model has three basic components: a sensory register, short-term memory store, and a long-term memory store. Information coming into various sensory systems is analyzed through a match–mismatch proc-

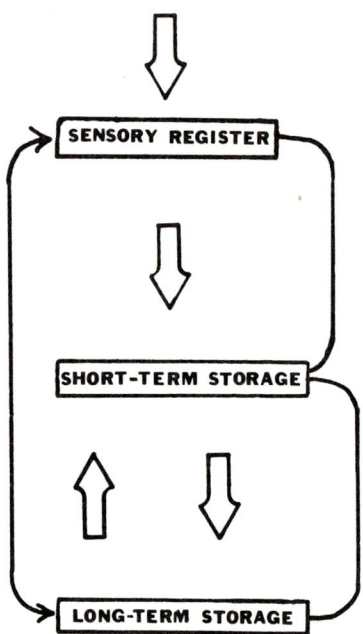

Fig. 1. Structure of the memory system.

ess between sensory input and long-term memory. This process is largely determined by past experience with the sensory information. Following analysis, *selective* information is transferred to a short-term memory store. The short-term memory store may be regarded as an individual's working memory. Information in short-term memory decays as a function of time unless rehearsal takes place. By rehearsal is meant that a subject either overtly or covertly repeats information thereby increasing its momentary strength in short-term memory or retarding its decay. Rehearsal not only maintains information in short-term memory but controls the transfer of information from short- to long-term storage. The long-term store is a permanent repository for information which is acquired through a consolidation process.

The effects of marijuana on memory have been interpreted in terms of this model (Abel, 1971; Darley *et al.*, 1973). The experimental paradigm used to test this model consists of a free recall task involving lists of words. The basic dependent variable is probability of recall as a function of position of word in the list or its "serial" position. A U-shaped function relating probability of recall to serial position of an item can be plotted.

Increased probability of recall for the initially presented words in a list is called the "primacy effect." An increase in the probability of recall for words in the last half of the list is termed the "recency effect." Research has suggested that the recall of items from the early portions of the list reflects retrieval from long-term storage while the recency effect is due to retrieval from short-term memory (Shiffrin and Atkinson, 1969).

Subjects presented with lists of words orally following treatment with marijuana show a decreased probability in recall of words from most positions in a list save the most recently presented two or three items. Abel (1971) concluded from these results that the major detrimental effect of marijuana is to retard the passage of information from short- to long-term memory. It is Abel's contention that under marijuana, subjects are less able to concentrate and hence rehearse information in short-term storage; hence, less information is consolidated. Unfortunately, no independent measure of rehearsal was taken, so it is difficult to pinpoint the exact locus of action of marijuana. Interestingly, recall is not affected if subjects acquire information *prior* to drug treatment even though recall occurs in the drug state.

It was noted that the recall of the most recent items in the list was not influenced by marijuana, suggesting that short-term memory as defined by the recency effect is not reduced (Abel, 1971; Darley *et al.*, 1973). The fact that terminal items of a list are remembered under drug and no-drug conditions suggests that marijuana does not inhibit the entry of items into short-term memory. However, on short-term memory tasks where a delay interval is interposed between presentation and recall, the decay process appears to be intensified by marijuana. For example, it has been shown that short-term retention of trigrams at different delay intervals is decreased, suggesting that the decay process is potentiated (Dornbush *et al.*, 1971; Zeidenberg *et al.*, 1973).

It is unlikely that facilitation of decay under marijuana is the only determinant of memory loss. It has been suggested that increased interference might occur under cannabis as a result of the enhanced stream of thought and imagery found during intoxication (Paton and Pertwee, 1973). Interference has been interpreted to have a postulated role in memory loss under other drugs, especially alcohol (Janes, 1970; Miller and Dolan, 1974).

A number of animal investigations have attempted to determine the action of marijuana on short-term memory. The most commonly employed method is the delayed matching to sample task. In the simplest variant of delayed matching, a subject is situated in front of three response keys. A press on the center of the three keys produces a visual stimulus (usually presented in a small window above the key). This visual stimulus disappears after a period of time and after a delay period is projected onto one of the side keys. The subject's task is to remember the sample stimulus and press the outer key which contains the same stimulus as the center key. The delay between stimulus sample offset and presentation of the comparison stimuli defines the length of short-term memory. The effect of cannabis on this task employing chimpanzees and monkeys has been evaluated by several experimenters (Scheckel et al., 1968; Zimmerberg et al., 1971; Ferraro and Grilly, 1973).

The first study on delayed matching in primates was performed by Scheckel et al. (1968) using THC. Rhesus monkeys were given extensive training on a delayed matching task and then administered low doses of Δ^9-THC intraperitoneally. A 4 mg/kg dose severely depressed responding on Day 1 of treatment; performance remained depressed for 7 days. Movements of all types seemed to be impaired including the instrumental response, and all monkeys appeared less motivated to perform. Because of the latter, these results are difficult to interpret in terms of a drug-induced disruption of short-term memory. It is likely that drug side effects played a significant role in performance decrements.

Zimmerberg et al. (1971) studied the effect of smoked marijuana on the performance of monkeys on a delayed matching task. Two monkeys were given access to 30 marijuana cigarettes a day (0.5 gm) during a 4 hour matching session. Delay intervals of 0, 5, and 30 second delay were employed. On control days monkeys were given access to regular cigarettes. Results showed that monkeys performed no differently during marijuana and control sessions at the 0 second delay, but were significantly impaired at the 5 and 30 second intervals.

In a second experiment, 4 monkeys were run on an oddity problem, having to choose the odd color among three colors presented. Four delay conditions were employed including 0, 2, 8, and 32 second delays plus a simultaneous matching condition. Monkeys were run up to 8 hours each day for water reward. Subjects received THC orally. Vehicle alone was given on control days. Accuracy was impaired by the 0.5 mg/kg dose at the 2 and 32 second delays, by the 1.0 mg/kg dose at the 32 second delay, and by the 2.0 mg/kg dose at the 0, 2, 8 and 32 second delays. The simultaneous procedure was not impaired by any of the doses of THC. Unlike the results of Scheckel et al., accuracy of performance was impaired over and above any decremental effect of THC on response rate.

Ferraro and Grilly (1973) trained chimpanzees on a color and form dimension with 0, 5, 10, 20, and 40 second delays. A 1 mg/kg dose of THC produced a significant decrease in correct responding at the 5, 10, and 20 second delays, but not at 0 and 40 seconds. There was no difference in the magnitude of the decrement at the three delays. Under a 4 mg/kg dose, some animals were unable to complete the experimental session and also displayed a reduction in appetite. No tolerance to the disruptive effects of THC on delayed matching was found.

The results of the latter two studies suggest that the actions of THC in primates certainly parallel results found in man on short-term recognition memory tasks.

Other investigations concerned with the effects of cannabis on various aspects of memory and acquisition have been mainly performed with rodents. Miller *et al.* (1973a) attempted to assess in rats the effects of Δ^9-THC on a memory task which was thought to be an animal analog of the goal-directed serial alternation task in man (Melges *et al.*, 1970, 1971). Rats were trained to traverse a runway for food reward on an alternating schedule of reinforcement.

After an extended period of training, an animal learns to run fast on rewarded trials and slowly on nonrewarded trials. This paradigm is termed nonspatial single alternation (NSSA), and the typical pattern of running which is found is reflected in the sawtooth pattern shown in Fig. 2. It should be noted that on this task no *external* cues are available which predict the occurrence of reward or nonreward. On this alternating schedule of reinforcement, reward and nonreward are thought to occasion distinctive *internal* stimuli, S^r and S^n. Following nonreward, S^n becomes conditioned to running because the elicitation of that cue is always followed by reinforcement on the following trial. On the other hand, S^r is always followed by nonreward; hence inhibition accrues to this internal stimulus, and response decrement results. Thus, in the presence of S^r, an animal will run slowly because this internal cue is predictive of nonreinforcement. The opposite prediction holds for S^n and therefore the animal will run fast.

The effects of graded doses of Δ^9-THC were compared with those of LSD-25 and scopolamine on this task. Tetrahydrocannabinol disrupted patterned running by decreasing running speed on R trials and increasing it on N trials. LSD disrupted alternation mainly by increasing speed on N trials, and scopolamine by decreasing speed on R trials. It was concluded that THC treatment may have resulted in an inability to recall or register internal cues which were operative following or prior to a goal box event that predicted whether reinforcement or nonreinforcement was due.

It was also suggested that THC might have interfered with NSSA performance through the distortion of time perception. That is, NSSA performance may be viewed as being dependent on the production of two incompatible responses (running fast or slow) which follow each other

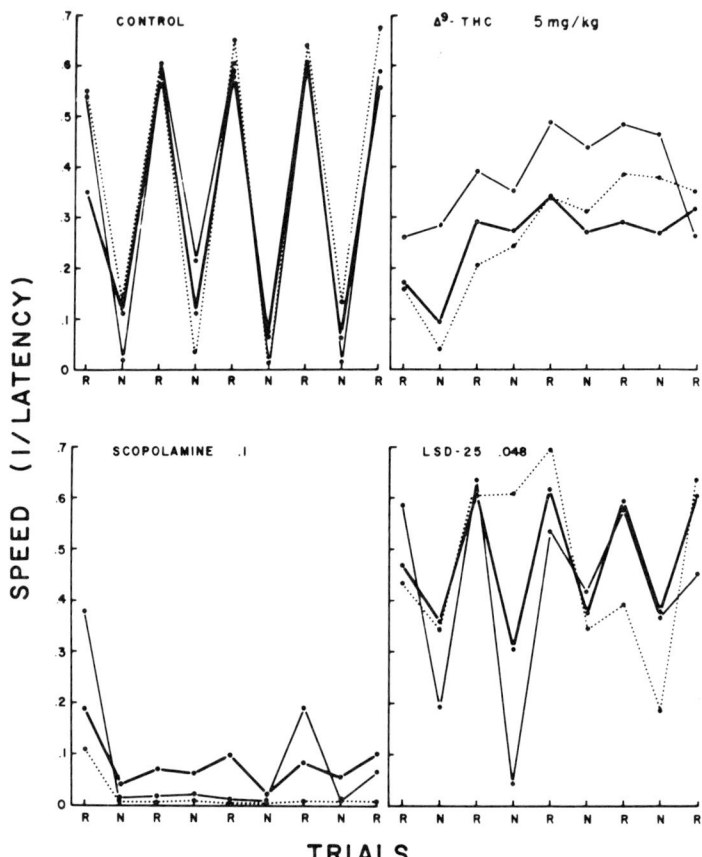

Fig. 2. Comparison of Δ⁹-THC, scopolamine, and LSD-25 on patterned running in the rat. The upper left quadrant shows typical control "sawtooth" pattern of NSSA obtained under no-treatment, saline, or 1% Tween 80–water conditions. Note fast speed on rewarded (R) and slow speed on nonrewarded (N) trials. Remaining quadrants show effects of selected dose levels of Δ⁹-THC, scopolamine, and LSD on NSSA. All doses are expressed as mg/kg body weight. In all quadrants, heavy dark lines represent the group mean pattern, whereas the thin dark lines and the dotted lines represent typical responding from two individual rats (from Miller et al., 1973a).

successively and are therefore appropriate at different points in time. If THC speeds up the "internal clock," the conditioned interoceptive cues which determine sequential responding might evoke running which is appropriate to the cues, but inappropriate for a given point in geophysical time.

Disruption of alternation under LSD was thought to be the result of interference with internal inhibition since running speed was disrupted mainly on nonrewarded trials. Scopolamine appeared to interfere with appetitive motivation since only speed on rewarded trials was altered. These findings are portrayed graphically in Figs. 2 and 3.

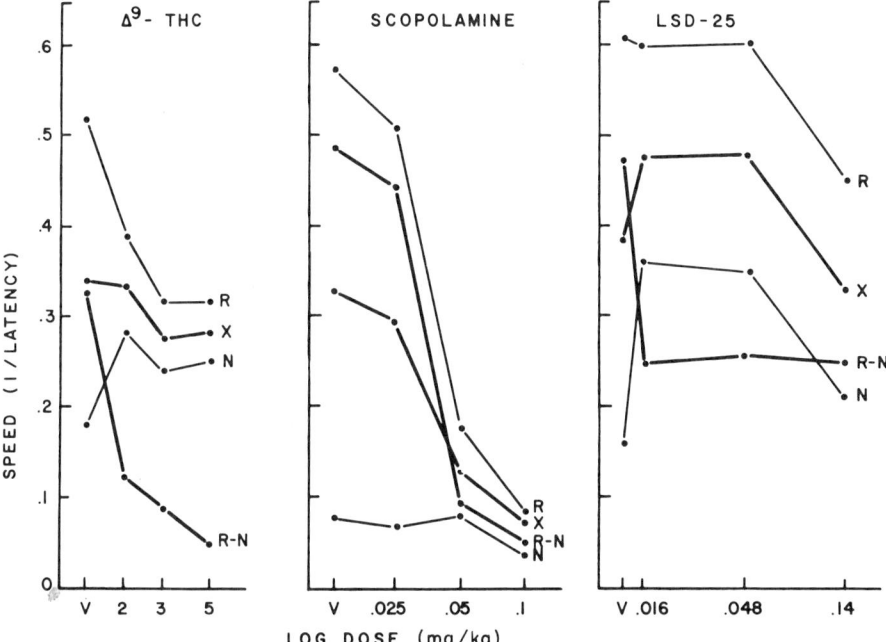

Fig 3. The effect of graded doses of Δ⁹-THC, scopolamine, and LSD-25 on specific components of NSSA responding. Mean running speed on reinforced and non-reinforced trials under each treatment condition are designated by the letters R and N, respectively. The difference in running speed between R and N trials is a measure of alternation (R-N). A higher score on the ordinate indicates superior discrimination of R and N trials (i.e., faster running on R trials and slower running on N trials). Mean running speed (X) was calculated by averaging running speed on R and N trials. The letter V refers to vehicle. For Δ⁹-THC the vehicle employed was a volume of 1% Tween 80–water which would theoretically deliver 5 mg/kg Δ⁹-THC. Saline was employed as vehicle for both LSD-25 and scopolamine, the amount administered being equal in volume to the largest dose of either drug (from Miller et al., 1973a).

A number of studies have attempted to ascertain the effect of cannabis on the acquisition and performance of maze behavior. Carlini and Kramer (1965) found that rats receiving 10 mg/kg cannabis extract displayed better performance than controls in acquiring a maze habit. Orsingher and Fulginiti (1970) in a partial replication of the Carlini and Kramer study obtained opposite results. Cannabis extract increased both the time to traverse the maze and number of errors. Carlini et al. (1970) indicated that Δ^9-THC disrupted well-established maze performance in a dose-dependent fashion. One factor which contributed to the different findings of these studies is that Carlini and Kramer tested their animals 3 minutes after injection and not at the peak effect of the drug. However, this would not account for the superior performance of the cannabis group.

The detrimental effects of cannabinoids on appetitive tasks has been thought to be possibly due to an anorexic effect of these agents especially with high doses of THC (Elsmore and Fletcher, 1972). Therefore, if cannabis produced similar decrements in acquisition and memory on nonappetitive tasks, this would lend support to the view that cannabis does exert disruptive effects on these processes independent of any actions on appetitive motivation. Unfortunately the findings in other areas have been somewhat disparate.

In a sequel to the Miller et al. study on nonspatial single alternation, Drew et al. (1973) compared the effects of Δ^9-THC, scopolamine, and LSD-25 on continuous, spontaneous alternation by rats in a Y-maze. In this paradigm an animal is allowed to freely explore the arms of the maze. Under normal conditions, a rat enters each arm successively. That is, the particular arm which is chosen is not one which was entered during the last two responses. Although spontaneous alternation is most often viewed as a simple form of exploratory behavior, it has often been employed as a measure of short-term memory. For example, Meyers and Domino (1964) have suggested that reduced alternation under scopolamine may be the result of a disruption in short-term memory.

The results of this study indicated that both scopolamine and LSD-25 reduced both the number of arm entries and percent alternation in a dose-dependent manner. Tetrahydrocannabinol reduced responsivity and percent alternation more at a lower dose (1 mg/kg) than at a higher dose (3 mg/kg). This result is difficult to reconcile with those of Miller et al. (1973a). But it is likely that spontaneous alternation is a better measure of exploratory activity than short-term memory, and hence the results are probably interpretable in terms of the dose-response and time action characteristics of THC on spontaneous activity (Drew et al., 1972).

Uyeno (1973) in an effort to clear up some of the discordant results of Carlini and associates concerning the action of cannibis on maze performance, and at the same time control for any effects of THC on appetitive motivation, examined the effect of graded doses of Δ^9-THC on the performance of rats in an underwater maze. Doses of 1, 2, 4, or 8 mg/kg THC were employed. Decrements in maze performance as a function of dose were reported with the peak action of the drug occurring about 2 hours after treatment, suggesting that THC interferes with performance independent of any side effects it might produce.

A number of different classes of drugs such as anticholinergics and phenothiazines, which are known to affect learning and retention, exert considerable influence on the acquisition and retention of passive avoidance. Miller et al. (1973b) subjected rats to a one-trial passive avoidance procedure under 5 mg/kg Δ^9-THC or vehicle.

Twenty-four hours after acquisition a retention test was given under drug or vehicle. Two retest procedures were used. In an active retest an animal was placed into the shock compartment and latency to enter the neutral compartment was recorded; in a passive retest an animal was placed into the neutral compartment and latency to enter the shock compartment was recorded. Δ^9-THC had no effect on acquisition and retention of passive avoidance and only affected retest latencies on the active retest if the drug was administered prior to testing. This study suggests that THC has some specific effect on performance rather than memory or habituation. In a second study, 15 mg/kg THC also had no important consequences on passive avoidance. Similar effects have been found in other studies with rats (Pandina and Musty, 1973) and mice (Goldberg et al., 1973). One study has found a disruptive effect of THC on retention of passive avoidance but this was a function of dissociation (Glick and Milloy, 1972). This study will be discussed in detail in a later section.

Perhaps the most studied area with infrahuman subjects and cannabinoids is avoidance learning and performance. Findings pertaining to the effects of cannabis and its derivatives on shuttle box acquisition have been mixed. Chronic treatment with THC has been found to facilitate acquisition with high doses (Goldberg et al., 1973; Pirch et al., 1972; Robichaud et al., 1973) and depress performance with low to moderate doses (Henriksson and Jarbe, 1971). Tetrahydrocannibanol appears to exert a biphasic effect on shuttle box avoidance with low doses having little effect, moderate doses depressing acquisition, and high doses (20 mg/kg and above) facilitating acquisition.

Depression and facilitation are correlated respectively with decreased and increased intertrial activity (Goldberg et al., 1973). The facilitation of avoidance is unlikely to be the result of hyperalgesia since THC actually decreases sensitivity to footshock (Parker and Dubas, 1973).

Inconsistent with the above results is the finding that cannabinoids depress well-established avoidance behavior in the shuttle box (Gruenfeld and Edery, 1969; Newman et al., 1972; Orsinger and Fulginiti, 1970; Pirch et al., 1972). Pirch et al. (1972) found that marijuana extract distillate (MED) increased the number of avoidance responses given by rats whose previous baseline level of performance was low and decreased performance in animals with high baseline levels of avoidance responding.

Operant avoidance studies have generally shown that THC increases response rate and often increases the number of shocks received. Sheckel et al. (1968) found that high doses of Δ^9-THC produced a 50% increase in responding in monkeys trained on a continuous bar press avoidance task. High doses appeared to cause hallucinations and to occasion unusual limb positions and bizarre movements. Excitation lasted 3 hours and was followed by marked depression and death in a number of animals. Low doses of Δ^8-THC increased responding, but higher doses did not produce the severe reactions seen with Δ^9-THC.

Both monkeys and rats also display an increase in responding and in number of shocks received on a Sidman avoidance schedule (Barry and Kubena, 1970; Webster et al., 1971). However, improved Sidman avoidance acquisition has been reported for rats treated with high doses of THC over an 8 day period (Barry and Kubena, 1971).

Virtually no comparisons of human and infrahuman behavior during avoidance following cannabis treatment can be made. Only one study has attempted to determine the effect of smoked marijuana on a visual–motor avoidance task in man, and no appreciable effects were noted (Hill et al., 1973).

An explanation of the actions of cannabinoids on both active and passive avoidance is elusive at this point. It seems that the finding of facilitated two-way active avoidance acquisition with high doses of THC and the lack of any effect on passive avoidance acquisition and retention are difficult to relate. As stated previously, the facilitation of avoidance under THC may be related to changes in spontaneous motor activity with high doses facilitating acquisition and increasing activity and intermediate doses depressing activity and avoidance acquisition. Hence, one might predict impaired retention of passive avoidance with high doses of THC since retention on this task has been shown to be dependent on level of activity. Interestingly, large doses of THC depress severely schedule-controlled responding (Miller and Drew, 1974).

One interesting avenue of research which might tie together some of these seemingly disparate findings concerns the finding that a 20 mg/kg dose of THC potentiates sympathetic nervous activity in stressed rats whereas the opposite is found in nonstressed rats (Ng et al., 1973). This finding might account for facilitated avoidance with high doses of THC if increased sympathetic activity is correlated with enhanced "fear." Other studies have suggested that THC might produce hyperemotionality (Jaffe and Baum, 1971; Potvin and Fried, 1972).

On the other hand, on appetitive tasks rats may be nonemotional in nature and hence THC might produce decreased arousal because sympathetic activity is reduced.

Unfortunately, the enhanced fear hypothesis receives little support from studies assessing the effect of cannabinoids on the conditioned emotional response (CER). In this paradigm, stimuli which precede an aversive event such as shock acquire the property of supressing some ongoing behavior of an organism. Drugs which ameliorate this supression apparently do so through the extinction of the effects of the conditioned aversive stimulus (Ferster and Appel, 1963). In the CER paradigm, cannabinoids attenuate behavioral supression, suggesting that this class of agents possesses *antianxiety* properties (Abel, 1969; Gonzales *et al.*, 1972).

The actions of cannabis on acquisition and retention in man are not at this point totally understood. In view of the ambiguous actions cannabinoids exert on numerous tasks including disrupted short-term memory as measured by delayed matching, poor maze learning and performance, facilitated active avoidance acquisition, and the lack of an effect on passive avoidance acquisition and retention, any conclusions concerning the behavioral mechanisms which might be influenced by this class of drugs must remain tentative. To state that cannabinoids simply affect acquisition and retention processes does nothing more than provide a description of behavioral alterations produced following treatment rather than providing an *explanation* of these effects.

The effects of cannabinoids on specifiable behavioral *antecedents* must be explored. For example, Barry and Kubena (1971) found that THC facilitated acquisition of avoidance in an operant chamber. To explain these results, the hypothesis was offered that THC reduced freezing behavior and this behavioral change mediated superior acquisition. Although they offered no independent evidence that this was actually the case, at least a direct measure of freezing can be made and correlated with avoidance performance.

Difficulties in interpreting much of the previously discussed data are probably less attributable to species differences than to a lack of task generality both between and *within* species. It may be that behavioral deficits on a series of tasks cannot be interpreted in terms of any single behavioral mechanism. Thus, it would not necessarily be predictable that cannabinoids would depress avoidance behavior in a variety of situations even if one were sure that this class of drugs generally depressed "acquisition and retention processes."

Other theoretical explanations might be sought in an effort to synthesize existing data. For example, cannabinoids might affect behavioral processes such as attention which are common to a variety of tasks. Marijuana has often been found to strongly influence time perception. Deficits in time perception may be related to cognitive changes. Finally, an important consideration in evaluating the effect of any drug on behavior is drug state change effects.

III. TIMING BEHAVIOR

It has been reasoned by Melges et al. (1970, 1971) that poor performance on the goal-directed serial alternation task (GDSA) is related to an impaired integration of current impressions with both preceding and subsequent experiences. The intoxicated subject makes errors on the GDSA because he has difficulty in serially coordinating and keeping track of information in immediate memory. The time line extending from past to present appears discontinuous to the intoxicated subject. As a result, time seems to pass more slowly. This is consistent with observations of Tinklenberg et al. (1972) that marijuana speeds up an "internal biological clock." It is possible that under marijuana there is an increase in the load of sensory information that reaches the central nervous system in a given period of *"objective"* time. In consequence, *"subjective"* time is altered in a manner which could be expressed as the "speeding up of the internal clock." Thus, an event that occurred recently in objective time is perceived as having occurred remotely in subjective time.

If this hypothesis proves to have experimental validity, this might account for the disruption of the consolidation process seen with marijuana (Abel, 1971; Darley et al., 1973). For example, a visually presented word cannot enter short-term storage until a long-term search and match process has identified the verbal representation of the visual image. An individual may retrieve an association from long-term memory by searching through numerous associations looking for one that has been elicited very recently.

Thus, an appropriate association may be identified by temporal position. Items in long-term store may carry what has been referred to as *time tags* which enable an individual to arrive at some decision as to the choice of an appropriate mediator. Coding on a temporal dimension would enable a subject to decrease the effective area of memory which must be searched at the time an association is made with some item in short-term storage.

Intoxication with marijuana might increase the search time necessary to choose an association in long-term storage for the purpose of matching it with information in short-term memory. This would result in information in short-term memory undergoing decay because relevant associations are not found quickly enough to block the normal decay process. While this hypothesis is speculative, it might account for a wide variety of memory disturbances under marijuana.

According to Paton and Pertwee (1973), three types of measurement of time perception have been made under marijuana. These methods differ in terms of whether "felt time" or "clock time" is the dependent variable. In a time estimation task, a subject is asked to report how long a specified interval of time seemed to him. The dependent variable is "felt time." In the time production task a subject is asked to state when a certain amount of time has passed by giving an actual clock estimate. Here "clock time" is the dependent variable. Like the time estimation task, an estimate of felt time in comparison to clock time is made. In time reproduction, the experimenter demonstrates a given time interval (i.e., present a tone of 30 seconds) and the subject has to reproduce it.

On tasks which require a subject to estimate the passage of time, there is a tendency to overestimate how much time has actually passed when intoxicated (Clark et al., 1970; Weil et al., 1968). For example, if 30 seconds has elapsed a subject might estimate that 40 seconds has gone by. In the time production task, normals tend to usually underestimate elapsed time. That is clock estimates fall short of actual elapsed time. Thus, a normal subject might state that a 30 second interval was actually 20 seconds on the clock. Under marijuana the underestimate is actually greater (Jones and Stone, 1970; Tinklenberg et al., 1972; Williams et al., 1946). With either time estimation or time production, the ratio of reported time to actual time is increased. On time reproduction tasks, marijuana apparently has little effect (Dornbush et al., 1971).

In studying time perception in infrahumans more subtle procedures have to be employed to assess timing efficiency for the lack of a verbal response. One procedure which has been used is a temporally controlled operant response or more specifically a differential reinforcement of low rate schedule (drl). Under a drl schedule, a response is reinforced only after a specified interval of time has elapsed since the preceeding response. If an interresponse time (IRT) occurs which is shorter than the specified interval, no reward is given. All IRTs which exceed the minimum interval are reinforced unless a limited hold (LH) condition is imposed. This latter condition sets an upper limit on the amount of time following the specified interval that an organism can wait before responding.

Conrad et al. (1972) trained chimpanzees on a multilink schedule of reinforcement. An animal had to respond to one button and then wait 60 seconds but no longer than 90 seconds (an LH is in effect) before responding on another. Then, 500 responses on the second button produced a reinforcement. Oral doses of Δ^9-THC (0.125–4 mg/kg) decreased work output and reduced the number of reinforcements with increasing doses. The reduction in reinforcement was due to a reduction in work output with higher doses of THC and a tendency to respond too early under low doses (chimpanzees tended to overestimate the passage of time). Biphasic dose-response functions have been demonstrated for THC in chimpanzees trained on drl schedules (Ferraro et al., 1971; Ferraro and Billings, 1972). Lower doses produced an increase in number of drl responses while higher doses produced a decrease in comparison to a control condition.

In rats, the effects of THC on drl responding have been somewhat more variable. Pradhan et al. (1972) found that 0.25–5 mg/kg THC increased the number of responses and decreased the number of reinforcements received on a drl 40 second schedule. This was interpreted as possibly being the result of disinhibition produced by the drug, a rate-dependent effect, or to timing inefficiency.

Unlike Pradhan et al., Webster et al. (1971) found that rate of responding on a drl 10 second schedule decreased with an increase in dosage of THC. Thus, the effect of THC on drl schedules may be dependent on the IRT requirement. Seemingly, the longer the interval between responses, the more likely that THC will produce premature responding.

A recent study with humans also indicates that a dose-related increase in premature responding occurs on a drl schedule after smoking marijuana (Cappell et al., 1972). Subjects were run on a drl 20 second schedule with a 4 second LH. A subject not only had to space his responses by 20 seconds but had to respond within 4 seconds after that 20 second interval in order to receive a reinforcement (three cents). A response after 24 seconds produced no reinforcement. Three doses of marijuana (0, 2, 4, or 8 mg/kg THC) and three doses of alcohol (0.48, 0.72, and 0.96 mg/kg) were compared for their effects on this schedule. Results indicated that while alcohol had little measureable effect on drl performance, marijuana produced a dose-dependent increase in premature responding and a decrease in the number of reinforcements.

Although the drl schedule has been linked to the ability to judge time, a more direct estimate has been made of time perception in monkeys and chimpanzees (Elsmore, 1972; Ferraro, 1972). In the Elsmore study, monkeys were trained to press the middle of three levers to produce a white light of a specific duration. Each subject was then required to press one of the other levers, the correct choice of which depended on the duration of the center light.

The effects of graded doses of THC on the above task and on an auditory discrimination task were assessed. Oral THC (1–16 mg/kg) decreased work output with higher doses and reduced accuracy at lower doses in one monkey and at the highest dose with a second. Tetrahydrocannabinol often produced an abrupt cessation of responding, and once monkeys stopped responding they never resumed working on the task. Before responding stopped, the accuracy of performance decreased. As far as the ability to estimate the duration of the center stimulus, contrary to expectation, monkeys tended to underestimate rather than overestimate its duration. In terms of performance, subjects were less likely to press the key normally associated with a long stimulus duration on the center key when a short duration stimulus was actually in effect. Ferraro (1972) performed a similar experiment with chimpanzees and obtained the expected overestimation of judged time. That is, the probability of making the long duration response was increased.

It is evident from the above experiments that animal investigators have attempted mainly to confirm the human data with regard to the actions of marijuana on time perception. Generally infrahumans as well as humans overestimate the passage of time following intoxication. To date, however, disturbances in time sense have not been related to deficits in other aspects of cognitive functioning in any systematic manner. Miller et al. (1973a) suggested that impaired performance on NSSA following treatment with THC might be due to impaired time perception.

Melges and associates also appear to feel that impaired immediate memory and time-sense disturbance under marijuana are somehow related, and there is evidence which suggests that this may be the case.

Adam (1971) in a review of the literature on the time sense suggested that disturbances in temporal experience are often correlated with memory disturbances in neurological and emotionally disturbed patients. Time perception disturbances have been found to accompany the amnesic syndrome (Spiegel et al., 1955). According to Piaget (1954) the development of the distinction between present, past, and future accompanies the development of free-recall memory.

An interesting set of data presented by D'Amato (1973) suggests that short-term memory can be regarded as a discriminative process in which "the major discriminative cues are temporal in nature." Thus, on a delayed matching task a subject has to decide which of two choice stimuli has been most recently presented as the sample stimulus. The probability of making the correct choice decreases with an increase in retention interval. This decreased probability is not only a function of the delay between offset of the sample stimulus and presentation of choice stimuli, but also how recently the sample or alternative choice stimuli have been presented as samples on previous trials. For example, say that a square serves as the sample stimulus on a given trial. On the subsequent trial, a triangle serves as the sample, with both the square and triangle serving as choice stimuli. The retention interval is 2 minutes and intertrial interval is 30 seconds. The square has been seen as the sample 4 minutes and 30 seconds earlier while the triangle was seen as the sample 2 minutes earlier. The "recency" ratio is slightly over 2 to 1. Reducing the retention interval to 15 seconds increases the ratio to 4 to 1 and, therefore, performance should improve. Thus consistent matching to sample performance may depend to a large extent on the ability to discriminate temporal intervals. Marijuana might depress matching to sample performance by making discrimination of temporal cues more difficult.

Time perception has been often related to body metabolism and physiological factors. For example, Pfaff (1968) found that higher body temperatures were correlated with a faster internal clock. It has also been suggested that changes in heart rate, respiration, and alpha rhythm may serve as a biological clock (Adam, 1971). Although the correlation between alterations in time perception induced by drugs and changes in various bodily functions has been studied infrequently, this might be an intriguing avenue of research with marijuana, especially with regard to heart rate increases.

In summary, marijuana does appear to produce a disintegration in thinking along a temporal continuum in humans, suggesting that memory loss may actually reflect a deficit in coding along a temporal dimension. This might account for the reduced consolidation which has been reported (Abel, 1971; Darley et al., 1973).

Infrahuman data confirm the time-sense disturbances found in humans, but this has not been related in any systematic way to changes in other "cognitive" operations.

IV. STATE-DEPENDENT LEARNING

A classic phenomenon produced by a number of different classes of drugs is state-dependent learning or dissociation (Overton, 1968). This refers to the finding that transfer of a learned response is reduced under conditions involving a change in drug state. Only after a particular condition (drug or no-drug) has been reinstated does transfer of training take place.

The two basic procedures used to evaluate the dissociative actions of drugs are transfer methods and drug discrimination paradigms (Overton, 1972). In the transfer design, usually four groups of subjects are placed into the cells of a 2 × 2 factorial design (Miller, 1957). Two groups of subjects acquire some response under drug or no-drug conditions, and then after a given interval of time (usually 24 hours) each group is split into two subgroups and retested in the same or different state. The basic format of such a design is shown in Table I. Dissociation is said to have

TABLE I

A Sample Design for Measuring Drug State Change Effects[a,b]

		Day 2 (retention)	
		Drug	Placebo
Day 1 (acquisition)	Drug	10	55
	Placebo	60	8

[a] Tabled scores are hypothetical error scores on Day 2.
[b] $n = 5$; $p < 001$ for change of state effect.

occurred if the state change groups (D-ND and ND-D) perform more poorly during the retest than groups (D-D and ND-ND) trained and tested in the same state. Evidence of dissociation is reflected in the interaction term of the factorial. If transfer of training is more complete in ND-D condition in comparison to the D-ND condition, asymmetrical dissociation has occurred.

In the drug discrimination procedure, subjects are required to perform one set of responses while drugged and another set when nondrugged or treated with another drug. A particular state acquires control over a specific set of responses. Employing both transfer and drug discrimination paradigms, state dependence under marijuana has been demonstrated in humans and animals.

Two human studies of the transfer variety have demonstrated dissociation under marijuana. Hill et al. (1973) tested Overton's (1972) notion that the abuse potential of various drugs parallel their tendency to produce dissociation. That is, if marijuana is a drug which is likely to be abused, it may produce state-dependent learning. Male subjects smoked marijuana containing 1.5 mg % Δ^9-THC through a spirometer. The design was 2×2 factorial with a 24 hour retention interval. The tasks included a word association test, a verbal learning task which required subjects to memorize word strings of varying degrees of meaningfulness, and a test which measured ordered recall. A visual avoidance task was also included which required a particular pattern of responding with the hands and feet. During retention testing, the pattern of responding on the avoidance task was reversed so that negative transfer was measured. Dissociation on a negative transfer task would be evident if the change of state groups made fewer errors than the same state groups.

The results of this study indicated that dissociation occurred for the sequential memory task and memory for a string of nonsense words. It was suggested that these tasks were more difficult to recall because the drug possibly influenced long-term memory for structure and meaningfulness. It should also be noted that demonstration of state dependence was task dependent.

Rickles et al. (1973) performed a study similar to Hill et al. but employed paired associate learning and a 10 day retest interval. Marijuana was smoked in cigarette form with the dose of THC similar to that used in the previous study (1.4% THC). Subjects learned a list of paired associates under drug or no-drug conditions and recalled it 10 days later. Following recall of the initially learned list, a new list was learned. It was found that marijuana interfered with acquisition during both sessions. Drug state change groups were more impaired than the same state groups during recall of the first list. State dependence was obtained even though subjects were overtrained on the paired associate list. Overtraining has been shown to reduce the probability of obtaining state dependence (Bliss, 1973).

Thus, two studies have shown that state dependence does occur under marijuana at similiar dose levels. However, the effect appears to be task dependent at least in the Hill et al. study.

A study of Klonoff et al. (1973) found no evidence for state dependence across a number of sensory modalities and a wide variety of tasks measuring concept formation, motor performance, and memory. These investigators employed two different doses of marijuana with the highest dose being similar to that employed by Hill et al. and Rickles et al., yet no dissociation was demonstrated.

Dissociation under cannabinoids has been demonstrated in animal studies under a variety of procedures in transfer and drug discrimination paradigms. The most utilized method of studying dissociation under cannabinoids is avoidance conditioning. One of the first demonstrations of dissociation was obtained by Barry and Kubena (1971). An 8 mg/kg dose of Δ^9-THC administered daily over an 8 day period was found to facilitate acquisition (reduce number of shocks received) on a bar-press avoidance task in rats. When rats receiving THC were switched to vehicle the number of shocks received increased. Rats trained under vehicle and switched to THC did not display impaired performance. Henriksson and Jarbe (1971) performed a shuttle box avoidance study similar in design to Barry and Kubena (1971). Contrary to these latter investigators, it was found that THC depressed acquisition over a 5 day period. However, following drug state change, dissociation was found to occur in both directions. Barry and Kubena (1971) found evidence only for asymmetrical dissociation.

Robichaud et al. (1973) tested the effects of THC on a number of different avoidance procedures including shuttle box avoidance, pit avoidance, passive avoidance, and conditioned fear. Low doses of THC disrupted pit avoidance while high doses of THC facilitated shuttle box avoidance when given chronically. Tetrahydrocannabinol had little effect on the acquisition of passive avoidance or conditioned fear. Evidence for asymmetrical state dependence was found only in the active avoidance situation. Further evidence for asymmetrical dissociation but not symmetrical dissociation in the shuttle box was found by Goldberg et al. (1973). Asymmetrical dissociation between THC and chlordiazepoxide (CDP) was also noted. That is, THC failed to prevent transfer deficits in mice trained under CDP and switched to THC. On the other hand, CDP prevented learning transfer failure in subjects trained under THC. This type of asymmetrical dissociation has been shown for scopolamine and Wy 4036, a benzodiazepine tranquilizer (Berger and Stein, 1969).

Herring (1972) failed to find any evidence for dissociation in a barpress discrimination avoidance paradigm. In a 2 day study, 4 mg/kg Δ^9-THC facilitated acquisition (reduced the number of shocks in comparison to controls) on Day 1. However, groups given THC on Day 2 received more shocks than the no-drug groups regardless of drug condition on Day 1. Thus drug state change did not necessarily produce poor performance; rather THC was thought to aid learning on Day 1, but impair retrieval on Day 2.

Glick and Milloy (1972) have demonstrated an unusual type of dissociation with THC in a passive avoidance paradigm. Mice were trained under 2, 4, or 8 mg/kg THC and retested 1 or 7 days later under vehicle. Only the 2 mg/kg group displayed a retention deficit when retested at 1 day. A retest at one week showed that both the 2 and 4 mg/kg groups were impaired, while the 8 mg/kg groups showed normal retention. It was reasoned that following higher doses more THC or its active metabolites would be present at retest at both retention intervals. The greater the interval between acquisition and retention test, the less THC present at the time of retest especially with low doses. Hence the greater the impairment in retention due to drug state change.

Another approach to the study of state dependence is through the use of drug discrimination procedures. According to Overton (1972) a major advantage of the drug discrimination paradigm is that weak dissociative effects can be measured. This is important because some drugs produce dissociation only at very high dose levels which may be debilitating to an organism. At lower dose levels, dissociative effects may be so weak as to not be noticed in the transfer paradigm.

The training method is similar to a sensory discrimination procedure. An organism learns one response while under the innuence of a drug and another while undrugged or under the influence of another drug or a different dose of the same drug. The basic dependent variable is the amount of training required to produce discrimination between two drug states. The more rapid the discrimination, the greater the dissociation. Subjects can also be trained to differentiate two drug states and then other drugs can be substituted to test for drug similarity. Thus, two drugs may have similar stimulus properties.

Another advantage of the drug discrimination procedure is that the development of physical tolerance can be distinguished from the development of behavioral tolerance. An improvement in performance with repeated administration of a drug could be the result of the development of physical tolerance or to a learned compensation for the drug effect (Barry and Kubena, 1971). However, in a drug discrimination procedure, if the discrimination breaks down or higher doses are required to maintain it, this would be evidence for the development of physical and not behavioral tolerance.

Initial studies with the drug discrimination procedure and cannabis were performed by Barry and Kubena (1972) and Kubena and Barry (1972). Rats were trained in an approach–avoidance conflict situation requiring them to press a bar on a fixed-interval schedule to receive food or shock. One-half of the subjects were trained under a drug condition for food and control condition for shock. The reverse held for the other half. The drug conditions included THC, alcohol, and atropine vs. vehicle. Under all three drugs an improvement in discrimination occurred with no substantial tolerance developing.

Transfer of the drug or control response to other conditions showed that lower doses of the same drugs elicited intermediate percentages of the drug response. When depressants, stimulants, or hallucinogenic drugs were substituted for THC, predominantly control responses were given. This indicated that cannabis may have a unique pharmacological profile.

Henriksson and Jarbe (1972) also found that rats could learn a position discrimination in a T-maze involving a swimming escape response on the basis of whether they were treated with THC or vehicle. The position discrimination reached 100% perfection in 11–13 sessions. Control of a given response (right or left turn) was easier to establish in the no-drug than drug state. There was no difference in acquisition rate between a 5 and 10 mg/kg dose of THC and no apparent development of tolerance.

A study by Bueno and Carlini (1972) employed the same rationale as Barry and Kubena (1972). Rats were trained in a two-level operant chamber on a fixed ratio schedule. Next they were trained to climb a rope. In a third phase one-half of the rats were administered 10 mg/kg cannabis extract while the other half remained undrugged. Rope climbing was continued. The extract depressed rope climbing initially but soon tolerance developed. The rats were then given bar-press discrimination training for 30 days along with rope climbing. Extract or vehicle were administered every other day. Under cannabis the left bar was active; under vehicle the right bar was activated. Results indicated that even when tolerance developed to the depressant actions of THC on bar pressing and rope climbing, the bar-press discrimination was learned on the basis of drug state.

Jarbe and Henriksson (1973) have argued that the dissociative effects found in avoidance paradigms could be the result of drug withdrawal rather than change of state per se. Therefore, it was of interest to demonstrate change of state effects where dissociation was reflected in enhanced rather than depressed responding. A reversal learning paradigm was employed in which rats were subjected to a change in drug state while reversal trained. If drug state change were an important determiner of performance, animals experiencing a change in drug state would learn the reversal faster than animals not experiencing a change. The paradigm was the swimming escape discrimination previously employed by Henriksson and Jarbe (1972). Rats were trained under drug (10 and 20 mg/kg Δ^8-THC or 5 mg/kg Δ^9-THC) or no-drug conditions on a position discrimination for 6 days. The vehicle groups received postsession injections during acquisition. Two retests were given in which subjects were put into the same drug state they experienced during original training and overtraining and exposed to a one-trial choice procedure. Results indicated that change of state groups made more correct responses during the reversal training phase than the same state groups. The most pronounced effect was seen with the highest dose of Δ^8-THC, and dissociation was in the symmetrical direction. The lowest doses of Δ^8-THC and Δ^9-THC were less potent in producing dissociation. When produced, it was in the asymmetrical direction. During the two retests only group D-ND displayed response control (swimming to the side associated with a particular state during original and reversal training). It should also be noted that pretreatment with THC during acquisition was necessary for the demonstration of a symmetrical dissociation.

Summarizing the results for state-dependent learning under cannabis, it has been found that (1) state-dependent learning has been widely demonstrated in humans and infrahumans with asymmetrical dissociation being the dominant result in the latter. Yet, asymmetrical dissociation has not been demonstrated in humans with marijuana. (2) Marijuana can exert differential control over responding in infrahumans as indicated by drug discrimination studies. (3) State dependence is obtained even when acquisition is facilitated and is independent of any depressant actions of cannabinoids on behavior or the development of tolerance.

It appears that cannabinoids do produce rather consistent state change effects in both humans and infrahumans. However, at this time broad comparisons across species are not possible since only a few human studies have been reported.

It is not clear why asymmetrical dissociation has been reported for infrahumans and not humans, but demonstration of this type of dissociation might be manifested as more human investigations are completed which sample a wide variety of methods and behaviors. Overton (1968) states that with a state-dependent learning model based on generalization decrement, asymmetrical dissociation would not be predicted. As Overton points out, a drug discrimination could not be learned on the basis of one-way dissociation since subjects would be equally likely to give drug or no-drug responses on drug trials. Yet drug discriminations develop rapidly under THC. It may be that task parameters and dosage play an important role in determining the direction of dissociation. Further research is needed to clarify this issue.

It is interesting to note that drug dissociation is most commonly found for active avoidance procedures but not in other types of avoidance procedures such as passive avoidance. Thus, if certain training effects transfer completely on one type of task, but not another, this suggests that cannabinoids do not produce dissociation in infrahumans solely through changes in sensory functioning.

V. ATTENTION AND HABITUATION

All behavior involves some discriminative process, whereby differential stimuli control selective behaviors. That is, an organism samples certain aspects of the environment to guide its behavior while ignoring others. The effective stimuli which exert control over behavior are those to which the organism *attends* (Bower and Trabasso, 1964).

Aspersion has been cast on the use of attention as an explanatory construct because many scientists consider the term to be vacuous. In recent years, however, there has been a resurgence of interest in this topic. The key to this renewed interest lies in the efforts of many behavioral scientists to explain discrimination learning (Sutherland and Mackintosh, 1971). Attention as a construct is no longer considered mentalistic; as a process, it can be empirically determined.

A number of studies in the marijuana literature have attempted to explain marijuana-induced deficits on particular cognitive behaviors as being a result of some effect on the process of attention. Tinklenberg et al. (1970) noted that speech patterns were often interrupted by episodic lapses in attention which were associated with intrusion of extraneous thoughts and percepts. One of the initial instances of the use of attention as an explanatory construct is the work of Abel (1970) who reasoned that impaired attention is largely responsible for reduced consolidation under marijuana. Galanter et al. (1973) have made a similar proposal. Unfortunately, no independent measures of attention were taken in these studies.

A study by Dittrich et al. (1973) obtained an independent measure of attention which consisted of a test which measured "the ability to concentrate on optical details." A significant impairment in attention was found under marijuana which was significantly correlated with a decrease in information input into long-term memory storage as well as with measures of depersonalization and temporal disintegration. The particular model proposed by Dittrich et al. encompasses the major findings of Melges et al. (1970, 1971) on depersonalization and temporal disintegration and Abel (1971) on consolidation.

A study by Casswell and Marks (1973) has taken a somewhat different approach in elucidating the action of marijuana on attention employing a divided attention task. This task appears to measure both vigilance and the ability to shift attention. Subjects were surrounded by lights and told to press a button every time they detected a break in the flashes. At the same time a peripheral light also flashed to which a subject was required to press a second button. Results indicated that significantly more central and peripheral light flashes were missed under marijuana than placebo.

Low et al. (1973) has employed a neurophysiological measure, contingent negative variation (CNV), as an indicator of attention. The CNV is a slow negative shift in baseline EEG recorded from the frontal vertical region of the cortex which occurs in a constant foreperiod between two successively presented stimuli, the second of which requires some response by a subject.

The generation of the CNV appears to be a function of the amount of attention directed toward the second stimulus (Tecce, 1972). In the Low et al. study, a flash of a strobe light was proceeded 1.4 seconds later by a tone to which subjects had to make a button-pushing response. Under a low dose of marijuana, there was a significant increase in CNV magnitude as compared with placebo. However, no significant change in the CNV was found with a more potent dose of marijuana. This suggested that during the intoxicated state, brain mechanisms underlying attentional processes were *enhanced* rather than diminished. These findings appear to be discordant with behavioral observations.

DeLong and Levy (1973) have developed a model of attention to account for the majority of effects that marijuana has on processes such as memory, time perception, and general cognitive ability. According to these authors, the major effect of marijuana is to alter resistance to distraction which is defined as the "degree to which one has resistance to non-volitional change in the focus of attention," and set shifting which is defined as "the capacity to voluntarily shift the focus of one's attention."

Recently, there has been a burgeoning of animal studies on attention (Sutherland and Mackintosh, 1971). However, pharmacological investigations of infrahuman attention are sparse. One study has attempted to obtain a measure of the effect of Δ^9-THC on attention and at the same time control for any possible disruptive actions the drug might have on appetitive motivation.

Miller and Drew (1973) ran rats in a latent learning paradigm which consisted of allowing the animals to explore freely a complex maze under the influence of THC and then testing them later in a drug-free state for the effects of this preexposure on the acquisition of a maze habit for food. While the rats treated with vehicle during maze exploration (groups LAT-ND) displayed a reduction in error scores compared with a group not given this exposure (groups CON-ND), THC-treated rats (group LAT-D) did not benefit from their familiarization period. Thus, THC nullified the latent learning effect. It was suggested that rats exposed to the maze under THC may have attended to fewer of its salient features and therefore learned less about the correct path to the goal. The results of this study are portrayed in Fig. 4. It is also possible that under THC erroneous response patterns were established during exploration and these carried over to acquisition. If THC blocks habituation, the probability of entering previously explored but incorrect blinds would remain high.

With regard to habituation under THC, an interesting study has been performed by Brown (1971). By habituation is meant that a behavioral response to a novel stimulus declines in strength with continued exposure to that stimulus. Mice given anticholinergics, Δ^9-THC, or vehicle were exposed to an experimental chamber for 15 minutes; 48 hours later all mice were water deprived for 24 hours and placed back into the chamber which contained a water bottle. Time was recorded from introduction to

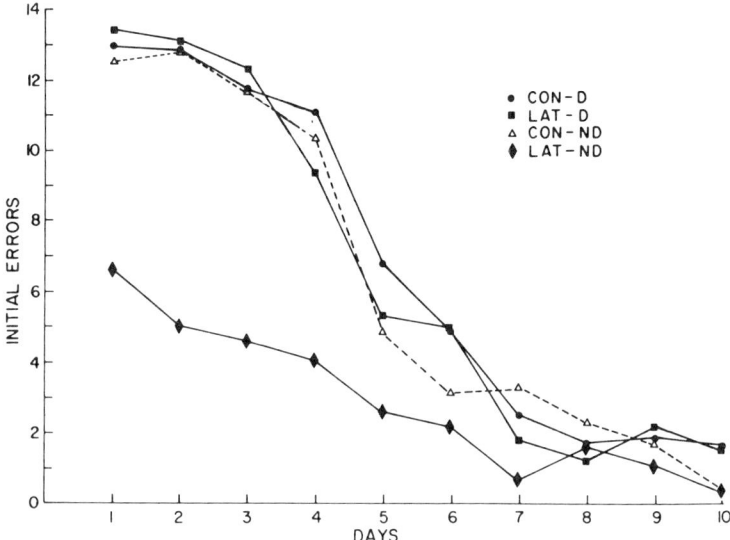

Fig. 4. Effects of Δ⁹-THC on the mean number of initial errors over 10 acquisition days (from Miller and Drew, 1973).

the chamber to the first lick at the drinking tube. Mice previously treated with anticholinergics and THC displayed longer latencies to make initial contact with the drinking tube when compared with controls, suggesting that these agents attenuated the effects of previous exposure to the chamber. Thus, the habituation of normal exploratory tendencies was blocked under THC and anticholinergics. Tacrine, an anticholinesterase, blocked this effect under both drugs.

Drew and Miller (1973) studied the effect of graded doses of Δ⁹-THC on the spontaneous activity of rats habituated or not habituated to activity wheels. A 6 mg/kg dose of THC significantly decreased the number of revolutions made by rats not previously exposed to the wheels when compared with controls. On the other hand, rats exposed to the wheels for 3 hour periods on three consecutive days displayed a significant increase in wheel activity when treated with THC. This increase in activity persisted for 24 hours following treatment with the highest dose. Thus, habituated rats became dishabituated under THC.

Studies with both humans and infrahumans suggest that attention and/or habituation are impaired following treatment with cannabinoids. Unfortunately, there are a number of methodological deficiencies in studies in this area especially with regard to attention. These include (1) few independent measures of attention along with a lack of agreement in defining the construct; (2) employment of both physiological and behavioral indices of attention neither of which necessarily correlate with each other; and (3) insufficient task generality across species.

To date, however, only a handful of studies have been performed in the area of attention, so any final conclusions concerning the affect of marijuana on this process would be unwarranted. It is well documented that an appreciation of the processes of attention and habituation are basic to the understanding of numerous types of behavior in both humans and infrahumans, and for this reason ascertaining the consequence of marijuana on these processes would facilitate the perspicuous dissemination of drug-behavior relationships.

At this point, the most fruitful approach to research on attention and drugs is a behavioral one. Assessing the action of any pharmacological agent on hypothetical neurophysiological correlates of attention may be premature inasmuch as behavioral indices of attention are not well defined. The employment of procedures which allow somewhat direct comparisons across species would be a salutary approach to the problem. For example, various operant techniques have been shown to be powerful methodological tools in the study of attention in both humans and infrahumans and therefore it would be advantageous to make use of these techniques.

VI. SUMMARY AND DISCUSSION

In this chapter comparisons between humans and infrahumans were made with regard to the action of cannabinoids on numerous aspects of behavior. Similarities and dissimilarities were noted along with methodological problems associated with making comparisons across species and tasks. Suggestions for future research were offered.

In concluding this chapter, some general methodological considerations should be uttered concerning problems associated with the comparative behavioral pharmacology of cannabinoids as well as other classes of drugs. It is evident that extrapolating from one situation to another is an arduous task not only behaviorally, but pharmacologically. Behavior not only varies across species, but various experimental parameters, especially dosage, may differentially influence similar behaviors in diverse species. For this reason, prudence is suggested in proposing behavioral explanations whose foundation is based on isolated dose levels, single behavioral parameters, and variable behavioral baselines. Furthermore, it should be realized that the demonstration of an impairment following drug treatment is not a sufficient condition for understanding its action; rather *selective*-impairment is the *sine qua non* of behavioral pharmacology. Awareness of these methodological considerations should promote more exacting research efforts with marijuana.

REFERENCES

Abel, E. L. (1969). *Psychon. Sci.* **16**, 44.
Abel, E. L. (1970). *Nature (London)* **227**, 1151–1152.
Abel, E. L. (1971). *Science* **173**, 1038–1040.
Adam, N. (1971). T.-I.-T.J. *Life Sci.* **1**, 41–52.
Ames, F. (1958). *J. Ment. Sci.* **104**, 972–999.
Barry, H., III, and Kubena, R. K. (1970). *Proc. 78th Annu. Conv. Amer. Psychol. Ass.* **5**, 805–806.
Barry, H., III, and Kubena, R. K. (1971). *Proc. 79th Annu. Conv. Amer. Psychol. Ass.* **6**, 747–748.
Barry, H., III, and Kubena, R. K. (1972). *In* "Drug Addiction: Experimental Pharmacology" (J. M. Singh, L. Miller, and H. Lah, eds.), Vol. I, pp. 3–16. Futura Publ. Co., Mount Kisco, New York.
Berger, B. D., and Stein, L. (1969). *Psychopharmacologia* **14**, 351–358.
Bliss, D. K. (1973). *J. Comp. Physiol. Psychol.* **84**, 149–161.
Bower, G. H., and Trabasso, T. (1964). *In* "Studies in Mathematical Psychology" (R. C. Atkinson, ed.), pp. 32–94. Stanford Univ. Press, Stanford, California.
Bromberg, W. (1934). *Amer. J. Psychiat.* **91**, 303–330.
Brown, H. (1971). *Psychopharmacologia* **21**, 294–301.
Bueno, O. F. A., and Carlini, E. A. (1972). *Psychopharmacologia* **25**, 49–56.
Burghardt, G. M. (1973). *In* "The Study of Behavior: Learning, Motivation, Emotion and Instinct" (J. A. Nevin, ed.), pp. 323–390. Scott, Foresman & Co., Glenview, Illinois.
Cappell, H., Webster, C. D., Herring, B. S., and Ginsberg, R. (1972). *J. Pharmacol. Exp. Ther.* **182**, 195–203.
Carlini, E. A., and Kraemer, C. (1965). *Psychopharmacologia* **7**, 175–181.
Carlini, E. A., Hamaoui, A., Bieniek, D., and Korte, F. (1970). *Pharmacology* **4**, 359–368.
Casswell, S., and Marks, D. (1973). *Nature (London)* **241**, 60–61.
Clark, D., Hughes, R., and Nakashima, E. N. (1970). *Arch. Gen. Psychiat.* **23**, 193–198.
Conrad, D. G., Elsmore, T. F., and Sodetz, F. J. (1972). *Science* **175**, 547–550.
D'Amato, M. R. (1973). "The Psychology of Learning and Motivation: Advances in Research and Theory" (G. H. Bower, ed.), Vol. 7. Academic Press, New York.
Darley, C. F., Tinklenberg, J. R., Roth, W. T., Hollister, L. E., and Atkinson, R. C. (1973). *Memory & Cognition* **1**, 196–200.
DeLong, F. L., and Levy, B. I. (1973). *Psychol. Rep.* **33**, 907–916.
Dittrich, A., Batting, K., and von Zeppelin, I. (1973). *Psychopharmacologia* **33**, 369–376.
Dornbush, R. L., Fink, M., and Freedman, A. M. (1971). *Amer. J. Psychiat.* **128**, 194–197.
Drew, W. G., and Miller, L. L. (1973). *Pharmacology* **9**, 41–51.
Drew, W. G., Miller, L. L., and Wikler, A. (1972). *Psychopharmacologia* **23**, 289–299.

Drew, W. G., Miller, L. L., and Baugh, E. L. (1973). *Psychopharmacologia* 32, 171–182.
Elsmore, T. F. (1972). *Psychopharmacologia* 26, 62–72.
Elsmore, T. F., and Fletcher, W. V. (1972). *Science* 175, 911–912.
Ferraro, D. P. (1972). In "Current Research in Marijuana" (M. F. Lewis, ed.), pp. 49–95. Academic Press, New York.
Ferraro, D. P., and Billings, D. K. (1972). *Psychopharmacologia* 25, 169–174.
Ferraro, D. P., and Grilly, D. M. (1973). *Science* 179, 490–492.
Ferraro, D. P., Grilly, D. M., and Lynch, W. C. (1971). *Psychopharmacologia* 22, 333–351.
Ferster, C. B., and Appel, J. B. (1963). In "Psychopharmacological Methods" (Z. Votava, M. Horvath, and O. Vinar, eds.), pp. 170–181. Macmillan, New York.
Galanter, M., Weingartner, H., Vaghan, T. B., Roth, W. T., and Wyatt, R. J. (1973). *Arch. Gen. Psychiat.* 28, 278–281.
Glick, S. D., and Milloy, S. (1972). In "Current Research in Marijuana" (M. F. Lewis, ed.), pp. 1–24. Academic Press, New York.
Goldberg, M. E., Hefner, M. A., Robichaud, R. C., and Dubinsky, B. (1973). *Psychopharmacologia* 30, 173–184.
Gonzalez, S. C., Karniol, I. G., and Carlini, E. A. (1972). *Behav. Biol.* 7, 83–94.
Gruenfeld, Y., and Edery, H. (1969). *Psychopharmacologia* 14, 200–210.
Henriksson, B. G., and Jarbe, T.U.C. (1971). *Psychopharmacologia* 22, 23–30.
Henriksson, B. G., and Jarbe, T. U. C. (1972) *Psychon. Sci.* 27, 25–26.
Herring, B. (1972). *Psychopharmacologia* 26, 401–406.
Hill, S. Y., Schwin, R., Powell, B., and Goodwin, D. W. (1973). *Nature (London)* 243, 241–242.
Hollister, L. E. (1971). *Science* 172, 21–29.
Jaffe, P. B., and Baum, M. (1971). *Psychopharmacologia* 20, 97–102.
Janes, L. (1970). University of Oklahoma, Norman (unpublished doctoral dissertation).
Jarbe, T. U. C., and Henriksson, B. G. (1973). *Psychopharmacologia* 31, 321–332.
Jones, R. T., and Stone, G. C. (1970). *Psychopharmacologia* 18, 108–117.
Kesner, R. (1973). *Psychol. Bull.* 80, 177–203.
Klonoff, H. K., Low, M., and Marcus, A. (1973). *Can. Med. Ass. J.* 108, 150–156.
Kubena, R. K., and Barry, H., III. (1972). *Nature (London)* 235, 397–398.
Low, M. D., Klonoff, H., and Marcus, A. (1973). *Can. Med. Ass. J.* 108, 157–164.
Melges, F. T., Tinklenberg, J. R., Hollister, L. E., and Gillespie, H. K. (1970). *Science* 168, 1118–1120.
Melges, F. T., Tinklenberg, J. R., Hollister, L. E., and Gillespie, H. K. (1971). *Arch. Gen. Psychiat.* 21, 564–567.
Meyers, B., and Domino, E. F. (1964). *Arch. Int. Pharmacodyn. Ther.* 150, 525–529.
Miller, L. L., and Dolan, M. P. (1974). *Psychopharmacologia* 35, 353–364.
Miller, L. L., and Drew, W. G. (1973). *Nature (London)* 243, 473–474.
Miller, L. L., and Drew, W. G. (1974). *Psychol. Bull.* (in press).
Miller, L. L., Drew, W. G., and Kiplinger, G. F. (1972). *Nature (London)* 273, 172–173.
Miller, L. L., Drew, W. G., and Wikler, A. (1973a). *Psychopharmacologia* 28, 1–11.
Miller, L. L., Drew, W. G., and Joyce, P. (1973b). *Behav. Biol.* 8, 421–426.
Miller, N. E. (1957). In "Psychotropic Drugs" (S. Garattini and V. Ghetti, eds.), pp. 83–103. Elsevier, Amsterdam.

8. Human and Infrahuman Comparisons

Newman, L. M., Lutz, M. P., Gould, M. H., and Domino, E. F. (1972). *Science* **175**, 1022–1023.
Ng, L. K. Y., Lamprecht, F., Williams, R. B., and Kopin, I. J. (1973). *Science* **180**, 1368–1369.
Orsingher, O. A., and Fulginiti, S. (1970). *Pharmacology* **3**, 337–344.
Overton, D. A. (1968). *U.S., Pub. Health Serv., Publ.* **1836**, 918–930.
Overton, D. A. (1972). *In* "The Biology of Alcoholism: Physiology and Behavior" (B. Kissen and H. Begleiter, eds.), pp. 193–217. Plenum, New York.
Padina, R. J., and Musty, R. E. (1973). *Proc. 81st Annu. Conv. Amer. Psychol. Ass.* **8**, 993–994.
Parker, J. M., and Dubas, T. C. (1973). *Int. J. Clin. Pharmacol. Ther. Toxicol.* **7**, 75–81.
Paton, W. D. M., and Pertwee, R. G. (1973). *In* "Marijuana: Chemistry, Pharmacology, Metabolism and Clinical Effects" (R. Mechoulam, ed.), pp. 287–333. Academic Press, New York.
Pfaff, D. (1968). *J. Exp. Psychol.* **76**, 419–422.
Piaget, J. (1954). "The Construction of Reality." Basic Books, New York.
Pirch, J. H., Osterhalm, K. C., Barratt, E. S., and Cohn, R. A. (1972). *Proc. Soc. Exp. Biol. Med.* **141**, 590–592.
Potvin, R. J., and Fried, P. A. (1972). *Psychopharmacologia* **26**, 369–378.
Pradhan, S. N., Bailey, P. T., and Ghosh, P. (1972). *Psychon. Sci.* **27**, 179–181.
Rickles, W. H., Jr., Cohen, M. J., Whitaker, C. A., and McIntyre, K. E. (1973). *Psychopharmacologia* **30**, 349–354.
Robichaud, R. C., Hefner, M. A., Anderson, J. E., and Goldberg, M. E. (1973). *Pharmacology* **10**, 1–11.
Scheckel, C. L., Boff, E., Dahlen, P., and Smart, T. (1968). *Science* **160**, 1467–1469.
Shiffrin, R. M., and Atkinson, R. C. (1969). *Psychol. Rev.* **76**, 179–193.
Sidman, M. (1960). "Tactics of Scientific Research." Basic Books, New York.
Spiegel, E. A., Wycis, H. T., Orchinik, C. W., and Frees, H. (1955). *Science* **121**, 771–772.
Sutherland, N. S., and Mackintosh, N. J. (1971). "Mechanisms of Animal Discrimination Learning." Academic Press, New York.
Tecce, J. J. (1972). *Psychol. Bull.* **77**, 73–108.
Tinklenberg, J. R., Melges, F. T., Hollister, L. E., and Gillespie, H. K. (1970). *Nature (London)* **226**, 1171–1172.
Tinklenberg, J. R., Kopell, B. S., Melges, F. T., and Hollister, L. E. (1972). *Arch. Gen. Psychiat.* **27**, 812–815.
Uyeno, E. T. (1973). *Proc. 81st Annu. Conv. Amer. Psychol. Ass.* **8**, 997–998.
Webster, C. D., Willinsky, M. D., Herring, B., and Walters, G. (1971). *Nature (London)* **232**, 498–501.
Weil, A. T., Zinberg, N. E., and Nelson, J. M. (1968). *Science* **162**, 1234–1242.
Weiss, B., and Laties, V. G. (1967). *Fed. Proc., Fed. Amer. Soc. Exp. Biol.* **26**, 1146–1156.
Williams, E. G., Himmelsbach, C. K., Wikler, A., Ruble, D. C., and Lloyd, B. J. (1946). *Pub. Health Rep.* **61**, 1059–1083.
Zeidenberg, P., Clark, W. C., Jaffe, J., Jr., Anderson, S. W., Chin, S., and Malitz, S. (1973). *Comp. Psychiat.* **14**, 549–556.
Zimmerberg, G., Glick, S. D., and Jarvik, M. E. (1971). *Nature (London)* **233**, 343–345.

Chapter 9

THE LONG-TERM EFFECTS OF CANNABIS USE

RHEA L. DORNBUSH

  I. Introduction 221
 II. Studies of Chronic Use in Man in Created Populations 222
III. Studies in Animals 226
 IV. Studies of Chronic Use in Man in Existing Populations 228
     A. Jamaica 228
     B. Greece 229
     C. Egypt 229
  V. Summary 230
     References 231

I. INTRODUCTION

The use of marijuana rose dramatically in the 1960's particularly among middle-class youth. Because marijuana was classified as a narcotic by the United States Government and it's effects poorly understood and subject to political and emotional misrepresentations, a large-scale national effort was undertaken to investigate the pharmacology of this substance. At this date, experimental information indicates that the acute effects of marijuana in moderate doses and under social or laboratory conditions, particularly on perceptual and cognitive functions, are minimal. There are only small performance decrements in the "higher cortical" functions and they are transient. Where decremental effects are obtained, they are usually related to higher dose, task complexity, and degree of experience with the drug (Hollister, 1971; Jones, 1973; National Commission on Marijuana and Drug Abuse, 1972; Commission of Inquiry into the Non-Medical Use of Drugs, 1972).

In summary the following has been determined about acute use through inhalation. The effects are very rapid in onset, changing during the course of measurement, and short lived (Dornbush et al., 1971). There is an increase in heart rate (Domino, 1971; Johnson and Domino, 1971); an increase in EEG alpha activity, and a decrease in mean (average) EEG frequency. Both EEG and heart-rate effects peak early in the postsmoking period and then taper off (Volavka et al., 1973). Performance on perceptual, cognitive, and motor tasks are mixed. Sometimes a decrement is obtained (Clark et al., 1970; Tinklenberg et al., 1972); often times there is no change (Dornbush et al., 1971; Tinklenberg et al., 1970). Short-term memory is perhaps the single most consistently affected function (Abel, 1971; Dornbush, 1974). Subjective effects are generally described as pleasant and tend to remain after objective changes have returned to baseline.

The acute effects of marijuana have been well defined. However, the eventual effects of repeated marijuana use are still not clear. Two approaches to studying chronic long-term effects have been taken. One has focused on creating chronic populations by administering marijuana daily for short periods (weeks). The second approach aims at identifying and studying already existing populations of very long-term users (years).

II. STUDIES OF CHRONIC USE IN CREATED POPULATIONS

In these chronic studies there were large differences in the populations, the laboratories, and the experimental conditions. However, the results were remarkably consistent particularly with regard to psychomotor performance, mental abilities, and some physiological measurements.

In one of the first studies in created chronic populations, Williams et al. (1946) initiated a 6-subject study with pyrahexyl compound which was judged qualitatively similar to marijuana. To avoid any questions concerning similarities in the two substances the authors included a 6-subject study using marijuana. The subjects were prisoners. They were the sole occupants of a research ward and confined to that ward. Subjects smoked marijuana *ad libitum* for 39 days preceded and followed by 7 nonsmoking observation days. The potency of the marijuana was not assayed. Early effects of exhilaration and euphoria were replaced after several days by lassitude and indifference. The authors doubted the establishment of physical dependence but observed evidence for tolerance development with both pyrahexyl compound and marijuana. After smoking marijuana, pulse rate increased for the first three weeks of the smoking period and then was no different than presmoking rates. This of course might not be tolerance but habituation. After the first week of pyrahexyl administration, effects appeared to be less and all subjects requested an increase in dose which was followed by a return of effects. In tests of various mental and psychomotor functions, comprehension and analytic thinking were made more difficult; in tests which required concentration and manual dexterity, there was an increase in speed but a decrease in accuracy. There were no adverse effects and no subject exhibited antisocial behavior. It is difficult to attribute the presence of lassitude and indifference in these subjects to marijuana use without an appropriate control group, particularly under the conditions of the experiment which included confinement, a limited selection of ward mates, and no diversions or activities.

Recent studies have employed more sophisticated techniques of measurement but similar designs, i.e., a pre- and post-nonsmoking period and a drug period. Most of these studies also required that subjects be confined for the duration of the observations. For example, the National Commission (1972) conducted studies on prolonged marijuana acquisition in 10 heavy and 10 casual users. The subjects were observed as inpatients. During a 21-day smoking period, subjects could work to obtain marijuana. The task consisted of accumulating points on a counter. Six-thousand points bought one marijuana cigarette. All subjects earned the maximum number of points every day, suggesting no relationship between marijuana use and decreases in motivation. Assessments included measurement of mood states, individual and group behavior observations, clinical psychological evaluations, psychomotor assessments, and physiological measurements. All effects were transitory. Generally, no impairment of performance on tests of cognitive and motor functioning were observed prior to, during, or following marijuana smoking. Rather, over time, there was an improvement in memory and psychomotor performance. Memory was assessed by digit-span performance, and improvement with practice normally occurs. The same is so for the psychomotor task, a "shooting gallery" event. Other tests included the Halstead Category test, tactical performance test, Seashore Rhythm test, finger tapping tests, and trail making tests. Practice effects occurred where expected. Other acute effects included decreases in anxiety and a general euphoria. Negative mood states were reported by casual users over the course of the experiment. It is difficult, however, to interpret these negative mood states; they may be more a function of ward conditions than drug effect.

Indeed, Dornbush et al. (1972) administered marijuana daily to detoxified heroin addicts. Dysphoria developed between the third and sixth day. The authors suggested that this effect may reflect boredom and other aspects of sustained hospitalization.

In the National Commission study (1972), tolerance did seem to develop but it did not follow classical definitions of the phenomenon. Some users smoked up to 200 mg Δ^9-THC during a daily administration (obviously implying a tolerance) but they did not require these large doses for an effect. It has been our experience that users who are unaccustomed to larger doses do experience undersirable, unpleasant, hallucinogenic-like states with a dose of 25 mg Δ^9-THC (R. Dornbush, J. Volavka, and M. Fink, personal communication).

Further evidence of tolerance may be suggested in the reduced acute heart-rate response with repeated administration. However, because there was no appropriate control group it is difficult to be certain that the cardiovascular response was not an habituation effect. There was no evidence of dependence or withdrawal.

There were differences between heavy and casual users. During daily marijuana administration, casual users did not increase their dose whereas heavy users did. Motivational differences between the two groups may account for this. Heavy users, who also tend to be multidrug users, may be seeking hallucinogenic effects to which tolerance develops rapidly. Casual users may seek only to enhance social effects.

In the Canadian Commission study (Commission of Inquiry into the Non-Medical Use of Drugs, 1972) the longest smoking period was 52 consecutive days. As in the National Commission Study, subjects worked for tokens which, in turn, were traded for desired objects, including additional marijuana. Subjects were confined during observation. Under mandatory drug conditions, subjects were increased from 16 to 30 mg Δ^9-THC. But when there were no mandatory doses and subjects were permitted free purchase, they smoked between 2 and 4 mg Δ^9-THC! The mandatory large doses were subjectively unpleasant. During free-purchase periods there was no attempt to increase marijuana intake over time. Initially, subjects who were permitted to smoke the more desirable smaller doses evidenced greater work productivity than those who received mandatory high doses. Tolerance to this effect may have occurred over the course of the experiment. At the end of the smoking period, differences in work productivity were minimal. The acute rise in pulse rate after smoking decreased progressively over the weeks of testing even with increased doses. There was no evidence of a withdrawal syndrome or signs of dependence.

Frank et al. (1973) conducted a daily administration study in healthy users who were hospitalized for the duration of the study. They smoked 7 mg marijuana (with either 1 or 2% Δ^9-THC) for 28 consecutive days preceded and followed by nonsmoking periods. An extensive array of medical, physiological, subjective, and behavioral measurements were assessed. All changes were transitory. There was some impairment in mental function and an elevation in mood. There were also significant effects on heart rate, blood pressure, and intraocular pressure. There was no evidence of cumulative effects, withdrawal effects or tolerance over a wide spectrum of physiological, psychological, and clinical laboratory parameters. A more extensive analysis of this data is forthcoming.

Dornbush et al. (1972) administered marijuana to users for 21 consecutive days. The test period was preceded and followed by drug-free periods. Users were not hospitalized. Fourteen milligrams Δ^9-THC were administered in a single dose. Assessments included EEG, heart rate, a mood scale, tests of short-term memory, and the digit-symbol substitution test (DSST). This study was considered preliminary and results were interpreted cautiously. However, they corroborated the data obtained in other chronic experiments. There was an improvement in short-term memory over days, after an initial decrement, and a consistent improvement in DSST. Because there was no control group it was difficult to attribute improvements in performance to practice or tolerance. Results, however, do indicate that marijuana does not inhibit a subject's ability to improve with practice, i.e., exhibit positive transfer. All subjects reported a sense of well-being and euphoria. However, there was a decrease in subjective effects during successive sessions, with the greatest changes occurring after the first week. This "tolerance" to subjective effects also has been reported in other chronic studies (National Commission, 1972).

As in other chronic studies, the initial acute increase in heart rate decreased progressively over the smoking period. With regard to the EEG, the immediate acute increase in alpha did not change over days, suggesting that tolerance to this particular effect of marijuana did not occur with this time and dose schedule. There were no signs of dependence or withdrawal.

In summary, in populations smoking daily up to 52 days there were no chronic changes that were not seen during occasional acute use. Effects were transitory. Subjects remained generally euphoric. There were no unpleasant or untoward effects except in instances where subjects were forced to exceed their want. Over time, performance on some cognitive, perceptual, and motor tasks showed improvement. Acute increases in heart rate decreased consistently over time. In all studies, because of inappropriate or inadequate design, it is difficult to attribute the diminishing heart-rate response and improvement in certain behaviors to tolerance. These changes could be the result of habituation and practice, respectively. There were no signs of dependence or withdrawal. Perhaps the surest sign of tolerance development was the ability of subjects to consume increasing doses of Δ^9-THC without ill effect.

On the other hand, Barratt et al. (1972) in preliminary studies conducted with a created chronic population of 5 subjects suggests that marijuana may, in fact, adversely effect behavior, but indirectly. These studies on sleep–wakefulness cycles indicate that the chronic use of marijuana leads to significant decreases in slow wave sleep and that this, in turn, results in dysphoria, lethargy, and less aggressive behavior (amotivation?) in every-day life situations. These investigators are currently studying the limits of dose and frequency within which these sleep changes occur, and they suggest that typical users may not approach these doses.

Perhaps one of the most limiting factors in these created chronic populations has been the need to confine individuals for the duration of observation. This also limits the subject population. Any dysphoria or lassitude which may have developed in any of these studies with repeated drug administration cannot be legitimately attributed to marijuana per se until appropriate nondrug groups are also confined and similarly observed. Dornbush et al. (1972) observed subjects as outpatients. They were observed in the laboratory in the morning and continued their normal activities during the afternoons and evenings. This was one of the few studies described where subjects did not report dysphoria.

III. STUDIES IN ANIMALS

Because of obvious ethical constraints there are few daily administration studies in man and even less using naive subjects. These constraints do not exist for animals, and indeed tolerance after prolonged repeated THC administration has been demonstrated in rats, dogs, pigeons, and chimpanzees (McMillan and Dewey, 1972). It is of course difficult to compare observations in animals with observations in man, but there are some effects in animals which are very similar to effects of marijuana in man and these deserve mention.

Grilly et al. (1973) trained chimpanzees on a delayed matching-to-sample task. In this task a visual stimulus was presented to the animal. After a delay, the chimpanzee was presented with three stimuli, one of which was identical to the previously presented stimulus. If the subject selected the correct (previously presented) stimulus it was reinforced with a banana pellet. The delays between the original stimulus and the three comparisons were 0, 5, 20, and 40 seconds. Under nondrug conditions there was a decrease in performance with increasing delays. Single administration of THC further disrupted performance. With repeated THC administration the drug effect on delayed matching-to-sample performance was reduced.

This task can be considered similar to the short-term memory task used by Dornbush et al. (1971, 1972) in human subjects. A nonsense trigram such as DKG was auditorially presented. After a delay, subjects were required to verbally recall that trigram. Dornbush et al. used 0, 6, 12, and 18 second delays. Under nondrug conditions, recall was decreased with increasing delays. After a single marijuana administration, recall was further decreased. With repeated marijuana administration, there was a reduced drug effect.

Under both drug and nondrug conditions, there was no deficit at 0 delay. Dornbush et al. and others (Abel, 1971) suggested that in human subjects this implies that marijuana does not effect input or output, that is, does not effect attention or the perception of stimuli or retrieval of stimuli from storage. Rather, the storage process itself must be affected by the drug as indicated by a performance deficit when a delay is introduced between presentation and recall. Remarkably, the same response is obtained in chimpanzees. There is no drug effect on performance at 0 second delay with either single or repeated THC administration. Grilly et al., unaware of the human data, also suggested that this implies that drug-induced impairments are not due to losses of attention or distortions in perceiving the stimuli. Tetrahydrocannabinol apparently effects storage. That the specifics of the response on higher level functions, such as memory, are so similar in chimpanzees and man is indeed remarkable.

McMillan et al. (1972) demonstrated tolerance in pigeons. Pigeons were trained on a specific schedule of reinforcement. Schedule-controlled behavior was disrupted after a single administration of Δ^9-THC. However, with repeated administration the disruptive effects of THC on schedule behavior disappeared, even when the dose was increased to 20 times its original level. Nontolerant pigeons given the increased dose died. Abrupt discontinuation of THC administration in tolerant pigeons had no effect on responding. The same results were also obtained with rats.

In other studies, Ford and McMillan (1971) demonstrated that pigeons continued to work for food after receiving 6000 to 18,000 times the minimally effective dose of THC. As will be discussed below, Greek subjects continued to perform with doses 4 to 9 times what may have been their starting dose and 4 to 9 times what Americans are administered.

In summary, apparently, tolerance to behavioral effects and some physiological effects of cannabinoids develops rapidly in animals and possibly in man. There is no evidence of disruptive behavior with repeated administration in either man or animal and there is no evidence of dependence or withdrawal syndromes in either man or animal.

IV. STUDIES OF CHRONIC USE IN EXISTING POPULATIONS

Admittedly, the studies on created populations, particularly in man, have limited applicability. They do, however, permit us to observe that "reefer madness" does not occur. There are no abnormalities or derangements in behavior. In fact, the individual remains competent in many of the areas investigated.

The question of the eventual and cumulative effects of long-term use remains. Because American populations of very heavy, very long-term users are not available, data on chronic long-term effects were obtained from users in other countries. Two foreign studies were undertaken, one in Jamaica and one in Greece. What is unique about these populations is that they have restricted themselves to only cannabis preparations. There is virtually no abuse or even use of other substances with the exception of tobacco and occasional social use of alcohol.

In Jamaica, 30 chronic users were compared with 30 nonusers. Chronic use was defined as daily use for not less than 7 years. Subjects reported that they smoked between 1 and 24 "spliffs" (cigarettes) a day with an average of 7. The samples contained a mean THC content of 2.96%. Assessments included psychiatric examinations and tests of physiological, sensory, cognitive, and perceptual performance. Results indicated no significant differences between groups in the incidence of mental illness or abnormalities of mood, thought, or behavior (Beaubrun and Knight, 1973). There was no indication of user impairment and there were no differences between the groups in any of the behavioral tests. There was no evidence of an abstinence syndrome.

Bowman and Pihl (1973) suggest that in studies of foreign populations many findings may be cultural artifacts rather than drug effects. They point to user expectation. Jamaicans expect and use cannabis to enhance thinking and memory. But as suggested in the short-term chronic studies done in this country, enhanced memory may in fact be a drug effect, perhaps indirect, and not an artifact. In chronic studies, it will be recalled, many higher cortical functions such as memory returned to normal levels over time. Indeed, what may be cultural and a function of length of experience is that aspect of the drug effect on which the user focuses.

The study on Greek hashish users (Fink and Stefanis, 1971–1974) is just being concluded and the data are not yet freely available. Forty users who had smoked hashish for over 10 years were compared with 40 nonuser controls. At the time of observation, subjects reported that they smoked an average of 3.1 gm of hashish a day. Analysis of samples indicated a THC content of 4–5%. Assessments included medical, neurological, psychological, psychiatric, and sociological measurements. Minimal differences between the groups were obtained. Studies of effects of acute use were carried out on the users in experiments which paralleled American experiments. Indeed, the physiological, behavioral, and subjective effects also paralleled American results: rapid onset of drug action, lability of drug effect during the course of measurement, and relatively short duration of drug action. The EEG profile in Greek long-term users was similar to the EEG profile in American occasional users: increases in alpha, decreases in beta, decreases in EEG frequency, and increase in heart rate.

Tolerance to large doses of Δ^9-THC (180 mg in a single administration) was demonstrated. However, marijuana effects were still obtained with considerably lower doses in these same subjects. Withdrawal effects are currently being evaluated.

A limitation in cross-cultural studies lies of course in the populations' comparability to American populations. While the similarity of acute effects in the Greek and American subjects is encouraging, it would have been considerably more relevant had Greek subjects been administered the smaller doses employed in American experiments, i.e., 20 mg Δ^9-THC.

A study of long-term hashish use in Egypt (Soueif, 1971) strikes the one discordant note among the data we have examined. In the over 800 users and 800 controls studied the following was obtained: Marked psychic dependence developed to the drug; the work capacities of the hashish users were significantly impaired in quality and quantity; and users were slow learners. However, a significant number of users also used other substances, especially opium, and it was demonstrated that users tended to seek agents acting on the central nervous system more than nonusers did. It is likely that this other drug use and the need for other drugs may be responsible for differences between users and controls, rather than the consumption of cannabis per se.

Recent reports of neurological impairment (Kolansky and Moore,

1971) and cerebral atrophy (Campbell *et al.*, 1971) attributed these changes to heavy cannabis use. But both populations were abusers of other substances, e.g., amphetamines and LSD. Appropriate documentation does not yet exist, but impression suggests that where deficits in behavior and mood do occur, they are associated with multidrug use and may be rooted in the personality and psychopathology of the individual rather than being due to direct drug effects.

V. SUMMARY

The use of animals has obvious limitations in the assessment of long-term drug effects in man. Chronic studies of daily marijuana administration in man for 21 days, 50 days, or even 90 days have limitations in evaluating the effects of 10, 20, or 30 years of daily administration. Likewise, studies on very long-term use in foreign populations limit comparability to American populations. Yet, results from these different categories of studies are somewhat consistent. Generally, the effects of marijuana are transitory. There may be behavioral, subjective, and physiological tolerance; there are no demonstrable deficits in intellectual abilities; there are no abnormalities of mood, thought, or behavior; there are no untoward effects and, there are no demonstrable dependence or withdrawal syndromes. Effects of acute use in very long-term users appear similar to acute use in occasional users.

Even though earlier studies lacked sufficiently sophisticated methodology and had multiple research deficiencies, results are also consistent with present knowledge. Prior to 1967 when the Center for Studies of Narcotic and Drug Abuse inaugurated its marijuana program the most extensive studies of chronic cannabis use were the Indian Hemp Commission, 1893–1894 (1969) and the LaGuardia Reports (Mayor's Committee on Marijuana, 1944). While these were mainly surveys, the LaGuardia Commission did undertake a clinical study. The subjects were prisoners from New York penitentiaries. The sample consisted of non-users, occasional users, and steady users. It was appreciated at that time that THC was the active component in marijuana but no estimates could be made on the potency of the drug administered. Despite the inadequacies and limitations in the research methodology, Farnsworth (Mayor's Committee on Marijuana, 1973) noted that the results of the report were remarkably consistent with information obtained nearly 30 years later by the National Commission on Marijuana and Drug Abuse (1972).

After reviewing the studies of chronic use, particularly in man, it has been concluded by the present author that at this time there are no cumulative detrimental effects of marijuana use.

ACKNOWLEDGMENT

This work was aided, in part, by a contract to the Department from the New York State Narcotic Addiction Control Commission. The author acknowledges the support and encouragement of Dr. Alfred M. Freedman, New York Medical College, and Dr. Max Fink, SUNY at Stony Brook.

REFERENCES

Abel, E. L. (1971). *Science* **173**, 1038–1040.
Barratt, E., Beaver, W., White, R., Blakeney, P., and Adams, P. (1972). In "Current Research in Marijuana" (M. F. Lewis, ed.), pp. 163–193. Academic Press, New York.
Beaubrun, M. H., and Knight, F. (1973). *Amer. J. Psychiat.* **130**, 309–311.
Bowman, M., and Pihl, R. (1973). *Psychopharmacologia* **29**, 159–170.
Campbell, A. M. G., Evans, M., Thomson, J. G., and Williams, M. J. (1971). *Lancet* **2**, 1219–1226.
Clark, L. D., Hughes, R., and Nakashima, E. N. (1970). *Arch. Gen. Psychiat.* **23**, 193–198.
Commission of Inquiry into the Non-Medical Use of Drugs. (1972). "Cannabis: A Report." Information Canada, Ottawa.
Domino, E. F. (1971). *Ann. N.Y. Acad. Sci.* **191**, 166–191.
Dornbush, R. L. (1974). *Trans. N.Y. Acad. Sci.* [2] **36**, 94–100.
Dornbush, R. L., Fink, M., and Freedman, A. M. (1971). *Amer. J. Psychiat.* **128**, 194–197.
Dornbush, R. L., Clare, G., Zaks, A., Crown, P., Volavka, J., and Fink, M. (1972). In "Current Research in Marijuana" (M. F. Lewis, ed.), pp. 115–128. Academic Press, New York.
Ford R. D. and McMillan, D. E. (1971). *Fed. Proc.* **30**, 279.
Frank, I. M., Epps, L. D., and Rickles, W. (1973). *Psychopharmacol. Bull.* **9**, 28–29.
Grilly, D. M., Ferraro, D. P., and Marriott, R. G. (1973). *Nature (London)* **242**, 119–120.
Hollister, L. E. (1971). *Science* **172**, 21–28.
Indian Hemp Drugs Commission, 1893–1894. (1969). "Marijuana," Report. Thomas Jefferson Press, Silver Springs, Maryland.
Johnson, S., and Domino, E. (1971). *Clin. Pharmacol. Ther.* **12**, 762–768.
Jones, R. T. (1973). In "National Commission on Marijuana and Drug Abuse," Vol. IV, pp. 168–180. US Gov't. Printing Office, Washington, D.C.
Kolansky, H., and Moore, W. T. (1971). *J. Amer. Med. Ass.* **216**, 486–492.
McMillan, D. E., and Dewey, W. L. (1972). In "Current Research in Marijuana" (M. F. Lewis, ed.), pp. 97–114. Academic Press, New York.

McMillan, D. E., Ford, R. D., Frankenheim, J. M., Harris, R. A., and Harris, L. S. (1972). *Arch. Int. Pharmacodyn. Ther.* **198**, 132–144.
Mayor's Committee on Marijuana. (1944). "The Marijuana Problem in the City of New York" (G. B. Wallace, chairman). Jacques Cattell Press, New York (Scarecrow Reprint Corporation, Metuchen, New Jersey, 1973).
National Commission on Marijuana and Drug Abuse. (1972). US Gov't. Printing Office, Washington, D.C.
Soueif, M. I. (1971). *Bull. Narcotics* **23**, 17–28.
Tinklenberg, J., Melges, F., Hollister, L., and Gillespie, H. (1970). *Nature (London)* **226**, 1171–1172.
Tinklenberg, J., Kopell, B., Melges, F., and Hollister, L. (1972). *Arch. Gen. Psychiat.* **27**, 812–815.
Volavka, J., Crown, P., Dornbush, R., Feldstein, S., and Fink, M. (1973). *Psychopharmacologia* **32**, 11–25.
Williams, E. G., Himmelsbach, C. K., Wikler, A., Ruble, D. C., and Lloyd, B. J. (1946). *Pub. Health Rep.* **61**, 1059–1083.

Chapter 10

CANNABIS INTOXICATION: THE ROLE OF PHARMACOLOGICAL AND PSYCHOLOGICAL VARIABLES

HOWARD CAPPELL AND PATRICIA PLINER

I. Introduction 233
II. Recent Evidence 235
   A. History of Cannabis Use 235
   B. Manipulations of Set and Setting 240
   C. Summary 242
III. The Experimental Program 242
   A. Marijuana and Motivation 243
   B. Environmental Influences on Intoxication 250
   C. Two Experiments on the Self-Administration of Marijuana 254
IV. Conclusions 261
   References 263

I. INTRODUCTION

In recent years, there has been a growing accumulation of research into the effects and mechanisms of action of cannabis as pharmacologists, psychologists, biochemists, psychiatrists, and others have applied their skills in response to a clear social demand for knowledge concerning this drug. Our own interests have been focused largely on the determinants and consequences of intoxication in man, with a view to sorting out the contributions of both pharmacological (e.g., dose and potency) and psychological (e.g., motivational set and environmental setting) variables to the experience of intoxication. We have also been interested in the role of history of exposure to cannabis, a variable which incorporates both pharmacological and psychological components.

It is widely accepted that the intoxication produced by a variety of recreationally used drugs is greatly subject to the influence of psychological factors. The reaction of investigators to this fact has been twofold. Some researchers (Weil et al., 1968) have been concerned with controlling for the effects of such variables as the experimental setting in order to get at the "real" pharmacological effects of the drug. At the same time, others (Jones, 1971a,b; Carlin et al., 1972) have shared our interest in *manipulating* psychological variables in an attempt to study their contribution to both subjective and objective aspects of marijuana intoxication. There is no conflict implied here, since it is often the case that what is "noise" for one investigator is a variable of interest to another. A particularly perceptive recognition of the joint contribution (no pun intended) of psychological and pharmacological variables to the experience of marijuana intoxication was elaborated in Becker's (1953) classic paper entitled *Becoming a marijuana user*, for which interviews with users provided the data. Becker presented a detailed analysis of the process by which these two factors may exert a profound influence on the marijuana user during his first contacts with the drug. The object of the analysis was to explain why the novice user usually fails to get "high" at the beginning of his career. The pharmacological consideration was rather mundane; the smoker may fail to become intoxicated because he lacks virtuosity in his smoking technique and fails to smoke "in a way which ensures sufficient dosage to produce real symptoms of intoxication." More interesting in the present context is the idea that even if the novice user ingests a pharmacologically adequate dose, the consequent state may not be experienced subjectively as a "high" because of a failure to recognize the symptoms produced by marijuana or to connect them with consumption of the drug. Thus physiological and psychological actions must coalesce to produce intoxication.

Although Becker's paper was widely read, his hypotheses about the importance of both pharmacological action and socially mediated learning in the marijuana experience had limited influence for the simple reason that experimental research on cannabis was virtually impossible until quite recently. In the absence of experimental data, one could be impressed by the persuasiveness of Becker's analysis, but a substantial empirical validation remained to be attempted. In the last few years, however, it has become increasingly evident that Becker was correct in emphasizing the dual determinants of intoxication by cannabis. The purpose of this chapter is to review recent data bearing on this issue and to present in more detail a series of relevant experiments completed in our own laboratory.

II. RECENT EVIDENCE

There is not an overwhelming amount of evidence to review, but there is certainly enough that a few generalizations are possible. The individual experiments do not fit neatly into categories since almost all involved the simultaneous manipulation of a number of pharmacological and psychological variables. In an attempt at providing some organizational structure to the material, we have grouped the studies into two major categories on the basis of the significant independent variables incorporated in them.

A. History of Cannabis Use

A variable that has received a considerable amount of experimental attention is the history of an individual's exposure to cannabis. The history of use of the drug may account for variation in drug response in two important ways. First, as Becker suggested, the user must go through a *learning process* whereby a set of physical symptoms comes to be recognized as a marijuana "high"; with repeated exposure, the user may become a connoisseur of the intoxicated state and acquire a number of attitudes and expectancies that can influence his future response to the drug. Repeated exposure to the drug provides the opportunity for psychological variables to operate, but at the same time raises the possibility of *tolerance* (Ferraro and Grisham, 1972; Harris *et al.*, 1972) of which an important component may be pharmacological. Without becoming embroiled in the complex argument about the mechanisms that might be operative, and at the risk of some oversimplification, we can say that psychology and pharmacology may act in opposition where use history is concerned. Experience may make a smoker more effective at becoming intoxicated, but at the same time an adaptation to the drug may take place such that its effects on some physiological and behavioral parameters are diminished. Our interest in this area has involved research into the relationship between use history and self-administration of marijuana.

In reviewing these studies, it must be emphasized that comparisons across experiments are difficult to make for all the reasons that this *caveat* generally applies. Moreover, although naive, frequent, and infrequent users have been compared in several studies, there has been no consistency in operationalizing these categories. All the studies have involved male subjects exclusively, and with one exception have used smoking as the route of administration.

1. PHYSIOLOGICAL EFFECTS

Although the learning component of the use history variable may have little to do with the physiological effects of marijuana once the technique of smoking has been mastered, it is nonetheless useful to summarize the relevant findings. The literature is characterized by inconsistencies. In a comparison of frequent and infrequent users, Jones (1971a,b) found that both pulse rate and salivary flow were affected in both groups but significantly less so among frequent users. Meyer et al. (1971) compared a group of frequent smokers quite comparable in use frequency to those of Jones to a group of infrequent users who smoked slightly more often than the ones in Jones' studies. Pulse rate was increased by marijuana in both groups, but not differentially as in Jones' research. In complete contrast to Jones' findings, Weil et al. (1968) observed that heart rate increased significantly *more* in a group of "chronic" users than in a totally naive group. Finally, Casswell and Marks (1972) found no difference at all in the pulse rate response of experienced and naive smokers of cannabis.

Thus, of the three possible outcomes relating physiological response to use history, all have occurred at least once. The probable reasons for the discrepancies are plentiful, since the studies differed considerably in a number of important respects, including drug dose and potency, absolute levels of experience, and instructions to the subjects concerning smoking technique. Thus we are still lacking in persuasive evidence on this issue. Consistent evidence in this area would have provided useful information about pharmacological tolerance in man as opposed to learned adaptation, since it seems unlikely that the latter factor would be generally operative where physiological functions are concerned.

2. EFFECTS ON PERFORMANCE

In this area, the data relating to use frequency are somewhat more uniform. Generally, the performance of infrequent users on simple perceptual-motor tasks has been adversely affected by marijuana while that of frequent users has been less impaired or relatively unchanged. Weil et al. (1968) found that the performance of naive smokers was impaired by marijuana in a Digit Symbol Substitution Task; in contrast, the performance of experienced users actually improved somewhat, resulting in a significant difference between the two groups. Although there were interpretational difficulties with this measure, comparable results were obtained when the task required performance on a pursuit rotor. However, the performance of neither group was affected by the drug on the Continuous Performance Test (CPT), a task requiring sustained attention to visually presented material. A similar pattern of results was obtained by Jones (1971a,b) who found that infrequent smokers exhibited a larger decrement in performance in both Digit Symbol Substitution and Complex Reaction Time than frequent smokers. Meyer *et al.* (1971) obtained an interaction between drug condition and use frequency using the CPT. Infrequent smokers made more errors following active marijuana than placebo, but the performance of frequent users was not affected by the drug. With regard to several other tasks (Hidden Figures, Digit Symbol Substitution, Color-Word Inference, time perception, and pursuit rotor), Meyer *et al.* observed that a "mild degree of impairment" was caused by marijuana regardless of use frequency. They suggested that the impairment was more pronounced among infrequent users, but the differences were not significant. Casswell and Marks (1972) found no difference in the impairment of experienced and naive smokers in a battery of tasks involving attention, memory, and arithmetic skills.

In summary, the preponderance of the data points to a relatively clear conclusion. With a good deal of consistency, it was the case that the significant differences involved an attenuated effect of marijuana in the case of more experienced users. The mechanism responsible for these differences is not clear, since it could involve pharmacological adaptation, behavioral adaptation (learned compensation), or even a combination of the two. It is interesting to note, however, that some of the results are consistent with the claims of some marijuana users that they can function effectively even though intoxicated. Indeed, some of our own data, to be presented later, are consistent with such claims. This of course begs the question of specifying an appropriate behavioral definition of "intoxication."

3. SUBJECTIVE RESPONSES TO ACTIVE DOSES OF CANNABIS

Research into the subjective experience of intoxication is crucial because it is presumably this consequence of marijuana use, and not a collection of behavioral and physiological effects per se, that provides reinforcement for smoking the drug. Although it seems clear that, as Becker hypothesized, use history is a significant variable in this context, it has not operated in a consistent manner. An outcome suggestive of tolerance was obtained by Jones (1971a,b) who asked his subjects to rate their subjective level of intoxication on a 100-point scale 30 minutes after smoking marijuana. Infrequent smokers rated themselves as more intoxicated than frequent users. In contrast, Meyer *et al.* (1971) obtained the opposite result when subjective intoxication was rated 30 minutes after smoking, although there was a nonsignificant reversal 90 minutes after smoking. Subjects in this study also completed the Subjective Drug Effects Questionnaire (SDEQ) developed by Katz and Waskow (Waskow *et al.*, 1970). Although a number of items in this exhaustive scale were sensitive to marijuana, there were no effects attributable to differences in frequency of use.

Weil *et al.* (1968) did not provide an adequate statistical analysis, but they did observe differences in the subjective response of their naive and chronic users of marijuana. All the latter group reported that they became "high," experiencing euphoria, distortion of visual or auditory perception, and confusion. Yet only 1 of 9 naive subjects appeared to enjoy a definite "marihuana reaction." Instead, the naive smokers "reported minimum subjective effects after smoking the drug, or more precisely, few effects like those reported by chronic users." Thus in the Weil *et al.* study, clear subjective effects were evident only among experienced smokers.

Casswell and Marks (1972) found significant, dose-dependent effects of marijuana on subjective level of intoxication, but failed to observe any difference in the response of naive and experienced users. Subjects in this study were also asked to rate themselves on a number of variables intended to measure changes in their state of consciousness. Once more, naive and experienced smokers did not differ in their response to marijuana on these dimensions, although experienced users tended to rate themselves as affected on more dimensions.

Especially when dealing with subjective effects, it is important to distinguish between totally naive subjects and infrequent users, since the former lack training in smoking technique. For example, the observations of Weil *et al.* were in accord with Becker's hypothesis that "the novice does not ordinarily get high the first time he smokes marihuana." Yet Casswell and Marks found comparable subjective effects in their naive and experienced subjects. There are at least two plausible accounts for this discrepancy. First, Casswell and Marks imposed a highly regulated smoking procedure which assured comparatively efficient inhalation whereas Weil *et al.* did not. Additionally, by using a rating scale explicitly mentioning behavioral phenomena often reported by experienced users, Casswell and Marks may have inadvertently sensitized naive users to the kinds of experiences that intoxication purportedly involves.

In the two relevant studies involving non-naive but infrequent smokers, the findings on subjective intoxication were contradictory, since frequent smokers have attained both lower (Jones, 1971a,b) and higher (Meyer et al., 1971) levels of intoxication than their less experienced counterparts. However, unlike some naive subjects, infrequent users in these studies never reported an absolute failure to achieve a "high." There is no ready explanation for this obvious discrepancy. Jones' interpretation of his results was that pharmacological tolerance had developed to THC among frequent users; if this is so, the Meyer et al. results are anomalous to the extent that subjects in the two studies may be compared.

It is interesting to note that within studies there has been relative consistency between the subjective and objective effects of marijuana. In Jones' work, infrequent users were both subjectively and objectively more sensitive to THC than frequent users. While otherwise at odds with Jones' findings, there was internal consistency in the observations by Weil et al. that frequent users were more affected both subjectively and objectively by marijuana. The results of Meyer et al. were somewhat mixed, but on all but subjective scaling of intoxication, frequent and infrequent users responded no differently on other subjective and objective indexes of intoxication. Finally, Casswell and Marks also found consistently equivalent subjective and objective effects comparing naive and experienced users.

4. SUBJECTIVE RESPONSES TO PLACEBOS

The importance of psychological factors in determining the subjective experience of intoxication becomes especially evident when responses to appropriate placebos are considered. The most impressive demonstration was reported by Jones (1971a,b) who found that frequent smokers rated themselves as significantly more "intoxicated" than infrequent smokers after consuming a placebo. Indeed, frequent smokers reported comparable levels of intoxication to both placebo and active marijuana containing 9 mg of tetrahydrocannabinol (THC). It may be recalled that the active dose had somewhat less subjective impact on frequent than infrequent users, leading Jones to postulate that tolerance developed to the subjective component of intoxication produced by active preparations of marijuana. Tolerance is irrelevant in the case of a placebo, but learning is not. Consequently, Jones argued that for frequent users, components of the intoxicated experience were elicited by the placebo through learned associations with such features of marijuana as its taste and smell. With fewer learning opportunities, such associations should be weaker; hence the difference between frequent and infrequent users. Meyer et al. (1971) also obtained data on the subjective intoxication produced by both placebo and active marijuana among frequent and infrequent users, but unlike Jones, found no evidence of differential placebo response between the two groups. Casswell and Marks did not obtain quantitative subjective ratings of intoxication in their experiments but they did report that after placebo, experienced subjects were more affected than their naive counterparts on dimensions of visual imagery, auditory imagery, and thought processes. Again this may reflect differences in conditioning history. Thus there is some evidence that experienced smokers may learn to respond subjectively to preparations of marijuana that are devoid of pharmacological activity.

B. Manipulations of Set and Setting

In a number of experiments, the modulating effect of behavioral set and setting on both subjective and objective components of intoxication has been examined. Again, both psychological and pharmacological factors have emerged as significant variables. In the most extensive of these investigations, Carlin *et al.* (1972) manipulated the response set of their subjects (a) by providing social influence in the form of an experimental confederate programmed to act either intoxicated or not and (b) by giving subjects a placebo pill with the instructions that it would potentiate or attenuate the effects of marijuana. These manipulations were applied in a mutually reinforcing manner such that subjects in an "up" condition were exposed to an "intoxicated" confederate and a "potentiating" pill while subjects in a "down" condition shared their experience with an "unintoxicated" confederate and took an "attenuating" pill. Within each of these conditions subjects smoked a placebo or marijuana cigarette calibrated to contain 15 mg of THC. Although marijuana had rather clear effects on subjective intoxication, ratings of potency, and a number of performance measures, there were no observable consequences of the manipulation of psychological set. Carlin *et al.* speculated that the failure of their manipulation was the result of the comparatively high dose of THC and proceeded with a very similar experiment which included an additional condition in which subjects were given marijuana containing only 7.5 mg of THC. As in the first experiment, the manipulation of set had no effect on ratings of potency of the marijuana or of subjective intoxication. Interestingly, there was no graded effect of dose on these measures, suggesting that they may have simply been insensitive. The set variable did, however, affect behavior in a number of the performance tasks and was particularly evident in the Hidden Figures Test. When subjects received the 7.5 mg dose and were exposed to a set that favored unintoxicated behavior, they performed as though they were not intoxicated, i.e., as well as subjects who smoked placebo and better than those who received either dose of active marijuana in the other conditions. When subjects smoked the 15 mg dose, however, the manipulation of set was without effect; in both the "up" and "down" conditions, performance was simply impaired relative to placebo subjects. The pattern of results was repeated in a Digit Symbol Substitution Test and in somewhat weaker form in a Color Naming Task.

In summary, Carlin et al. clearly demonstrated that a behavioral set could offset "intoxication," at least when the dose was comparatively low. The fact that the effect was restricted to the lower dose demonstrates that both behavioral and the pharmacological considerations were important. It was particularly interesting that the effect of set was not apparent in the subjective measurements, since a priori one might expect subjective state to be even more prone to behavioral manipulation than performance in a task. This outcome does not accord with some of our own results, as will be seen later.

One relevant experiment is distinguished from the others discussed here in that an oral cannabis preparation was used. In this study, Waskow et al. (1970) manipulated the psychological environment by having subjects experience the effects of placebo or active THC in the presence or absence of recorded music. In general, THC produced ratings on the SDEQ indicative of somatic discomfort. With one of the scales (Scale 3: tense and unsteady with less control of the body) there was a significant interaction such that a drug–placebo difference was evident only in the presence of music. Somewhat surprisingly, marijuana also produced feelings of relaxation and well-being in addition to discomfort. Once more, this effect was most pronounced when music was played, but the difference was not statistically significant. In two measures of performance drawn from the Mental Control section of the Wechsler Memory Scale, significant differences between drug and placebo were observed such that performance improved under placebo and deteriorated following THC. Although the drug and music interaction did not attain conventional levels of significance, the author noted that "these effects were especially marked in the music condition." In yet another instance then, there was an interaction between a behavioral and a pharmacological manipulation.

Finally, a setting variable was incorporated into a segment of Jones' extensive work. In this segment of the research, subjects smoked marijuana on two occasions separated by a week. During one session the subjects smoked in a freely interacting group of 5 and during the other they smoked in isolation. In keeping with Jones' expectations, ratings on the SDEQ were substantially different in the two settings. Subjects who smoked alone reported significantly less euphoria, perceptual change, and thinking change than when they smoked in the group. Unfortunately, the absence of placebo controls renders this outcome equivocal, since the results might well have reflected a main effect of the group, independent of intoxication.

To summarize, it seems clear that intoxicated behavior is significantly influenced by environmental variables. Moreover, this influence appears not to be confined to subjective response alone, but can modify performance as well.

C. Summary

Notwithstanding the inconsistencies in the literature, some generalizations appear to emerge. Although the direction of its effects is not entirely uniform, cannabis use history does seem to be a significant variable. The most regularity was evident in tests of performance; when use history made any difference, it appeared to mitigate the effects of the drug. However, the question of mechanism remains open. The differences could reflect behavioral compensation, pharmacological tolerance, or both. Through the variable of use frequency the potential importance of learning was manifested. In two studies, there was evidence that a marijuana placebo could actually elicit a marijuana-like subjective response among frequent users. Additionally, there was quite persuasive evidence that both subjective and objective consequences of marijuana were subject to modulation by the psychological variables of instructional set and social setting, at least within limits. A limiting factor appeared to be pharmacological, since Carlin *et al.* found that pharmacological considerations were paramount at a relatively high dose* of THC.

III. THE EXPERIMENTAL PROGRAM

Research into the effects of marijuana in man has been in progress in our laboratory since late in 1970. Several experimental issues have been addressed:

(a) To what extent can individuals voluntarily offset the effects of marijuana on performance?

---

* It is evident that we have not mentioned the doses of marijuana used in most of the experiments reviewed. This stems not from a lack of concern about dose, but from the belief that this information is limited in its usefulness because of the absence of standardized procedures of administration. Thus we hesitate to invite comparisons among the essentially noncomparable doses used in the various studies.

(b) To what extent does the psychological environment modulate subjective response to marijuana? If such a phenomenon occurs, is it, as Carlin *et al.* found, dose-dependent?

(c) Our most significant interest has been in the variables controlling the self-administration of marijuana. Can subjects titrate their intake according to potency in seeking to achieve a constant subjective effect? Is there such a thing as a social dose? Does a history of frequent exposure to THC lead to an escalation in the amount required to achieve an acceptable subjective state? To what extent is self-administration subject to cognitive effects?

A. Marijuana and Motivation

Among the claims of many users of marijuana (cf. Tart, 1971) is that it is possible to exert volitional control over intoxication level in both the "up" and "down" directions. Indeed, this can be postulated as one of the mechanisms whereby the variable of use frequency operates to modulate the effects of cannabis. However, we have only self-report data (Tart, 1971) that changes in the quality of intoxication, and in particular *performance* changes, can be self-controlled in the intoxicated state. Our first hint of the possibility of such a phenomenon came from two experiments designed simply to provide a comparison of the effects of alcohol and marijuana on a behavior involving temporal control of responding (Cappell *et al.*, 1972). The major behavioral task involved a drl (differential reinforcement of low rate of responding) schedule in which subjects were required to space key-presses at particular temporal intervals in order to receive a small monetary reinforcement. Subjects became quite proficient at this task by the second of their three training sessions. The interesting result occurred when the "placebo effects" of alcohol and marijuana were compared. Table I describes the performance of the subjects on their final training session and when they were tested with an

TABLE I

Percent of Reinforcements Obtained following Alcohol and Marijuana Placebos

	Experimental condition	
Drug condition	Final training session	Placebo
Alcohol	54.5	54.1
Marijuana	55.6	64.6

alcohol or marijuana placebo. Responses could occur prematurely, late, or on schedule; only the latter responses were reinforced. There was no difference in performance from the last training session to the placebo session in the alcohol experiment; in both instances subjects were reinforced for approximately 54% of their responses. However, when placebo marijuana was smoked, there was a 9% increase over the training baseline in the number of reinforcements obtained. Thus subjects did significantly *better* ($p < 0.01$) after the placebo than in the final training session, even though performance had stabilized by the next-to-last training session. There was no question that subjects in the alcohol and marijuana experiments were evenly matched, since performance during the final training session was quite similar in both experiments. As far as the actual drug effects were concerned, doses of alcohol up to 0.96 gm/kg had no effect, but marijuana in doses up to 16 mg of THC per subject reduced the number of reinforcements earned. The different placebo effects suggested the possibility that different sets of motivational dispositions were engaged by alcohol and marijuana. Perhaps as some researchers have suggested (Crancer *et al.*, 1969) the subjects may have been predisposed to show that marijuana is innocuous. Consequently they may have been challenged to exert sufficient extra effort after smoking such that when placebo was administered, this motivational boost resulted in better than "normal" performance. If the subjects had no special axe to grind where alcohol was concerned, they would not invest the same effort in the task.

However, in the absence of research explicitly designed to manipulate this variable we could only speculate on the role of volition in altering the effects of marijuana on performance. The issue justified further experimental work for a number of reasons:

(a) From a purely practical standpoint, there is the question of whether intoxicated individuals can compensate for the impairment of performance that marijuana clearly produces. Whether or not subjects can exert self-control over intoxicated behavior has obvious implications for the issue of traffic safety, which has been of major public concern in connection with marijuana; indeed, a number of subjects passing through our laboratory have proudly claimed to be exemplary drivers while "high."

(b) It has been conjectured (Crancer *et al.*, 1969) that marijuana users may be biased to make the drug appear relatively innocuous, presumably by volitionally overcoming its effects in experiments. If this is generally true, and we have already cited some evidence consistent with this possibility, much behavioral work with human subjects would be suspect.

(c) Independent of the practical and methodological concerns, an examination of subjects' ability to exert volitional control over drug-induced disturbance is scientifically intriguing in its own right.

Our strategy (Cappell and Pliner, 1973) was to address the issue with a rather straightforward experiment in which motivation was directly manipulated. The subjects were 20 males, all who claimed to be experienced users of marijuana. They were recruited in order to "study some behavioral effects of marihuana." On arrival at the laboratory, a subject was briefed about the experimental procedures. A 30 second sample of pulse rate was then obtained, followed by four behavioral tests. In a time estimation task, subjects were asked to estimate the duration of 9 passages of recorded music. Next came a memory task consisting of two lists of 40 words presented aurally via recordings. This was followed by a series of arithmetic problems and a task which required subjects to recall lists of digits in reverse order of their presentation. Pulse rate was again measured after completion of the reverse digits task. Although the content and order of the tasks were uniform across subjects, no individual subject was exposed more than once to a specific content or order of presentation of material on more than one trial within a task. This testing procedure took about 40 minutes to complete.

When the tasks were completed, a subject smoked a single 1 gm marijuana cigarette or a marijuana placebo. An experimenter supervised the smoking to ensure that the material was properly consumed. The instructions were to smoke the cigarette down to a line drawn 10 mm from the end of the 70 mm cigarette. The marijuana preparation contained 12 mg of Δ^9-tetrahydrocannabinol (THC) and the placebo was an equivalent amount of marijuana from which the THC and other cannabinoids had been exhaustively extracted. The dose was chosen as one that would be likely to affect the behaviors under investigation. Although a full dose-response study would have added useful parametric information, the single-dose study was justifiable on the grounds that we had the limited goal of demonstrating volitional control *in principle*. A total of approximately 15 minutes was allowed for smoking. After finishing a cigarette, the subject was asked to rate his level of intoxication on a 200-point scale anchored at 0 (not at all intoxicated) through 100 (the highest you have ever been) to 200 (unlabelled). A second pulse rate sample was then taken.

Following the pulse rate sample, the major experimental manipulation was introduced in the form of instructions. The 10 subjects in the High Motivation condition were told:

> Before we repeat the tasks, there are a few things I would like to mention. It has been our experience that marihuana can have a detrimental effect on the efficiency of performance on tasks like the ones we are using. What we are

particularly interested in in this experiment is whether subjects can overcome these detrimental effects. Therefore, what I would like you to do is try as much as you are able, using whatever methods are best for you, to overcome the interfering effect of the drug. We are interested in any mental exertion you can put forth, but no physical exertion like running on the spot or pinching yourself. I'd like to mention one more thing. For experimental reasons, the other experimenter doesn't know the purpose of experiment. For this reason, I'll ask that you don't ask her any questions about the experiment, unless of course, you have any questions specifically related to the tasks. If any other questions arise, you can ask me at the end. Is everything clear?

Subjects in the Low Motivation condition were simply told: "Now we are going to repeat the tasks again. Is everything clear?" These instructions were delivered in both drug and placebo sessions.

Once the instructions had been delivered, the four behavioral tests were repeated in the same order as before. Alternate forms of the tasks were used in order not to repeat material presented earlier. When the tasks were completed, intoxication was rated for a second time and a final pulse sample was obtained.

Each subject served twice in the same motivational condition, once in a placebo session and once in an active drug session. Within each motivational condition, equal numbers of subjects were tested in the placebo–drug and drug–placebo orders. The behavioral tests and pulse determinations were supervised by a nurse who was blind to drug condition, motivational condition, and to the purpose of the experiment generally. Smoking was supervised by a second experimenter who was blind to drug dose. At the end of the second session, each subject was asked "Did you make any special effort to overcome the effects of the drug on your performance?" Responses were recorded on a scale ranging from 0 ("no effort at all") to 100 ("a great deal of effort").

In evaluating the results, the first order of business was to check the effectiveness of the manipulation of motivation. The effort ratings are shown in Table II. The only significant effect was that of motivational condition ($p < 0.001$); thus the instructions had the intended effect on effort expended.

Marijuana failed to have any effect on performance in either the arithmetic or reverse digits tasks. Therefore, the test of the ability to "come down" from the drug was confined to behaviors for which drug consumption had reliable consequences. Figure 1 illustrates the results of the time estimation task. The scores represent changes in time estimation from pre- to postsmoking determinations. Discrepancies for each of the 9 determinations were simply summed to provide the unit of analysis. It is clear that in the high motivation condition, drug and placebo effects were

TABLE II

Mean Self-Ratings of Effort to Overcome Drug Effects[a,b]

Drug condition	Motivational condition	
	Low	High
Placebo	29.6	75.8
Active marijuana	28.1	74.8

[a] All but 3 subjects gave identical ratings for placebo and marijuana sessions.
[b] From Cappell and Pliner (1973). Copyright by the American Psychological Association, 1973. Reprinted with permission.

quite similar ($p > 0.20$), but there was a significant drug-induced increase in time estimates in the low motivation condition ($p < 0.001$). The direction of this effect was in keeping with expectation (Cappell *et al.*, 1972). High and low motivation discrepancies in estimate did not differ when placebo was smoked, but the increase in time estimation was greater in the low than in the high motivation condition following active marijuana ($p < 0.001$). Thus it was fairly evident on this task that sub-

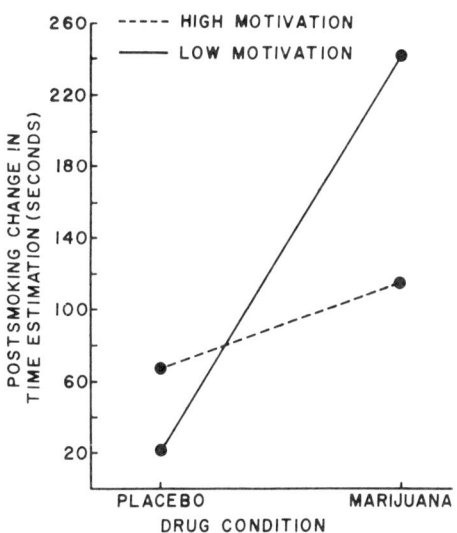

Fig. 1. Mean discrepancies in time estimates from pre- to postsmoking determinations. (From Cappell and Pliner, 1973.) Copyright by the American Psychological Association, 1973. Reprinted with permission.

jects could volitionally control an effect of marijuana on performance. That this ability was task specific is illustrated in Fig. 2. There was a

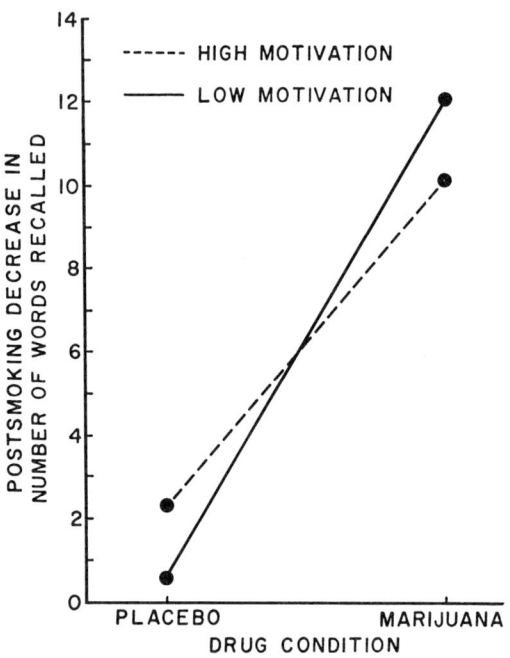

Fig. 2. Mean discrepancies in number of words recalled before and after smoking. (From Cappell and Pliner, 1973.) Copyright by the American Psychological Association, 1973. Reprinted with permission.

significant drug effect ($p < 0.01$) since marijuana impaired recall of words. However, the motivational manipulation had no modulating effect on drug-induced impairment. A similar result was obtained when subjective intoxication was the dependent variable. Table III contains the mean self-ratings of intoxication and changes in these ratings. Marijuana clearly produced greater subjective intoxication than placebo ($p < 0.01$), and intoxication waned from the postsmoking to the postexperimental measure ($p < 0.01$). However, the motivational condition had no effect on subjective ratings.

In summary, our data lent some support to the claim that individuals can voluntarily "come down" from a marijuana "high." However, this ability was restricted to the time estimation task and was not at all evident in the memory task. In the former case, motivation completely overrode the "normal" effect of marijuana, which is to increase estimates of

TABLE III

Mean Self-Ratings of Intoxication[a]

		Motivational condition	
Drug condition	Time of rating	Low	High
Placebo	Postsmoking	38.0	52.8
	Postexperiment	24.5	35.0
	D	13.5	17.8
Active marijuana	Postsmoking	68.2	71.5
	Postexperiment	62.7	58.4
	D	5.5	13.1

[a] From Cappell and Pliner (1973). Copyright by the American Psychological Association, 1973. Reprinted with permission.

elapsed time. In the latter, the normal effect on memory, which is impairment, was unaffected. Since little is known of the mechanisms which may mediate the various behavioral effects of marijuana, we can only speculate on the discrepancy in outcomes with the different tasks. One possibility is that the memory task was in some sense more difficult than time estimation, and that consequently the naturally impairing effect of the drug could not be overcome as readily. Relevant to this suggestion is the interesting hypothesis of Ferraro and Grilly (1973), which was developed in the course of studying tolerance to THC. Using chimpanzees as subjects, they failed to find evidence of tolerance in a task involving a memory component, although tolerance has been shown using other behaviors (Ferraro and Grisham, 1972). Because of the consistency with which THC disrupts memory in man and other primates, they conjectured that tolerance failed to develop because of a lack of "compensatory responses" where memory is concerned. Perhaps then it is the case that time distortion is more easily compensated for than memory distortion. However, this hypothesis is totally speculative, since we cannot specify the nature of "compensatory responses." We are thus left with some challenging data in search of a mechanistic explanation.

One of our expectations was not fulfilled when the manipulation of motivation failed to affect the subjective report of intoxication. The surprise was due to the fact that subjects in previous studies often complained that having to perform was adversely affecting their "high." Perhaps such an effect was maximal even in the low motivation condition, but it is interesting that there was no subjective consequence of the motivational manipulation even though there was a clear objective consequence. However, this is certainly not the first instance of a discrepancy in outcomes using subjective and performance indices of intoxication (cf. Carlin et al., 1972).

What can we conclude from these data? One thing which seems clear is that subjects are *capable* of controlling their intoxicated behavior to some extent; at the same time, the implication of the drl experiment notwithstanding, it seems that subjects are not likely to purposely distort the outcome of an investigation in order to present a particular (i.e., favorable) impression of marijuana use. Only when specifically instructed to do so did they demonstrate such a capability. Moreover, the capability was task specific. Finally, although we now know that volitional control of marijuana intoxication is possible *in principle,* it will take further experimental tests to determine whether this control applies to such vital everyday behavior as driving an automobile.

B. Environmental Influences on Intoxication

It is by now a cliché to say that the effect of a psychoactive drug may be greatly influenced by the setting in which it is consumed. Particular cognizance of this fact has been taken where marijuana is concerned. For instance, Weil *et al.* (1968) went to some lengths to maintain a "neutral" laboratory setting in their work on the grounds that previous researchers had "succumbed to the temptation to have subjects take drugs in 'psychedelic' environments." When their work was published, this concern was based more on conjecture than empirical observation. More recently, however, evidence has accumulated to suggest a drug–environment interaction in the case of THC (Carlin *et al.*, 1972; Jones, 1971a,b). Our specific interest was to test derivations having Schachter's (Schachter and Singer, 1962) theory of emotion as their origin. Although the theory was designed to make predictions about the relationship between autonomic arousal and the cognitive determination of the quality of emotional experience, it can be readily generalized to yield predictions about the environmental modulation of drug effects. Essentially, Schachter's theory predicts that cognitive cues will determine the quality of an emotion, but only to the extent that autonomic arousal is present. Our derivation was that the sensory environment would influence the degree of subjectively experienced marijuana intoxication, but only to the extent that a pharmacologically active substance was administered. To test this derivation, one group of subjects was observed in a "neutral" environment and another in a "psychedelic" environment.

Subjects were invited to the laboratory on the pretext of participating

10. Cannabis Intoxication

in an experiment on some biochemical effects of marijuana. All accepted the explanation without question. The pretext was supported by collecting urine samples at various stages of the experiment. The basic manipulation consisted of varying the environmental setting in which the drug effects were experienced. Twelve male subjects were exposed to a "neutral" environment and 12 to a "psychedelic" environment. Subjects returned at weekly intervals until they had smoked a placebo and three different doses of THC, always in the same environment. The doses were 0 (placebo), 4, 8, and 16 mg per subject, available as two 1 gm cigarettes of equal potency. A Latin Square design was employed to control for order effects. As in all of our research, the subjects were experienced with marijuana.

Prior to smoking on the first visit, the ostensible purpose of the experiment was explained. Subjects were informed in advance about what the session would be like. Thus those in the psychedelic environment knew that they would be able to listen to music, be free to move about in the room, etc., in advance of the actual application of the manipulation. Similarly, those to be exposed to the neutral environment had advance knowledge of the comparative lack of stimulation that they could expect. However, no subject knew that there was an environment other than the one to which he was to be exposed.

The site for both environments was a spacious, carpeted room located in a laboratory suite. When decorated as the psychedelic environment the room was furnished with several brightly colored posters, a mobile suspended from the ceiling, and a bright Indian style rug draped over a psychiatrist's sofa. On one side of the room was a table on which were a game requiring motor coordination in guiding a marble through a number of hazards, reading material, a kaleidoscope, a prism, playing cards, and some candy. A ring toss game was on the floor nearby. The subjects could choose from a wide variety of musical selections played on a tape recorder which they were taught to operate; when functioning, the tape recorder controlled a multicolored "light show" which pulsed in sympathy with the frequency and intensity of the music. Throughout the session the room was comparatively dark, illuminated only by a shaded 60 W lamp located in one corner. Thirty-five minutes into the session, a nurse entered. She remained for the remaining 10 minutes of the 45 minute exposure in the environment and engaged in small talk with the subject if he chose to do so.

When the room served as a neutral environment, most of the above mentioned items were removed. All that remained were the comfortable upholstered chair in which the subject was required to remain, some reading material, a table, and the psychiatrist's couch, unadorned. The subject remained seated for 45 minutes after which time the nurse entered.

Prior to being issued their cigarettes, subjects in the neutral environment were told: "You should remain seated, but you may read if you wish. It has been found that activity and excessive stimulation affect some of the biochemical indices we are monitoring, so in order that our measurements not be disturbed, we must restrict your behavior." In contrast, subjects in the psychedelic environment were told: "We thought the experiment would be more meaningful if we simulated, as best we can, the way people normally experience the effects of marijuana. For this reason there will be several activities available to you."

Prior to introducing the environmental manipulation, each subject was given two cigarettes to be consumed over a 20 minute period. Within this restriction, subjects could smoke at their own rate. During smoking, normal room illumination was maintained and all subjects were required to remain seated. The paraphernalia of the psychedelic environment were present during smoking but inoperative. All subjects smoked in isolation. Exposure to the different environments lasted for 45 minutes after the completion of smoking.

The basic dependent variable was the self-rating of intoxication obtained using the 200-point scale described earlier. It was administered once immediately after smoking and again right after the 45 minute period of exposure to the environment.

Our first test of the hypothesis was based on the second self-rating of intoxication. To review the hypothesis, as was predicted that the environment would affect intoxication only to the extent that an active drug (i.e., not placebo) was smoked. At a first inspection the pattern of the data generally conformed with our expectation. Intoxication ratings were quite similar at the placebo dose, but higher in the psychedelic than in the neutral environment when active marijuana was consumed. Regrettably, our pleasure on first viewing the results was not sustained by the statistical analysis, which revealed significance of neither the main effect of Environment nor of an Environment × Dose interaction. However, an inspection of the raw data suggested that statistically stronger results might be obtained by constructing an index based on the ratings taken both before (Intox 1) and after (Intox 2) exposure to the environments. The index was calculated as (Intox 2 − Intox 1)/Intox 1 and multiplied by 100 to provide a percentage change score. This index adjusts somewhat for the individual differences, which were considerable, in the use of the rating scale. The product of this analysis is shown in Fig. 3. Following the placebo treatment, intoxication ratings fell regardless of the

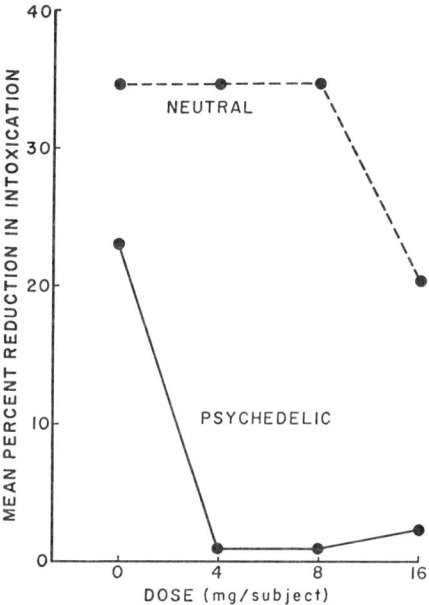

Fig. 3. Mean reduction in self-rated intoxication.

environment, reflecting a loss of "intoxication" with the passage of time. Although the drop was somewhat greater in the neutral environment, the changes in the two environments did not differ significantly. At all the active dose levels, there was virtually no change in intoxication during 45 minutes of exposure to the psychedelic environment, but a reduction occurred at all doses when the environment was neutral. The differences between experimental conditions were significant ($p < 0.02$ in each case) at the 4 and 8 mg doses, but not at the 16 mg dose.

Thus we were able to provide some support for our derivations from Schachter's theory, albeit only after an internal analysis of the data. As predicted, the environmental manipulation was without effect when placebo was administered, and enhanced the level of intoxication at the two lowest active doses. However, the manipulation was comparatively ineffective at the highest dose. This latter finding, although unanticipated, has interesting parallels in both drug and nondrug contexts. Carlin et al. (1972) found significant effects of their social manipulation only when they administered a comparatively low dose (7.5 mg of THC per subject); when the dose was high (15 mg per subject), the drug effect "clearly overwhelmed the effects of the social manipulation." Analogous results have been reported by Nisbett and Schachter (1966) in an experiment in which emotion was cognitively manipulated. They were able to alter the experience of emotion cognitively when they produced a relatively modest state of physiological arousal (induced by electric shock), but cognitive effects were absent when a high level of arousal was produced. Thus in general it appears that strong physiological states are less subject to cognitive manipulation than weak ones. Such an hypothesis is also implicit in Jones' (1971a,b) theorizing about the psychosocial determinants of marijuana intoxication.

C. Two Experiments on the Self-Administration of Marijuana

By now it should be clear that the pharmacological effects of administered doses of marijuana are quite subject to modification by variables which are traditionally outside the realm of pharmacology per se. This point has been strongly emphasized by Jones in his research. Indeed, he (Jones, 1971a) went as far as asserting that much of the existing behavioral research on THC in man may be "irrelevant" because the importance of psychosocial variables has not been sufficiently recognized. Jones' concern was based on the suspicion that researchers have tended to use doses of THC which are probably much larger than those used in "real life." One of his more intriguing findings was that many subjects rated their level of intoxication quite similarly whether they smoked placebo or a fixed dose of active material. Such a result calls into question the very role of a fundamental feature of marijuana, namely, its potency, in determining its intoxicating effects. Jones ultimately concluded that socially relevant doses of marijuana are drawn from the low end of the range, since these were sufficient to produce intoxicated behavior. One of the limits of Jones' research was that marijuana of only a single potency was made available to his volunteers. This could well have acted as an artificial constraint on the total doses that subjects self-administered.* Thus in the context of an experiment on titration of intake, we first attempted to determine the contribution of the potency of marijuana to its self-administration (Cappell et al., 1973). Our reasoning was that good titration would provide evidence of the ability to respond to the crucial variable of potency. On the other hand, relatively poor titration would suggest a lesser role for strictly pharmacological activity as a determinant of the amount consumed during social use of marijuana. The Canadian report of the Commission of Inquiry into the Non-Medical

---

* This was not an explicit experiment on self-administration. Subjects were issued cigarettes which were standard in size and concentration of THC, but there were few if any constraints on how they were to consume the drug.

Use of Drugs (1972) simply stated that "great variations in the potency of different samples are usually accommodated by the experienced user through a 'titration' of dose (intake is reduced or stopped when the smoker reaches a preferred level of intoxication)." However, no data were offered in support of this assertion. In this experiment we were also interested in the objective consequences of subjectively "relevant" doses. To this end, a number of behavioral and physiological tests were included.

The experiment consisted of 5 sessions spaced at weekly intervals. Except for the first, each session involved exposure to a battery of tests, a smoking period, and a repetition of the test battery. In Session 1 subjects were familiarized with the tests and procedures but did not smoke. Session 2 was a "standardization" session during which all subjects were exposed to material of the same concentration of THC (0.4%). This provided a reference point against which the 12 subjects were to titrate intake on subsequent occasions. In a Latin Square design, each subject smoked marijuana in concentrations of 0.2, 0.4, or 0.8% on the 3 remaining sessions. The subjects were not aware of the fact that titration was the major interest; they were led to believe that the sole purpose of the study was to examine various behavioral and physiological effects of marijuana. When issued their cigarettes, the subjects were in all cases simply asked to smoke until they reached an "optimal" high. They were explicitly told to use their experience of Session 2, on which they had been asked to achieve this level with the 0.4% potency. All cigarettes contained a total of 1 gm of material and were issued one at a time on demand. It was stressed that subjects were to smoke at their own rate and that they were not to consume more than necessary to achieve the specified level of "high," even if this meant discarding a portion of a cigarette. An observer recorded the details of smoking behavior using a polygraph and collected the noncombusted residue once the subjects had attained the intoxication criterion. All the subjects, it should be added, claimed to be experienced users of marijuana.

The data describing smoking behavior are shown in Table IV. None of the indices of consumption were significantly related to drug concentration save the estimated weight of material consumed. This quantity was determined by weighing the noncombusted residues of smoked cigarettes on a scale sensitive to variations as low as 0.01 gm and then subtracting this amount from the total given to the subject. The amount consumed was inversely related to potency ($p < 0.001$). The increase in the estimated weight of material consumed from the highest to the lowest potency was approximately 36%. Subjects accurately discriminated the

TABLE IV

Means of Marijuana Consumption Indices in the First Experiment on Self-Administration[a]

Index	Standard (0.4%)	THC concentration		
		0.2%	0.4%	0.8%
Total time with smoke in lungs (seconds)	325.15	356.95	320.70	284.81
Number of puffs	43.08	53.33	40.50	39.58
Mean duration of puff (seconds)	8.25	7.25	8.95	8.26
Mean interval between puffs (seconds)	20.48	20.17	20.32	20.62
Estimated weight of material consumed (gm)	1.47	1.88	1.50	1.38
Potency rating (100-point scale)	56.33	44.50	58.16	66.40

[a] From Cappell et al. (1973). Reprinted with permission.

various potencies, as the significant ($p < 0.001$) linear relationship between actual and rated potency attested.

The major question of this experiment was: To what extent can subjects titrate intake in pursuit of an "optimal" high? A decision on this issue must ultimately involve a judgment, since statistical analysis offers only a limited guide here. Though somewhat consistent with such a process, the quantitative indices offered far from compelling evidence that the subjects were generally capable of effective titration. Even though the potency of the weakest and strongest material varied by a factor of 4, the mean consumption of the least potent material exceeded that of the most potent by only 36%. Given the reasonable assumption that the proportion of THC delivered was independent of potency (Johnson and Domino, 1971), the weight index indicated that the effective dose delivered by the high potency material was approximately three times that of low potency marijuana. That the effective dose was higher as concentration increased was independently confirmed in the behavioral and physiological data. Without going into detail, Table V gives an idea of the behavioral and physiological effects of the self-administered doses. In the case of reaction time, pulse rate, and diastolic blood pressure, the effects increased significantly as a function of concentration. Nonetheless, the subjects equated these varying doses on the subjective dimension which is presumably one of the significant regulators of intake, namely, the ability of a particular quantity of drug to produce a desired level of "high."

It appeared from the first experiment that even experienced users of marijuana were relatively insensitive to the potency of marijuana in regulating their intake to achieve a subjective effect. However, there

TABLE V

Summary of Major Effects of Marijuana on Behavioral
and Physiological Indices in the First Experiment
on Self-Administration[a]

Index	Drug effect	p value
Pursuit rotor	Impairment	<0.01
Reaction time	Impairment	<0.05
Recognition	Impairment	<0.01
Recall	Impairment	<0.01
Pulse rate	Increase	<0.001
Conjunctival injection	Increase	<0.01
Diastolic blood pressure	Increase	<0.05

[a] From Cappell et al. (1973). Reprinted with permission.

were a few methodological limitations of the first experiment which could have influenced the outcome. Possibly, titration would have been more effective if a different range of potencies had been sampled. However, a limitation that we found more compelling was the possibility that there might be an essentially learned constraint on titration as a result of a tendency among some subjects to consume all of a cigarette once it was begun. The development and frequent use of devices such as "roach holders" to obviate the waste of material attests to the strength of this habit. Moreover, a number of subjects commented that a frequently observed "stop" mechanism for regulating intake of cannabis socially was indeed the efficient completion of all prepared material. If such a tendency exists, it would obviously interefere with pharmacologically based intake regulation. Thus in a subsequent study, we attempted to examine this issue by varying the fineness of the units of consumption in the form of cigarettes of different size. Just as a more finely calibrated ruler produces more accurate estimates of length, the smaller the unit, the smaller should be the error contributed by a tendency to complete all of a cigarette once it has been started. To further explore the importance of drug potency, the potency range was extended to include material roughly twice as strong as the most potent of the first experiment.

Methodological improvements were, however, not the sole aim of the additional research. A controversial issue in the marijuana literature (cf. Nahas, 1973) involves the extent to which a high level of exposure to marijuana results in tolerance to the reinforcing effects of the drug, with the consequence of an escalation in consumption to achieve the same effects. Nahas has simply asserted that this is the case, saying that "tolerance to cannabis gives a physiologic basis to the necessity for the frequent smoker to increase dosage, or to use more potent psychotropic drugs such as other hallucinogens or the opiates." One of the important bits of evidence cited in favor of this argument was that frequent users of marijuana in Jones' experiments reported a lower level of intoxication to a fixed dose of marijuana than did a group of infrequent users. That tolerance may develop to some of the effects of marijuana is not in dispute here. What is in dispute is the drawing of inferences about *self-administration* in the absence of data from an experiment in which this is the dependent variable.

In this experiment[*] we opted for a $2 \times 2 \times 3$ factorial design in which a subject served only once in a given treatment combination. The observational procedures and instructions were quite like those of the original experiment, except that subjects were asked to achieve a "nice high" rather than an "optimal" one. Cigarette size was varied by including "joints" containing either 500 or 1000 mg of material. The length of the smaller cigarettes was 45 mm compared to 70 mm for the larger ones. The THC concentrations were 0.36, 0.73, and 1.45%. Subjects were selected on the basis of their self-reported use of marijuana during the period covering at least 6 months preceding their appointment. The self-reported use frequency of the group of 30 frequent users averaged 18.2 cigarettes per week (range 9 to 35 per week), while the use frequency of the 30 infrequent users averaged only 2.3 cigarettes per month (range 0.25 to 6 per month). Five subjects were assigned to each of the 12 cells generated by the design. Pulse rate was obtained to provide an objective index of the drug's effect. This was measured at rest, when a subject reported experiencing the first symptoms of intoxication, and finally when the criterion of intoxication was reached.

The amounts of marijuana consumed, expressed as milligrams of total material per kilogram of body weight, are contained in Table VI. As in the previous experiment, the total material consumed increased significantly as its potency decreased ($p < 0.001$); the means for the high, medium, and low concentrations were 13.34, 15.57, and 21.36 mg/kg, respectively. Subjects issued large cigarettes consumed 19.16 mg/kg compared to 14.34 mg/kg for those issued small cigarettes ($p < 0.005$). However, the 17.53 mg/kg consumed by frequent users did not differ significantly ($F < 1.00$) from the 15.97 mg/kg required by infrequent users. There was no tendency for titration to vary depending on the size of cigarettes; the interaction between the variables, concentration and cigarette size, was trivial ($F < 1.00$). When self-ratings of intoxication were

---

[*] Cappell, H., and Pliner, P. (1973). Regulation of the Self-Administration of Marihuana by Psychological and Pharmacological Variables. Unpublished manuscript.

TABLE VI

Amount of Marijuana Consumed (mg/kg) in the Second Experiment on Self-Administration

Cigarette size	Frequent users			Infrequent users		
	0.36%	0.73%	1.45%	0.36%	0.73%	1.45%
Large	25.49	16.80	18.08	23.98	16.27	14.33
Small	17.08	18.29	9.45	18.87	10.89	11.47

analyzed, it was the case that ratings increased significantly as a function of drug potency. This was most likely the result of the actual *dose* consumed increasing sharply as a function of potency. This finding was potentially embarrassing, since it suggested that subjects smoking cigarettes of different potency did not achieve comparable levels of intoxication as demanded by the instructions. Happily, this was not a serious problem; when self-rating of intoxication was held constant in a covariance analysis, the direction and magnitude of all the experimental effects remained unchanged.

The index of the objective effect of the self-administered doses was pulse rate. As shown in Fig. 4, marijuana exerted its usual effect of in-

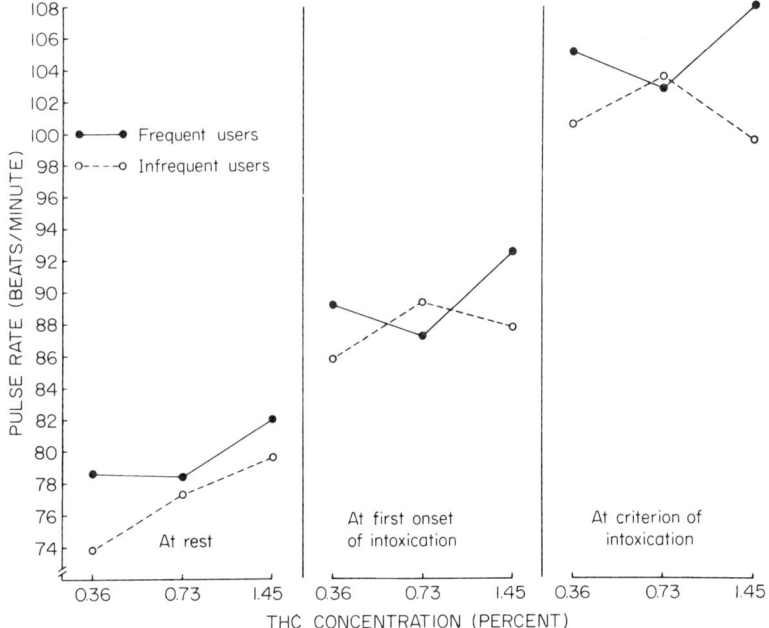

Fig. 4. Effects of self-administered marijuana on pulse rate.

creasing pulse rate. Most important, however, was the fact that pulse rates of frequent and infrequent users did not differ in response to the drug.

For a second time then, we were able to show statistically reliable titration of intake according to potency. Yet also for a second time, even with the increased range of potencies, the compensation was much smaller than the actual variation in potencies. In this case, subjects consumed approximately 60% more of the weakest than the strongest material. The consequence of this was an *effective dose* at the highest potency that exceeded the *effective dose* of the lowest potency by roughly 2½ times. Apparently there is a strong tendency for subjects to ingest more THC, *while attempting to attain the same subjective level of intoxication,* the more potent the available material. Evidently, there is no such thing as a particular "social dose" of marijuana; the dose required to produce reinforcing subjective effects appears to depend greatly on the potency of the available material. Importantly, doses equated in their ability to produce a satisfying "high" had quite different objective consequences in the first titration experiment. What this implies is that for no apparent gain in subjective reinforcement, subjects are exposed to more extreme physiological and psychomotor effects as drug potency increases. Moreover, if any of the effects of THC are hazardous over the long term, the chronic user may be more at risk to the extent that he has access to potent material, even though there may not be a commensurate gain in reinforcement.

As with any unanticipated outcome, only a speculative explanation can be applied in an attempt to account for the effect of the variable of cigarette size. The interaction which should have occurred if titration were finer with finer units of measurement did not materialize. Yet this variable had a substantial main effect; indeed an appropriate analysis revealed that it accounted for almost as much variance in self-administration as did the variable of potency. A possible explanation for the outcome is that because of learning outside the laboratory situation, many smokers have acquired an idea of the maximum number of "joints" needed to produce an acceptable "high." Given the obviously unreliable nature of somatic feedback in controlling marijuana intake, the development of such a "stop mechanism," based on more concrete external data, is at least plausible. Of course, in order to explain our results, we would have to argue further that this habit operates to an extent independently of the size and potency of a cigarette. Clearly, no definitive account of this result is possible, but one implication of it seems vital. An essentially cognitive variable accounted for nearly as much variance in self-administration as a key pharmacological feature of the drug. There can be little doubt then that in addition to their effects on the nature of the intoxicated state produced by a fixed dose, cognitive variables play a significant part in determining self-administration as well.

The most important result of this experiment was that the subjects' history of use did not affect self-administration of the drug in any measurable way. Frequent users did not consume more drug, they did not titrate any more or less effectively, nor were they any differently affected by the cognitive variable of cigarette size. Although drawing conclusions from negative results is always a dubious practice, the experiment was sufficiently rigorous to justify conclusions in this case. The discrepancy in frequency of use was extreme and applied for a period of at least 6 months prior to the experiment. Moreover, the discrepancy far exceeded that employed by Jones in demonstrating apparent tolerance to the subjective experience of intoxication. The negative outcome is at odds with Nahas' (1973) assertion that frequent exposure to cannabis will ultimately result in an escalation of dosage to maintain an acceptable level of reinforcement. That tolerance to some effects of cannabis develops is not the issue here (cf. Ferraro and Grisham, 1972) even though there was no evidence of this in our pulse rate data. What is in question is the dubious practice of making predictions about the consequences of the development of tolerance for the behavior of *self-administration*. To show that a fixed dose of a drug may have a progressively diminishing impact on some feature of behavior is not to show that the reinforcing action of the drug, whatever its mechanism, will be affected. If there is one thing that has been evident in our research it is that the experience of marijuana intoxication is subject to many vicissitudes having little to do with pharmacological action. Perhaps then we should not be surprised if a totally plausible prediction about self-administration and drug history was not confirmed. The one thing of which we are certain, however, is that statements about self-administration should be restricted to data based on this behavior and not on indirect inference, however plausible.

IV. CONCLUSIONS

Our series of experiments has further confirmed the general hypothesis that the subjective and objective consequences of cannabis consumption are subject to the influence of both pharmacological and psychological variables. Perhaps this is not surprising in view of the fact that the actions of numerous psychoactive drugs are similarly affected. But beyond reinforcing this generalization, some new and potentially significant findings emerged. For instance, it does appear to be the case, as many users of marijuana claim, that some behavioral consequences of the intoxicated state are subject to volitional control. Clearly, however, one must be careful not to overgeneralize in this regard. Even in the context of a single experiment, the motivational manipulation was not universally effective. Moreover, there may be dose levels at which compensation is totally impossible. The only certainty is that claims of self-control are plausible. For the relevance of this finding to be more than theoretical, it would be necessary to show that it applies to such socially significant behaviors as driving.

We were also able to confirm that the immediate environment may contribute to the subjective experience of intoxication. Apparently, Schachter's theory concerning the interaction of physiological states with cognitive determinants applies equally when the state is induced by marijuana. The mere act of consuming a cigarette resembling active marijuana was not sufficient to engage an environmental effect; rather a *bona fide* pharmacological manipulation was essential. In this sense, no placebo effect was observed. By the same token, a pharmacological excess also appeared to mitigate the contribution of the environment to subjective intoxication. In this, the results corroborated those of Carlin and his associates. However, our findings were also discrepant in that Carlin *et al.* had little success with their subjective index of intoxication. On balance though, the similarities in our findings seem to outweigh the differences.

If we have taken a novel direction, it is in using the self-administration of marijuana as a dependent variable. Gratifyingly for our general theoretical orientation, both psychological and pharmacological factors proved to be important in these studies as well. Although pharmacological regulation undoubtedly occurred, this ability was obviously limited even among the most sophisticated of users. Indeed, a seemingly minor cognitive manipulation was almost as important a determinant of intake as potency itself. Our results strongly suggested that there is no single quantity of THC which can be described as a "social dose." Even though the instructions were strongly worded to encourage subjects to consume just such a dose, this quantity had no meaning independent of the potency of the available material. Finally, only by incorporating a measure of self-administration of THC was it possible to comment validly on the role of use frequency in the regulation of intake. When this was done, no evidence was found to support Nahas' contention concerning the putative relationship between frequency of exposure to THC and the need to escalate dose to maintain a constant level of reinforcement.

ACKNOWLEDGMENTS

The marijuana used in the experiments reported here was provided by the cooperation of the Food and Drug Directorate of the Department of National Health and Welfare, Ottawa, Canada. A host of individuals were indispensible in providing technical assistance, medical examinations, urinalyses, nursing supervision, and general research assistance. We are deeply grateful to the many people who generously provided this help.

REFERENCES

Becker, H. S. (1953). *Amer. J. Sociol.* **59**, 235–242.
Cappell, H., and Pliner, P. (1973). *J. Abnorm. Psychol.* **82**, 428–434.
Cappell, H., Webster, C. D., Ginsberg, R., and Herring, B. (1972). *J. Pharmacol. Exp. Ther.* **182**, 195–203.
Cappell, H., Kuchar, E., and Webster, C. D. (1973). *Psychopharmacologia* **29**, 177–184.
Carlin, A. S., Bakker, C. B., Halpern, L., and Post, R. D. (1972). *J. Abnorm. Psychol.* **80**, 132–140.
Casswell, S., and Marks, D. F. (1972). *Science* **179**, 803–805.
Commission of Inquiry into the Non-Medical Use of Drugs. (1972). "Cannabis." Information Canada, Ottawa.
Crancer, A., Jr., Dille, J. M., Delay, J. E., and Haykin, M. D. (1969). *Science* **164**, 851–854.
Ferraro, D. P., and Grilly, D. M. (1973). *Science* **179**, 490–492.
Ferraro, D. P., and Grisham, M. G. (1972). *Physiol. & Behav.* **9**, 49–54.
Harris, R. T., Waters, W., and McLendon, D. (1972). *Psychopharmacologia* **26**, 297–306.
Johnson, S., and Domino, E. F. (1971). *Clin. Pharmacol. Ther.* **12**, 762–768.
Jones, R. T. (1971a). *Ann. N.Y. Acad. Sci.* **191**, 155–165.
Jones, R. T. (1971b). *Pharmacol. Rev.* **23**, 359–369.
Meyer, R. E., Pillard, R. C., Shapiro, L. S., and Mirin, S. M. (1971). *Amer. J. Psychiat.* **128**, 198–204.
Nahas, G. H. (1973). *Bull. Narcotics* **25**, 9–39.
Nisbett, R. E., and Schachter, S. (1966). *J. Exp. Soc. Psychol.* **2**, 227–236.
Schachter, S., and Singer, J. E. (1962). *Psychol. Rev.* **69**, 379–399.
Tart, C. (1971). "On Being Stoned: A Psychological Study of Marihuana Intoxication," Chapter 17, pp. 191–206. Science and Behavior Books, Palo Alto, California.
Waskow, I. E., Olsson, J. E., Salzman, C., and Katz, M. M. (1970). *Arch. Gen. Psychiat.* **22**, 97–107.
Weil, A. T., Zinberg, N. E., and Nelsen, J. M. (1968). *Science* **162**, 1234–1242.

Chapter 11

MARIJUANA USE AND PSYCHIATRIC ILLNESS

JAMES A. HALIKAS

- I. Statement of the Problem 265
- II. Pitfalls in Marijuana Research 267
  - A. Psychiatric Questions 267
  - B. Marijuana Questions 274
- III. Psychiatric Syndromes Described in Association with Marijuana Use 277
  - A. Introduction 277
  - B. Panic Anxiety Reaction 279
  - C. Marijuana Acute Brain Syndrome 281
  - D. Intercurrent Psychiatric Illness 285
- IV. Correlations of Marijuana Use with Psychiatric Illness 289
  - A. Review of the Literature 289
  - B. A Systematic Study of Marijuana Use and Psychiatric Illness 292
  - C. Other Systematic Studies 295
- V. Conclusion 297
- References 299

I. STATEMENT OF THE PROBLEM

The question of the relationship between marijuana use and psychiatric illness is complex and controversial. Is marijuana use, alone, sufficient to cause psychiatric illnesses? If so, how much use, how often, in what circumstances, in what proportion of users, and by what mechanism? Which users are spared psychiatric consequences, and why? If marijuana use, alone, is not sufficient to produce psychiatric consequences, then will such consequences occur to any users, and if so, under what additional circumstances, to which users, and why? If marijuana use does not cause psychiatric consequences, might it be related in other ways to psychiatric illness? Are some users of marijuana already ill before first use of the drug; does it alter the natural course of their illness? Or, is there perhaps no higher incidence of psychiatric illness among marijuana users than among comparable nonusers? Perhaps, there is no relationship between marijuana use and psychiatric illness. Diverse and mutually contradictory conclusions have been reached in the literature. How is one to evaluate the work available that has led to such startlingly different opinions by researchers in the field? If these questions can be answered, then the relationship between marijuana use and psychiatric illness would become clear.

Every exogenous chemical produces physiological consequences in an organism. These changes are sometimes beneficial, sometimes harmful, sometimes trivial, and sometimes important. Physiological consequences are related to several complex separate factors, including intrinsic properties of the chemical, intrinsic properties of the organism, details of administration such as dosage, route, and frequency, previous experiences of the organism, and subsequent challenges to the organism by other conditions in the environment. Beneficial or harmful consequences can be either short term and immediate or long term and delayed. As such an exogenous chemical, marijuana will produce characteristic physiological consequences in an organism. The elucidation of these pharmacological and physiological consequences characteristic to marijuana intake is of prime importance in understanding marijuana effects in man.

As part of the physiological consequence of intake of exogenous chemicals, psychiatric effects and psychological and behavioral consequences are for man often prominent. For marijuana use, the psychiatric consequences are of importance in large part because of the widespread use of marijuana as a social intoxicant. While psychiatric consequences of alcohol use (the other historically significant social intoxicant of mankind) are relatively well described and agreed on, psychiatric effects of cannabis remain controversial and inadequately examined. Current controversy is in part the result of this vacuum of knowledge, and in part due to the social controversy which involves marijuana use symbolizing other behavior as discussed by Kaplan (1970). To deal with the question of marijuana use and psychiatric illness, problems not germane to the question must first be considered.

II. PITFALLS IN MARIJUANA RESEARCH

A. Psychiatric Questions

In every society historically, attempts have been made to explain the meaning and cause of human behavior. In modern day psychiatry, attempts have become codified as a variety of psychological theories attempting to explain individual growth and development, awake and asleep mentation, interpersonal behavior, and group and societal movements. These theories are based on the belief that every behavior must have meaning unique for the individual but also recognizable and generalizable to other individuals. For psychodynamic theories, the content of behavior has significance in light of the individual's past experience, interactions, thoughts, and feelings, which can only be judged and interpreted against a theoretical framework.

Psychodynamic theories that have been developed to explain human behavior have never been adequately tested for validity. More importantly, all such theories have focused on explaining the meaning of current behavior in light of some theoretical analysis of past intrapsychic or interpersonal conflicts or adaptational techniques. This preoccupation with developing an attractive theoretical formulation first and then interpreting empirical data for concordance with that formulation later has deterred the accumulation of objectively valid descriptions of human behavior. Thus, speculations on the theoretical importance of various techniques of toilet training are far more abundant in the psychiatric literature than are empirical studies of just how toilet training is achieved in various population samples of youngsters. The development of all-encompassing *a priori* theories to explain human behaviors led to a progressive lack of precision in recognizing and accurately describing aspects of behavior. With increasing emphasis on interpretation, some specific symptoms of previously outlined clinical syndromes took on increased importance and overshadowed other aspects of clinical appearance and clinical course. Diagnostic imprecision soon followed.

1. DEFINITIONS

A descriptive term should be able to communicate precisely what was seen and heard in words that have explicit meanings requiring no additional information about that patient in order to comprehend that behavior. A conclusion in the form of a diagnosis is then derived from the concordance of the observed cluster of behaviors in this patient with an earlier predetermined compilation of behaviors (symptoms) drawn from studies of other patients. In interpretive psychiatry the use of a descriptive term often connotes a conclusion based on that behavior or in some instances implies a specific diagnosis. The use of the descriptive term "loose associations" in some centers defines the patient as being schizophrenic whether or not the patient fulfills any other criteria. Such a symptom-equals-diagnosis approach forces observers to modify their description of a patient's behavior in light of the entire clinical picture as they perceive it. At the same time, in other centers "loose associations" may not imply any preordained diagnosis. The error therefore is to describe a patient's behavior in terms of his illness, rather than to describe his illness in terms of his behavior.

There are unfortunately few terms in psychiatry which connote the same behavior to different readers. Case histories summarized in the literature must use terms therefore which are subject to various interpretations based on the reader's own beliefs. Also, many different terms may be used by different observers to describe the same observed symptoms. Even physiological vegetative changes may be described differently by different observers. For example, substantially slowed motor activity by a patient may be variously described as psychomotor retardation, catatonic posturing, or adynamic mutism.

There are terms which by casual use have lost much of their meaning in psychiatry. "Psychosis" and "psychotic" for some clinicians are administrative terms, which describe the patient's inability to care for his own needs temporarily; for others, they may be equivalent to the diagnosis of schizophrenia. These terms may mean any loss of reality-testing or reality-modification of behavior; or the presence of any irrational thoughts, feelings, or actions; or they may mean regression to a more primitive state of ego integrity as a reaction to current environmental events which trigger an earlier unresolved or maladaptively resolved intrapsychic conflict. Hallucination may mean a subjective sensory experience which has no basis in reality, or it may include subjective misinterpretations of poorly recognized sensory input. The concept of the "marginal" or "borderline" personality, in some psychiatric centers, implies a constellation of personality traits and defense patterns which, given the right environmental stress, will trigger a "psychotic reaction." In other centers this term describes patients who have had in the past a psychotic episode and then recovered; other investigators use it only retrospectively when faced with an instance of psychosis to indicate that the patient indeed had a poor premorbid personality, but which was not obvious; in still other centers the term may not be used at all because of being considered so diffuse as to signify nothing.

Thus, there is as yet no commonality of language, no agreed on set of definitions for terms used in the field. Therefore, communication of descriptive information concerning a patient's status becomes a tenuous and cautious activity.

2. DIAGNOSTICS

Ideally a diagnosis in psychiatry just as in all other branches of medicine is a succinct way of communicating a great deal of information about a patient's condition. Information communicated by a diagnosis should include etiology of the condition, the clinical appearance of this condition in a majority of similar patients, the expected laboratory and diagnostic test results of such patients, the natural course or history of this syndrome in similar patients under both treated and untreated conditions, and the prognosis or predictive expectations for the future status of this patient based on previous experience with other similar cases.

Rarely in medicine is the etiology determined early in the historical development of a syndrome. Rather, meaningful studies into the etiology of a condition can only be made after the development of a consistent clinical description which accurately parcels out patients with common characteristics who can then be studied more precisely. In psychiatry, the validity of a clinical diagnostic category requires confirmation from several different types of research perspectives. A first approximation is the development of a homogeneous clinical description of the disorder based on the study of large numbers of patients having common clinical, laboratory, and demographic characteristics. Tentative diagnostic criteria based on this clinical description are then set forth as a group of signs and symptoms which must be present before such a diagnosis can be made. Meaningful exclusion criteria must also be determined that can separate patients with this condition from patients with other overlapping or similar clinical syndromes. The clinical syndrome is then validated by a later follow-up investigation of the originally described patients to determine the common characteristics and description of the natural history of the disorder. If at follow-up several different clinical pictures are found, each of which is already subsumed under some other existing diagnosis, or varied outcome states per se are found, the validity of the described syndrome should be in question.

A clinical description that can be tested and confirmed by other investigators must consist of objective behavioral characteristics and patterns of behavior explicitly described. In interpretative psychiatry, objective clinical description of gross behavior and patterns is clouded by microscopic analysis of subjectively selected bits of verbalizations and feeling tones. Further, theoretical approaches have tended to obscure not only the investigator's ability to objectively describe behavior, but also have caused gross behavior patterns and natural history descriptions to be ignored. By focusing on certain aspects of a putative syndrome which fit some theoretical formulation, psychiatrists have come to equate the presence of one symptom with the presence of the syndrome in which that symptom is theoretically appropriate. It is now clear from many descriptive studies that there is no single pathogneumonic symptom which determines the presence of a single specific psychiatric diagnosis. However, this focusing on particular symptoms enlarged many diagnostic categories to include several clinical pictures, several different clinical courses, and several different outcome states, thereby negating whatever descriptive and predictive value the original diagnostic label may have contained.

The problem of diagnostic variations in psychiatry was clearly demonstrated by Kendell et al. (1971) in their study of American and British diagnostic approaches. Psychiatric diagnostic nosology, its contradictions and limitations, has also come under recent scrutiny by Fitzgibbons and Hokanson (1973), Strauss (1973), and Panzetta (1974).

Though not in widespread use in psychiatric research as yet, descriptive diagnostic criteria for major syndromes in psychiatry have been developed and validated by consistency of clinical appearance and follow-up studies. One such set of criteria has been presented by Feighner et al. (1972). Additionally, descriptions of the appearance and natural course of each syndrome as well as an exposition of the descriptive diagnostic approach is now available in *Psychiatric Diagnosis* by Woodruff et al. (1974). Though these diagnostic criteria were derived from repeated descriptive studies of different inpatient and outpatient populations, varieties of control groups, extensive family studies, and thorough follow-up investigations, they are still tentative and flexible and may be modified and refined further by additional systematic studies. They are based on clusters of descriptive psychiatric symptoms and gross behavior patterns as they affect various life areas. Such a diagnostic formulation is not predicated on any etiological postulation and makes no assumption about the causes or meaning of the behaviors noted. This set of diagnostic criteria for various psychiatric syndromes, a sample of which is about to be presented, will be used later in this chapter to assess reports in the literature linking marijuana use with psychiatric disorders.

Objective criteria are used to evaluate each symptom. The symptom must have interfered with the patient's normal life functioning in some way; or the patient must have sought some sort of professional assistance for the symptom; or the symptom caused the patient to take medication on more than one occasion; or in the absence of the preceding responses, the clinician evaluating the symptom must feel it is of such overwhelming clinical importance as to be scored positive anyway. Symptoms are not scored positive toward a psychiatric diagnosis if they can be explained on the basis of a known medical illness which the patient has.

a. Primary Affective Disorder—Depressed Type. For this diagnosis, a subject must report an episode of dysphoric mood, characterized by feeling depressed, sad, despondent, blue, hopeless, discouraged, worried, etc., plus five of the following eight symptoms for a "definite diagnosis" or four of the following for a "probable" diagnosis: (1) unplanned change in weight or appetite; (2) sleep difficulty including initial, interval, terminal insomnia, or hypersomnia; (3) loss of energy; (4) agitation, irritability, internal restlessness, or psychomotor retardation; (5) change in libido, withdrawal, or loss of interest in usual activities; (6) alteration in thinking, memory, or ability to concentrate; (7) suicidal ideas or explicit death wishes; and (8) inappropriate self-depreciatory ruminations, self-reproach, or guilt. The cluster of symptoms must have lasted at least 2 weeks and not be explainable on the basis of medical illness or social activity. The subject must have been free of any preexisting psychiatric illness. This cluster of symptoms must be different from the patient's usual premorbid psychosocial adjustment.

b. Primary Affective Disorder—Manic Type. For this diagnosis, a patient must report an episode of euphoria or irritability lasting at last 2 weeks with no preexisting psychiatric condition (excepting the possibility of a past history of depression), plus at least 3 of the following 6 symptom categories: (1) hyperactivity, which includes motor, social, and sexual activity; (2) push of speech, which includes the sensation of a pressure to keep talking, increased rate, rhythm, and amount of speech; (3) flight of ideas including racing thoughts and loosening of associations; (4) grandiosity which may be delusional; (5) decreased sleep; and (6) distractibility.

c. Antisocial Personality, or Sociopathy. Here, objective behavioral characteristics as developed by Robins (1966) are used, rather than subjective, interpretative criteria proposed by Cleckley (1964). Sociopathy is a chronic disorder with onset prior to age 15 requiring antisocial behavior in at least 5 of the following life areas: (1) school problems, demonstrated by recurrent truancy, suspension, expulsions, or fighting and other problems which required parental or principal's involvement; (2) overnight runaway prior to age 16; (3) police trouble as a juvenile or stealing as a child; (4) recurrent or significant police trouble as an adult; (5) fighting after the age of 18; (6) vagrancy or wanderlust; (7) multiple job firings; (8) multiple marital problems; (9) military service discipline difficulties; (10) pathological lying; and (11) sexual misconduct including promiscuity, repetitive venereal disease, pimping, or prostitution.

d. Schizophrenia. For this diagnosis, the patient must present a chronic illness symptomatic for at least 6 months prior to the evaluation without return to premorbid level of functioning; there must also be an absence of symptoms which would be sufficient to qualify for the diagnosis of affective disorder or probable affective disorder. Additionally, the patient must demonstrate either (a) delusions or hallucinations *without* significant associated perplexity or disorientation or (b) verbal production which makes adequate communication difficult because of lack of logical or understandable organization. And further, for a diagnosis of schizophrenia, 3 of the following manifestations must also be present: single; poor premorbid social adjustment or work history; family history of schizophrenia; absence of alcoholism or drug abuse within 1 year of onset of current symptom complex; and onset of illness prior to age 40.

e. Organic Brain Syndrome. For this diagnosis the patient must have at least 2 of the following: impairment of orientation, impairment of memory, and deterioration of other intellectual functions. This diagnosis may also be made if a patient has at least one of the aforementioned manifestations and also a known probable cause for organic brain syndrome. Clincal characteristics of this illness as determined by Wolff and Curran will be described more fully later in this chapter.

Similar objective diagnostic criteria have been developed for alcoholism, secondary affective disorder, anxiety neurosis, obsessive-compulsive neurosis, hysteria, phobic neurosis, homosexuality, transsexualism, and anorexia nervosa. Other diagnostic systems in use at this time lack objective clinical descriptions necessary for even preliminary validation of their approach. The absence of such objective criteria in the marijuana literature have severely diluted the value of case reports and populations collected of impaired marijuana users, as will become apparent.

3. LIMITATIONS OF PSYCHIATRIC RESEARCH

Limitations of research in psychiatry fall into two broad categories: first, constraints caused by real methodologic difficulties; and second, limitations caused by internal diagnostic and definitional controversy within the profession. An ideal theoretical research design studies a behavior by manipulation of select variables. This model presupposes a knowledge of the prevalence of that behavior in different populations, an understanding of the types of variables which could be expected to alter that behavior, and a psychophysiological understanding of that behavior such that experimental conditions can be sufficiently controlled to rule out unconsidered factors; none of that knowledge or capability currently exists in psychiatric research.

A second research formulation is that of generalizing from individual cases. Much psychiatric research has consisted of summarizing the experiences of a given patient and selectively interpreting the life experiences in concordance with a theoretical framework. The intrapsychic theoretical framework, which is most frequently used in such a context, admits of no null hypothesis and therefore cannot be tested. Further, because samples are small and rarely accompanied by control groups, statistical analysis for significance cannot be performed which would demonstrate that the findings are other than a chance occurrence.

Descriptive research in psychiatry is beset by its own group of problems. The selection of which aspects of a behavior are to be recorded is often as subjective and biased in descriptive studies as in those using a theoretical framework. Having once made this critical determination, however, the descriptive researcher must then find a suitable population to study. For example, the possibility exists that marijuana use is associated with a unique chronic psychosis. To demonstrate this, a clinical syndrome would have to be described having several common features among those patients thought to be suffering from it with exclusion criteria which clearly delimit the new syndrome from other known and recognized psychiatric disorders. Sampling limitations on the syndrome thus described which may or may not be significant would include use of other drugs, age, sex, race, socioeconomics, education, ethnicity, religion, and regional factors which are perhaps peculiar to this sample. To determine whether this clinical description is limited by any of these sampling factors, other selected marijuana-using and non-marijuana-using populations would similarly be studied. Later, follow-up studies of patients suffering from this new disorder would have to demonstrate that this is a homogeneous group having a common natural course. Ideally, patients thought to have this new syndrome should be free of preexisting psychiatric illness, have a negative family history for psychiatric illness, be free of other drug use, and occur in sufficient numbers as to demonstrate that this is not an idiosyncratic drug reaction, e.g., as was the allergic marijuana reaction described in one patient by Liskow et al. (1971). Finally, to accurately estimate the frequency and distribution of this hypothetical syndrome or any proposed psychiatric syndrome in the general population, a representative sample of the entire population would need to be studied, correcting for all sources of possible sampling error. Such systematic studies with respect to marijuana syndromes have not been done. Further, the epidemiology of accepted psychiatric illnesses and behaviors has not been delineated adequately as yet. Data on incidence and prevalence of psychiatric syndromes remains tentative, partly because of methodological sampling difficulties and partly because of diagnostic variability. Information is limited describing the natural course of illnesses, the clinical variations amongst different populations, and the constitutional and environmental factors which may affect psychiatrically important behavior. Because of these epidemiological limitations, also, attempts to correlate psychiatric problems with various human behaviors must be viewed cautiously.

Thus: if you cannot agree on what it is you think you are looking for, in whom you should be looking for it, how you aim to find it, and what the value of the tools you are using are, then how are you going to agree about what it is, and what it means, after you think you have found it.

B. Marijuana Questions

1. WAYS OF GETTING AT MARIJUANA DATA

The ideal method of studying the relationship between marijuana use and psychiatric illness would be to collect a representative sample of all marijuana users in the society, interview and test them in a double-blind manner, then compare them against a carefully matched control group of nonusers similarly studied. This ideal epidemiological study has never been done with marijuana users or with any other psychiatric, medical, or social subgroup in the society. Several other methods have been developed to attempt to gather data concerning the relationship of marijuana use to psychiatric illness.

Anonymous questionnaires, either mailed or filled out in large groups, have been used repeatedly with selected populations to study marijuana use. Usually this has occurred in a high school or college setting or in the military. With such surveys, accuracy of data collected cannot be determined; questions cannot be clarified if misunderstood; no information can be obtained concerning that proportion of the sample which does not respond; nor can the cooperation of those who do respond be estimated. In such large scale surveys, control groups are not matched in any systematic fashion, but rather are usually all the respondents who are not self-admitted marijuana users. With this technique, basic demographic data have been collected which attempt to characterize marijuana users in general terms and to describe patterns of changing drug use.

Another method by which data concerning marijuana use and psychiatric illness have been accumulating is that of anecdotal reports. Because of the invariably small size of the populations being presented, the absence of control groups, the absence of information concerning the size and type of population from which the cases have been drawn, the failure to present diagnostic criteria used by the reporter, and the inherent distortion present in drawing conclusions from one or two cases, case reports are of quite limited value. Since most psychiatric syndromes described in association with marijuana use have been in the form of anecdotal reports, these will, however, be presented at length in the next section.

Where and how a study sample is obtained can in large measure preordain the results. If marijuana users are chosen from a population having had police contact as a consequence of their marijuana use, results will show a high correlation with criminality; if psychiatric patients who are also marijuana users are studied, a high correlation with psychiatric illness would be found. When such samples are studied, they may not even be representative of the larger population from which they were drawn, but rather may be skewed samples. Because there may be other drug users in those same populations who have remained anonymous and are therefore totally uncharacterized, it is not possible to determine how representative the found users are of the larger groups.

Samples collected of volunteers, such as those presented by Goode (1969), and this author, are limited in analogous ways. The phenomenon of volunteering for participation in a study has not adequately been investigated itself. Additionally, since the focus of both mentioned works was the study of marijuana use, an illegal activity, how can one evaluate those who would volunteer for such participation? How did they differ from their counterparts who were also approached and chose not to volunteer? Were they more zealous, more naive, more trusting, more impulsive, more scientifically minded, or a host of other possible factors? A similarly obtained control group might provide valuable comparisons to the volunteer user sample, but since it too may be unrepresentative for similar reasons, such a control does not necessarily allow generalizations to any larger populations. Thus, volunteers cannot be known to be representative of the larger group from which they sprang, and the larger group itself cannot be evaluated as to representativeness of the entire population of marijuana users. Even with extensively studied large volunteer populations, therefore, all conclusions drawn must be considered quite tentative.

2. PROBLEMS OF INTERPRETING MARIJUANA-RELATED BEHAVIOR

With any study evaluating marijuana use and its effects, there are inherent social and investigative biases which determine what is studied and what is ignored. Usually information is collected about problems possibly related to marijuana use but less frequently to assets or benefits derived from marijuana use. The observer, trained though he may be, is bound by social expectations, prejudices, and biases, so that his observations and expectations are less than objective. The differing expectations of the user, based on prior experience or heresay, which each brings to his marijuana experience and to his research evaluation, may alter considerably the data collected. Thus, one subject may consider tachycardia an exhilarating experience while another may perceive it as evidence of an impending heart attack and thus report it as an unpleasant side effect. Marijuana studies are further complicated by the question of just what behaviors are indeed primary drug effects or related consequences and what behaviors are secondary coping behaviors of the individual in response to either drug effects or social consequences of drug use.

Among the problems of interpreting behavior arise the cross-cultural questions. In societies where marijuana use is condoned but limited to the lowest social classes, studies find associations between marijuana use and poverty, ignorance, societal disenfranchisement, criminality, medical and psychiatric illness, and hopelessness. In societies where marijuana use is illegal, associations are found with deviant or disapproved behavior of other types. In both instances, should marijuana use spread to other segments of society, these sociologically bound characteristics of the users may diminish. Studies in other cultures have limited applicability, also, because of differing priorities in mental health, different training systems for psychiatric personnel, different diagnostic constructs, different environmental and social factors which cloud psychiatric pictures, differing culturally bound attitudes, and differing drug usage patterns. Thus, time, place, situation, and investigative bias limit research attempts.

3. PROBLEMS OF INTERPRETING DATA OBTAINED

Studies of marijuana users are almost invariably tainted by the fact that these users have also used other drugs, both licit and illicit. Thus, it is virtually impossible to determine which consequences or behaviors were the effect of one drug or another drug or of any drug. Additionally, since marijuana remains an illicit substance obtained by indirect means relative to its point of origin, it is impossible to determine what is in fact being used which is purported to be marijuana or its derivatives. Thus the question of an unknown dose of an unknown substance hangs over all studies of acute effects. Further, laboratory controlled studies using known quantities with known strengths have not as yet surmounted methodological questions of absorption, metabolism, and breakdown sufficient to generate a reliable dose-response curve correlating clinical response to absorbed dose of the putatively active cannabinoid.

Finally, we must contend with what may be the most crucial and yet most vexing methodological question: causation versus coincidence. There is an old medical adage that a dog can have both lice and fleas. Thus having found psychiatric problems among some marijuana users, the investigator must still demonstrate whether and what sort of association exists between marijuana use and the psychiatric problem. Does the problem predate marijuana use and could it be the explanation for the later use? Is the effect a direct consequence of marijuana use? Or, are both contingent on some third unconsidered variable? Or, is there perhaps no relationship between the two behaviors? Coexistence does not prove association, and association does not prove causation.

III. PSYCHIATRIC SYNDROMES DESCRIBED IN ASSOCIATION WITH MARIJUANA USE

A. Introduction

There is a large anecdotal literature describing adverse reactions to acute marijuana introxication. Each report describes a limited number of cases; many are encumbered by diagnostic controversy and by questions of definition; few describe the clinical material fully. There are, also, in the literature many reviews of adverse reactions, usually promoting a particular classification of these reactions. All classifications attempted must be viewed cautiously in light of previously discussed diagnostic and methodological problems. However, within the limitations discussed, the classification to follow seems logical and provides a framework within which the presently available data can be evaluated and explained.

Any drug used may result in perceived pleasant effects, perceived unpleasant effects, a combination of both pleasant and unpleasant perceived effects, or no perceived effects. Effects which occur usually or regularly during most occasions of marijuana use by regular users may be considered normal effects of marijuana use. Most of these effects presumably would be considered subjectively pleasant or one would expect use to cease in the absence of physical addiction. Some subjectively unpleasant effects may be viewed as inconsequential though frequent occurrences. Additionally, there may be a wide range of effects which occur infrequently, which again may be perceived as pleasant or unpleasant. The precise combination of particular effects on a given occasion of use will determine the perceived nature of that particular experience. Just as with social use of alcohol, there are average or unremarkable experiences, particularly pleasurable occasions of use, and particularly unpleasant occasions of use.

Some of the determinants of pleasurable versus unpleasurable experiences of marijuana use have been tentatively described. They include the expectations of the user, the current psychological situation of the user, the potency of the drug used, the social situation during the use, in short, "the set and setting." Similar factors influence the social alcohol use experience. An attempt was made to systematically determine the frequency of occurrence of 105 described effects during and after marijuana intoxication by this author (Halikas et al., 1971). A questionnaire of 105 acute emotional and intellectual effects, acute physical effects, and hangover effects was filled out by 100 regular users of marijuana as part of a larger study. Acute effects which "usually" occurred to more than 50% of the group were high feeling, relaxation, keener sound sense, peaceful, increased sensitivity, increased hunger, time slowed down, increased thirst, and dry mouth and throat. Aftereffects noted by the majority of the group to occur on a "usual" basis were calm feeling, mind clear, and more restful sleep. Though no single effect considered adverse by the investigators occurred on a "usual" basis to more than 5 of the 100 subjects, 16% did report the "usual" occurrence of at least one of the following unpleasant effects: acute effects—anxiety or fearfulness, brooding or morose feelings, sadness or despondency, aggressive feelings, amnesia, confusion and bewilderment, hearing voices, seeing visions; postintoxication effects—depression, driving badly, unreasonable fears, hearing voices or seeing visions, and "anxiety flashes."

A wide variety of effects occurred at least "occasionally" to a majority of the 100 subjects. Among the effects considered adverse that were noted as an "occasional" experience by a majority of the users were separation from self, separation from reality, anxious or fearful, less self-confident, as well as such unpleasant physical effects as clumsiness and unsteadiness of walk. Among these experienced users, it appeared that the random marijuana intoxication could include a wide variety of acute and postintoxication effects, most of which were probably pleasant but some of which were probably not. A similar questionnaire checklist of 150 regular users, reported by Tart (1970), noted that 80% of the users acknowledged paranoid and suspicious feelings among the negative effects. *The Medical Letter* (Anonymous, 1967, 1970) presents a summary of psychological and physical effects though without indicating frequency of occurrence. These normal variations in the marijuana high among different subjects are described well by Goode in his monograph, *The Marijuana Smokers* (1970).

Allentuck and Bowman (1942, and in the LaGuardia Report, 1944), Siler *et al.* (1933), Chopra (1969), and Weil *et al.* (1968) using marijuana, Clark *et al* (1968) and Waskow *et al.* (1970) using synthetic tetrahydrocannabinol, and Williams *et al* (1946) using parahexyl all reported the clinical reproduction of a similar assortment of pleasant and unpleasant effects. In addition, as Miras (1970) has noted, placebo effect and the possibility of self-hypnosis cannot be excluded as accounting for some of the subjective experiences of marijuana users since there is great variability in the potency of illicitly obtained marijuana. Thus, there is a wide range of normal effects which can possibly occur during any given intoxication and, depending on the set and setting at the time, these normal effects may occasionally be mildly to significantly disturbing.

There have been several reviews attempting to organize a reasonable classification of marijuana untoward effects. Bialos (1970) considers the question of expectations in describing outcome; he supports the contention that a reaction is not adverse unless the subject considers it unpleasant or untoward. Bromberg (1939) and Weil (1970) both also considered the question of a continuum between effects perceived as either pleasant or unpleasant. All assume that the significant factors causing such an alteration in perceptions of those effects are set, setting, dosage, expectations, and immediate psychological state of the subject. Recently, Paton *et al.* (1973) have catalogued adverse reactions to marijuana as reported in the literature without attempting to reevaluate the cases, accepting the interpretive conclusions of the authors and listing the cases accordingly. Alternatively, a reevaluation and reclassification will now be presented.

B. Panic Anxiety Reaction

The panic reaction has been noted by several reviewers to be the most common adverse reaction to marijuana use. Most of the signs and symptoms found are distortions or enlargements of the normal marijuana effects as described by users. The panic reaction is usually described as consisting of most of the following prototypical symptoms: (1) psychological—anxiety, apprehensiveness, panicky feelings, paranoid feelings and/or verbalizations with insight, depersonalization complaints, misperceptions or misinterpretations of perceptions, emotional lability, and groundless fears such as fears of losing one's mind and fears of having a heart attack: (2) physiological symptoms of anxiety including tachycardia, dizziness, hyperactivity, chest tightening or chest pains, subjective respiratory insufficiency, paresthesias, and, often, difficulty walking, speech impediments, and trembling: many of these physiological symptoms having been initiated as part of the normal marijuana intoxication. Insight or partial insight into the situation is present though it may be overwhelmed by the panic and fears; orientation and memory are intact. This reaction is self-limited, lasting from several minutes to several hours. It is said to occur most frequently in novice users, ambivalent users, highly suggestible users, users in a strange or threatening situation (such as a clinical laboratory), and in regular users receiving an unexpectedly large dose. The frequency of occurrence of this reaction as with all other adverse reactions with marijuana to be presented is unknown.

CASE MATERIAL

a. From Persyko (1970). A 22-year-old white female brought by police to hospital on New Year's Eve. On admission was highly apprehensive, crying and laughing alternately, and refusing to be interviewed. A companion reported that the patient suddenly became disturbed and began screaming uncontrollably after smoking two marijuana joints. Patient was trembling and expressed fear of dying. After supportive care and sedation the patient fell asleep. She awoke the next morning free of symptoms and with a clear memory for the episode. She related that she had been afraid she would die. Following the first joint, while watching her face in the mirror, she noticed it was white, as if she were dead. She became more frightened following the second joint when she observed the bulbs on her Christmas tree moving; she became fearful of being left alone and of losing control of herself and she began screaming. The patient had used marijuana on two prior occasions with no ill effects; she had no prior psychiatric history.

b. From Talbott and Teague (1969). A 26-year-old white male, second lieutenant, registered nurse in Vietnam with no history of psychiatric difficulties, immediately after smoking his first marijuana cigarette, became aware of a burning, choking sensation in his throat. He went to a civilian bar where he shortly began feeling apprehensive, anxious, and suspicious; he became fearful that the Vietnamese Nationals meant him harm; he fled in terror to his quarters. When examined he was anxious and disoriented to time but not as to person and place; his anxiety and fear of harm by Nationals seemed to intensify and decrease in wavelike fashion, and at its peak this fear was thought to be delusional. He was unable to identify the nature of the harm he feared. Affect was labile but appropriate; thinking was rapid and disjointed, as if unable to follow a line of thought and experiencing a wide variety of thoughts rapidly and dissimilar except for a common apprehensive quality; he concentrated poorly; no hallucinations were noted; and judgment and insight were considered impaired. A generalized impairment of coordination was demonstrated by heel-to-toe walking and finger-to-nose testing; Romberg sign was positive; conjunctivae were injected; reflexes were hyperactive; and a general psychomotor agitation was noted. Patient was treated with sedation and discharged within 36 hours asymptomatic.

In addition to the representative cases presented, there have been several case reports describing what appear to be panic anxiety reactions among cases collected by Wikler (1970), Milman (1969), Marten (1969), Grossman (1969), and Baker-Bates (1935). Some of these cases have been considered by the presentors as being other syndromes; often the case presentations had limited descriptions and are therefore difficult to interpret; rarely are the descriptions free of inferences drawn without indicating the objective basis for that inference. The cases presented above and referenced, however, fulfill the general criteria described for this clinical picture: prominent anxiety and panic features; prominent physiological concomitants of anxiety; psychological and physiological symptoms of intoxication; a relatively clear sensorium; and relatively short-lived.

C. Marijuana Acute Brain Syndrome (Toxic Delirium)

The Acute Brain Syndrome secondary to marijuana toxicity has been reported frequently in the literature in the form of anecdotal reports. Usually this syndrome has been called by other names; toxic psychosis, marijuana psychosis, hemp psychosis, acute psychotic reaction, or acute schizophrenic decompensation. On the basis of descriptions presented, however, it seems clear that the syndrome described is a classic acute brain reaction to an exogenous toxin, in this case marijuana. The syndrome fulfills characteristics described by Wolff and Curran (1935) in their review of 106 cases of delirium present in 27 different toxic situations both endogenous and exogenous.

Characteristic clinical features of the marijuana acute brain syndrome are similar to those of other toxic acute brain syndromes and include the following: impaired mentation demonstrated by disorientation, absent, or fragmentary memory of the condition, emotional lability, fluctuating sensorium, absence of insight, loss of higher thinking processes and reality testing, clouding of consciousness, poor concentration and attending, rambling verbalizations, increased suggestibility, inappropriate fearfulness and apprehension, misinterpretations, illusions and fragmentary hallucinations, poorly organized delusional ideas, and paranoid misinterpretations; and physiological dysfunction indicated by restlessness, tremors, slurred speech, failure in rapid movements, staggering gait, difficulty swallowing, and sleeplessness.

Spencer (1970) has summarized his observations with regard to the marijuana-induced acute brain syndrome as seen in the Bahamas. He described the onset as sudden and probably continuous with drug effects, amnesia dating from prior to the onset of the clinical syndrome until after treatment has begun, psychomotor overactivity, pressure of thought, flight of ideas, general restlessness, ceaseless change of activities, passivity feelings, ideas of influence and reference, delusions of grandeur, incongruous and labile elation, clouded sensorium which cleared rapidly, and the absence of insight during the acute phase. In his clinical experience, hallucinations did not occur as part of the syndrome. Bey and Zecchinelli (1971), reviewing 20 cases of American soldiers in Vietnam, noted hyperalertness, irritability, suspiciousness, fearfulness, ideas of reference, persecutory delusions, disorientation, confusion, combativeness, hallucinations, and delusions. In their series these symptoms subsided within 24 to 48 hours and patients were then able to present a logical chronologic history. Chopra and Smith (1974) reviewed features common among 200 acute adverse reactions to marijuana and found, most commonly, the sudden onset of confusion, garrulousness, delusions, visual hallucinations, emotional lability, temporary amnesia, disorientation, depersonalization, and paranoia; the amnesia was noted to last from several hours to several days and to resemble the alcoholic black-out. The 200 cases included 34% with no psychiatric history, 61% with a previously noted nonpsychotic personality disorder, and 5% with a previous history of overt psychosis. In this series, as in others reported, symptoms of the acute brain syndrome rapidly cleared, usually within a few days. Klee (1969) has presented an excellent description of such an acute brain syndrome from marijuana in a thorough and well-detailed case report.

CASE MATERIAL

a. From Bloch (1969). A 26-year-old black male American soldier in Vietnam who had had prior behavioral problems was referred for admission because of violent behavior and inappropriate speech from that morning. No meaningful history could be obtained from the patient at the time. He was unshaven, agitated, with vague and disjointed speech, and markedly loosened associations. Severe impairment of attention span, recall, and orientation were noted. There was posturing with religious connotations; he acknowledged direct communication with God. He was extremely suspicious, had apparent ideas of reference and influence, and struck the psychiatrist, thinking an experiment was being performed on him. Following 48 hours of sedation, symptoms abated and a history of marijuana use the day prior to admission was obtained. Prior psychiatric history revealed behavioral problems and difficulties with civilian authorities prior to military service.

b. From Talbott and Teague (1969). A 24-year-old black male American soldier in Vietnam was transferred from another hospital with a history of having smoked a pipeful of "strange tasting tobacco" 2 days previously: After initially feeling lightheaded and "funny," he subsequently developed feelings of depersonalization and derealization and thought his mind was split into good and evil parts. The patient had expressed the morbid preoccupation that he was dead, had admitted to unusual illusions or hallucinations (clouds pulling him in, bright lights coming out of a cloud toward him), and had expressed frightening fears that he would kill someone or be killed by someone. He was disoriented, confused, and forgetful. He was sedated and 2 days later transferred to the psychiatric facility. There, on admission, he was apprehensive, worried, and preoccupied with fears, sensations, and impulses. His restlessness, tremulousness, agitation, and rapid speech alternated with staring, mutism, and inability to complete his thoughts. He continued to express the belief that his mind was split, but denied hallucinations or delusions. He seemed adequately oriented. Past history was noted with excessive drinking, job problems, and aggressive outbursts in adolescence. Symptoms cleared rapidly with chlordiazepoxide.

Talbott and Teague, in their review of 12 cases that they considered to be acute marijuana brain syndromes, noted the definite toxic, organic quality which included impaired cognitive functioning in each soldier. They also found impairment of orientation, severe impairment of primarily recent memory, impaired intellectual functioning with confusion, short attention span and difficulty concentrating, tangential and disjointed thinking, and impaired judgment. This impairment of cognitive functioning is crucial for the diagnosis of Acute Brain Syndrome to be made, of whatever etiology.

Wolff and Curran (1935) described at length the characteristic features of the Acute Brain Syndrome, including this crucial clouding of higher cerebral functions. Their work is so trenchant in the context of this review of marijuana-induced reactions as to merit an extensive summary. In their series 106 patients were studied. Alcohol, bromide, barbiturates, or heavy metal toxicity accounted for 46 cases; infectious states accounted for 19 cases; and other systemic pathological conditions (e.g., renal failure and eclampsia) accounted for 41 cases. For three-fourths of the cases, the duration of "maximal disturbance" was approximately three weeks. What was most clearly found was that variability was the most consistent feature. Within short periods of time, patients would vary widely in their range of impairment. Also it was felt that many of the disturbances seen may have been brought on by leading questions of the investigators.

General physical symptoms of dysfunction and prostration were almost always present in these severely ill patients including restlessness, tremors, and poor sleep. In addition, physiological symptoms reflecting the psychological state of the patient were present, including sweating, pallor, tachycardia, flushing, nausea, diarrhea, and constipation. Slurred speech was common, motor incoordination, staggering gait, difficulty swallowing, pupillary changes, and inconsistent changes in deep tendon reflexes were found. The occurrence of all these somatic changes bore no specific relation to the etiological agent, but rather were related to the degree of general disturbance.

In every case there was clouding of consciousness. The extent of this impaired mentation varied from patient to patient and from moment to moment in the same patient. Common clinical features were gross disorientation at some time, poor attention span, decreased concentration, disconnected thinking, diffuse and rambling answers to questions, poor recent memory with relatively intact remote memory, poor retention, poor calculations, and increased suggestibility. Restlessness was invariably present. Mood was characteristically labile and frequently would alternate rapidly between a dreamlike state and one of elation, depression, irritability, panic, anger, anxiety, perplexity, or suspicion. Suicidal verbalizations and attempts occasionally occurred during these toxic states.

Simple misinterpretations of activities around them frequently became the basis of delusional beliefs, the specific content of which was contingent on the patient's past life and personality make-up. Usually these beliefs were transient and poorly systematized; at some point every patient verbalized paranoid fears of persecution. Visual hallucinations were experienced by 72 of the patients and auditory hallucinations by 44, often devoid of personal implication and triggered by a misperception. Confabulation was common and occasionally prominent.

Unique features of this syndrome seen in individual patients were derived from the specific etiological agent, the physical condition of the patient, the specific situation of the patient's care, and the patient's own personality. This "individual equipment and experience" formed the basis for the content of the hallucinations and delusions experienced; for the quality of the misperceptions and misinterpretations prominent; for the content of the confabulations; for the dominant mood state; and for the relative importance and content of sexual, religious, and occupational themes noted in such conditions. In addition to outstanding personality qualities, intelligence and important life problems contributed to the individual variation found during such a condition. As described by Wolff and Curran, the occurrence of an acute brain syndrome in the presence of an intercurrent psychiatric illness or in patients with a history of a past psychiatric episode sometimes caused a transient recrudescense of that illness or took on many of its features. Whether that is the etiology of prolonged psychiatric consequences following an acute toxic reaction to marijuana as described in the literature is speculative, though possible. They also noted that experiences during the clouded condition occasionally were remembered by patients long after recovery as events which they were convinced either did occur or might have occurred, thus remaining as residual false beliefs. Such residual false beliefs could easily be misinterpreted by an overly zealous psychiatrist as evidence of chronic residual impairment.

D. *Intercurrent Psychiatric Illness*

In addition to the relatively short-lived panic reaction and marijuana acute brain syndrome as adverse effects of marijuana use, several authors have attributed an etiological role to marijuana in precipitating an enduring psychiatric illness, i.e., an illness lasting more than several days. Schizophrenia, depression, mania, and at least one new illness, the "amotivational syndrome," have been attributed to marijuana. Case reports drawing such conclusions, as those in earlier sections, have presented scant descriptive data and lacked diagnostic criteria to justify such diagnostic decisions. Here, most acutely, are felt the limitations of the case report. It is impossible to know what information was sought, what was elicited, and what was ignored; only what is reported. It is not possible therefore to apply any systematic criteria to these cases to verify the diagnostic decision.

There are three possible etiological relationships between marijuana use and the apparent precipitation of an enduring psychiatric illness: (1) Psychiatrically well individuals who use marijuana may develop psychiatric illness. (2) There may be borderline ill individuals whose use of marijuana alters their psychiatric illness from a "latent" form to an overt one. (3) Psychiatrically ill individuals who use marijuana may have an exacerbation or alteration in their illness. In any of these groups, to demonstrate that marijuana use can precipitate *de novo* a new psychiatric syndrome or a known disorder such as schizophrenia, depression, or mania, sufficiently large numbers of such users must be studied, along with nonuser controls carefully matched to show that a significantly higher prevalence of psychiatric illness occurs in these users over the nonusers not accounted for by other factors held constant. With one exception to be discussed later, such controlled systematic studies have not been performed. Rather, record reviews, uncontrolled collections of patients, and case reports have linked marijuana use with psychiatric disturbance. In the absence of systematic studies it is not possible to demonstrate a causal relationship between marijuana use and psychiatric disturbance in previously well populations. The concept of the "borderline" or "marginal" personality itself has not as yet been defined sufficiently to be useful in marijuana studies; it is therefore impossible to evaluate its importance with regard to possible precipitation of illness by marijuana use. In the remaining group, the previously ill individuals, though it is possible to describe clinical modifications of the illness by drug use, it is extremely difficult to demonstrate that a recrudescence of the illness was precipitated by drug use. What literature exists linking marijuana use with intercurrent known psychiatric disorders will now be reviewed.

Bernhardson and Gunne (1972) reviewed admissions to all Swedish mental hospitals involving habitual cannabis users for the period 1966 to 1970. Of 66 cases found, 46 were evaluated where marijuana was the dominant drug used, though in only 10 was marijuana the only drug used. They found that in 16 of the 46 cases signs of psychosis preceded drug abuse. Twenty-four suffered from a brief psychotic episode, of which 16 resembled schizophrenia, 6 were called mania, 1 depression, and 1 confusional state. Enduring psychoses were found among the other 22 patients of which 14 were already psychotic prior to drug use and 8 were not. Of these 22, 20 were diagnosed as schizophrenia and 2 as manic depressive. Campbell (1971) found that among 13 marijuana users with psychosis, 3 had a schizophrenic picture, 4 had a psychotic depression, 2 had amotivational syndrome, and 4 had transient psychoses. There is no indication in Campbell's work of premorbid mental state, of family history information, or of diagnostic criteria. Gaskill (1945) reviewed 150 marijuana using American soldiers seen while stationed in India and Burma during the Second World War. He felt that habitual users were soldiers who had a major personality defect, i.e., "melancholic, mentally deficient, early schizophrenic, psychopathic." Chopra *et al.* (1942) reviewed 600 cases of "hemp drug insanity" collected during a 10 year period. Acute disorders lasting from a few days to a few weeks thought to simulate all forms of insanity and usually marked by "an extreme vehemence of mania" were described as "confused, excited, bright shining eyes (congested), shouts, sighs, violent, aggressive, may run amuck": patients recovered completely and were afterwards oblivious to things which took place during the period of intoxication. Such acute disorders accounted for more than three-quarters of the total cases presented. Although in the absence of diagnostic criteria it is impossible to elucidate the meaning of the diagnostic categories which were used, something of the quality of the syndromes may be obtained from the terms chosen: mania of confusional type 33%, maniacal condition of explosive form 7.5%, toxic hallucinosis 12.5%, melancholia 12%, depressive mania 2%, and recurrent toxic mania 10%. Chronic conditions found were chronic toxic mania 15%, schizophrenia 5%, and dementia 3%. It is of note that of the 600 cases, one-third were complicated by other drug use, factors of heredity, or prior psychiatric illness. Since marijuana use was then endemic in India, it can be suggested that in Chopra's material many of the cases of mania were unrelated to the coincidental use of marijuana. Colbach and Crowe (1970) and Grossman (1969) have also each included among their case reports apparent episodes of possible mania concurrent with marijuana use. Harding and Knight (1973) discuss this question of mania complicated by marijuana use in presenting 4 such cases where they felt the drug altered the clinical manifestations of the manic syndrome to include schizophreniform symptoms.

Milman (1969) described 11 adolescent patients, 7 of whom had sought psychiatric help prior to drug use and all of whom were multiple drug abusers. Almost all were considered to have become chronic schizophrenics subsequent to their marijuana use. No diagnostic criteria are presented and it is impossible to confirm that diagnosis based on the 6 case histories as presented; rather, diagnoses of depression, antisocial personality, and acute brain syndrome seem more applicable. Depression has been described in association with marijuana use. The "amotivational syndrome," when described clinically, as by Smith (1968), Keeler (1967), and Scher (1970), seems quite similar to depression seen in comparable non-marijuana using young adults. Thurlow (1971) described 5 students with symptoms of depression who responded to antidepressant medication promptly, but who, because of marijuana use, were each called amotivational syndrome. Kolansky and Moore (1971), Davison and Wilson (1972), Kaplan (1971), Tylden (1967), George (1970), and Perna (1969) have all described among their reported cases patients with clinical syndromes of apparent depression concurrent with marijuana use. Kupfer et al. (1973), using a questionnaire psychological test with college students who were all marijuana users reinforced the suggestion that the amotivational syndrome is synonymous with the clinical picture of depression in a college population. Thus it would seem that many authors may have attributed an etiological role to marijuana use in precipitating or explaining known intercurrent psychiatric syndromes that is not justified on the basis of current information.

CASE MATERIAL

a. Possibly Depression—From Kolansky and Moore (1971). A 16-year-old girl with no prior psychiatric problems used marijuana regularly for 2 years. She began to lose interest in academic work and became preoccupied with political issues. From a quiet and popular girl, she became hostile and quite impulsive with inappropriate verbal attacks on teachers and peers. She dropped out of her senior year of high school and was referred. She showed inappropriate affect and developed paranoid ideas. She refused to discontinue marijuana use and eventually became so depressed that she attempted suicide by hanging. After withdrawal from the drug, her depression and paranoid ideas slowly disappeared, as did her outbursts of aggression. Ten months later, she continued to show impairment of memory and thought disorder, marked by her complaint that she could not study or transform her thoughts into written or spoken words as easily as previously.

b. Amotivational Syndrome, Possibly Depression—From Smith (1968). A 22-year-old second year medical student was brought by his parents because he was doing quite poorly in his studies and was considering dropping out of medical school. After having quite successfully completed his first year, he had begun smoking marijuana with friends prior to his second year and had gotten sick of the "phony struggle for grades." After much debate, he moved home, discontinued marijuana use, continued in school, and seemed reasonably happy with his future career in medicine 1 year later.

The possibility exists that what has been described is the coincidental use of marijuana with intercurrent psychiatric illness. Until several controlled studies have confirmed the type of association marijuana may have with psychiatric illness, it is as premature to attribute etiological significance to the use of marijuana as to suggest that only because of preexisting psychiatric problems are people drawn to its use. In light of methodological and psychiatric research questions raised earlier, accurate reevaluation of cases reported in the literature is impossible. However, as Guze (1970) has pointed out, a "toughminded" attitude is essential to the improvement of knowledge in the area of psychiatric research. To accept facilely the notion that any life activity can cause a recognized psychiatric syndrome whose clinical course has been previously characterized merely by indicating a temporal relationship is to obfuscate rather than clarify the question of psychiatric etiology. Some clinical features will vary amongst differing subgroups of patients having the same clinical syndrome as a function of demographic, social, ethnic, religious, and educational differences, as well as differing social habits. In the absence of controlled studies, it is imprudent to create new classifications based on a few possibly irrelevant or coincidental variables, such as marijuana use, when the clinical cases might be comfortably and accurately subsumed by already existing psychiatric diagnoses. As will be discussed in the next section, the association of psychiatric illness with marijuana use as determined by systematic studies is by no means clear.

IV. CORRELATIONS OF MARIJUANA USE WITH PSYCHIATRIC ILLNESS

A. Review of the Literature

Populations of marijuana users have been studied for antecedent personality characteristics and behavioral events. These studies can now be scrutinized, cognizant of the methodological and diagnostic pitfalls. Soueif, in Egypt (1967), found among young cannabis users as motivations for first use conformity, euphoria, curiosity, and to be "real men." Compared to matched nonusers, users were considered to have been neglected by their fathers; to have had parental conflicts during their upbringing; and to be impulsive, suggestible, and shy. Boroffka (1966), studying marijuana users in Nigeria, found them to be emotionally, mentally, or socially unstable. They wanted to "cheat destiny." In 1946 Bromberg and Rodgers in a study of Navy offenders, found no positive correlation between aggressive crime and marijuana use, deciding that marijuana usage was but an aspect of some type of "mental disorder or personality abnormality." Charen and Perelman (1946) studying 60 soldier users in 1945, of whom 51 had been referred for psychopathic behavior, found that most had come from broken homes with dis-social fathers and strict mothers, most had a poor work history, 10 had civilian arrests, and most were considered at the time of study to be sullen, resentful of authority, and to lack motivation. Similarly, Marcovitz and Myers in 1944 studied

35 soldier marijuana "addicts," 34 black and 1 white, and found that their backgrounds were heavily loaded with adverse familial, social, economic, criminal, and delinquent factors.

Freedman and Wilson (1964) decided that drug addiction in the young came from a multiplicity of factors and felt that something predisposed an individual to addiction. "The younger the boy involved with drugs, the greater the deviation and pathology in social and personal areas." Keeler (1968) studied 54 white college marijuana users who had made contact with the psychiatry health service. The main reasons for initial drug use were curiosity and "desire to go along"; continued use was attributed to tension relief, release of inhibitions, desire for euphoria, and desire for psychotomimetic experiences. Similar findings came from Hogan et al. (1970) studying college students with a questionnaire and psychological inventory who felt that users and nonusers were indistinguishable with regard to prior schooling, but that marijuana users were socially more skilled and broader in outlook. Also, they were more adventuresome, more impulsive and nonconforming, and more concerned with the feelings of others. When compared to principled nonusers who were considered responsible, considerate, conventional, but lacking spontaneity and verve; the users were poised, self-confident, narcissistic, and had an overconcern with personal pleasure, diversion, and self-aggrandizement. Also, Norton (1968) studied 13 users who saw a psychiatrist for some legal reason. After psychological testing he concluded that the users had good education, conventional jobs, expressed a preference for aesthetic values, and had a high degree of extraversion.

Other investigators have found more substantive differences between users and nonusers. Thus, Harmatz et al. (1972) using personality tests felt that users showed more "psychiatric impairment" than nonusers. McAree et al. (1969) using the MMPI and a questionnaire studied three college drug using groups. Multiple drug users separated easily from the other groups on the basis of abnormal MMPI findings, but marijuana-only users could not easily be differentiated from controls. The multiple drug users had more withdrawal, aloofness, and inability to express emotions than marijuana-only users and nondrug users. Robbins et al. (1970) using self-administered drug surveys in two colleges reported that marijuana users had looser religious ties than nonusing students, were less likely to be at the top of their class, and were more dissatisfied with school. In this survey, users of any drug were more likely to be anxious, bored, cynical, disgusted, impulsive, moody, rebellious, or restless than the nonusers. In King's report of his questionnaire survey (1970), marijuana users were found to be more opposed to external controls and to view marijuana as a specific agent for tension relief and relaxation. Recently, Kupfer (1970), using a survey of upperclassmen, compared heavy marijuana users (more than three occasions of use per week) with less heavy users and with 50 psychiatric patients. Most of both drug using groups had used other drugs in addition to marijuana. No differences were found between the two drug using groups regarding grade point averages, work adjustment, or personality changes. Among the heavy marijuana users, Kupfer did find more depression and organicity than among the psychiatric patients, but less anxiety. It was concluded that psychiatric symptoms increased with increased drug use. Several symposia have speculated about motivations for use and personality types of users, including the UCLA Interdepartmental Conference (1969) which considered that heavy marijuana users had "severe underlying psychological disturbances" and that marijuana use was a surface symptom functioning as an anxiety-relieving mechanism (also, the Committee on Youth, 1969; Joint Session of the Mental Health Association and Orthopsychiatry Association, 1967).

Marijuana "flashbacks" have been described anecdotally in the literature. As presented by Keeler et al. (1968a), the flashback is a "spontaneous recurrence of unusual somatic or visual sensations originally experienced during the drug reaction." As Keeler found, such recurrences may be subjectively considered adverse or pleasant, may be linked to current psychopathology rather than to drug effect, or may be linked to some residual improvement in perceptual awareness. The existence of this phenomenon with regard to marijuana by other than case reports has not as yet been documented. Whether it exists as an independent primary event, whether it is the spontaneous recollection of an emotionally significant event, i.e., an important memory, or whether it is the coincidental occurrence of anxiety symptoms falsely linked to earlier irrelevant marijuana use is unknown. If flashbacks with regard to marijuana use do exist separate from the above-mentioned considerations, their explanation, incidence, and significance are unknown.

The existence of physiological tolerance to marijuana in man is controversial. Tolerance in rats was found by Carlini (1968) and in pigeons and other animals by McMillan (1970; McMillan et al., 1971) using intramuscular administration of THC. This author (Halikas et al., 1972a) found among some experienced marijuana users the development of "reverse tolerance," i.e., the production of a subjectively comparable level of intoxication using less marijuana; this "reverse tolerance" in some and tolerance in others has also been noted by Smith and Mehl (1970). Physiological addiction as indicated by the appearance of a stereotyped withdrawal syndrome has never been demonstrated either in animals or man. Psychological habituation [defined by Jaffe (1970) as when drug effects or the conditions associated with its use are necessary to maintain an optimal subjective state of well being impelling use of the drug] theoretically exists at least among some regular marijuana users if not in the United States, possibly in societies where daily marijuana use is traditional.

Thus attempts to determine the association between marijuana use and psychological factors have produced limited and often contradictory results. A systematic attempt, using a random population of marijuana users and a comparable control group of nonusers, to determine the association of marijuana use with psychiatric illness performed by this author will now be presented.

B. A Systematic Study of Marijuana Use and Psychiatric Illness

In 1969 and 1970 a total of 100 regular marijuana users and 50 nonuser friends were interviewed by this author (Halikas *et al.* 1972b) using a systematic structured interview. All subjects were at least 18 years old and white. The users had to be self-defined as regular marijuana users and to have used marijuana on at least 50 occasions during at least 6 months of use. This criterion was designed to obtain a sample population that viewed themselves not as experimenters or casual, social users, but as regular, committed users; to assure an extensive experience in its use; and to assure a sufficient time period of use during which psychiatric, social, or legal consequences might have occurred.

Subjects were obtained through the creation of word-of-mouth chains of referrals beginning with three "source" people known to have access to different drug using groups in the community, without either financial remuneration or personal participation for themselves. Each volunteer was assured of anonymity and paid $10.00 for his participation. Interviewed subjects were then requested to tell their friends, both users and nonusers, about the study; up to 9 generations of referrals were obtained in an arborization effect. No attempt could be made to obtain information about people contacted who chose not to participate. The use of nonuser friends as a control group was chosen to have some analogous population group against which to make comparisons, based on the untested hypothesis that friendship selection is a process reflecting internal traits, that "birds of a feather flock together."

The interview was primarily a systematic current and lifetime psychiatric evaluation. In addition, childhood experiences, parental habits and rearing practices, educational background and experiences, chronological development and social landmarks, medical history, family history, and personal drug use including alcohol and tobacco were all explored by structured and open-ended questioning. Extensive information was also obtained from the users concerning their marijuana use and its consequences. Interviews lasted from 2 to 4 hours for users and from 1 to 2 hours for controls. Diagnostic criteria used in the study consisted of specific psychiatric symptoms and life patterns as described earlier in this chapter. No separate diagnoses of drug dependence were made nor were direct consequences of drug abuse considered as contributing to diagnostic criteria of other psychiatric illnesses.

Both samples studied were in general well educated, of upper middle-class background, and young (mean age of users, 22; of nonusers, 23). About two-thirds of each group were males. Among the users, the average duration of marijuana use was slightly more than 2 years. Their checklist description of marijuana effects was noted earlier in this report; other aspects of their marijuana use have been previously described (Halikas et al., 1971, 1972a,b). All but 16 of the 100 users had also used other drugs; among the self-selected nonuser controls, about half had tried marijuana, averaging 7 trials each.

There was a strikingly high lifetime incidence of psychopathology found in both groups. Approximately half of both the regular marijuana users and the control group of nonuser friends fulfilled criteria for a definite or probable psychiatric diagnosis. About one-third of each group received a diagnosis of primary affective disorder. Sociopathy was found in 12% of the users compared to none of the controls ($p = <0.05$). Anxiety neurosis and hysteria were more frequent among the nonusers, and homosexuality or other sexual deviance were more common among the users, but these differences were not significant. No subject fulfilled criteria for a diagnosis of schizophrenia in either group.

An additional one-quarter of each group reported past psychiatric manifestations of significance which, however, did not fulfill diagnostic criteria. For both users and nonusers, a past depressive period was the most frequently reported problem. Antisocial activity, multiple homosexual experiences, and problems from drinking all occurred substantially more frequently among the marijuana users, but only the difference in early antisocial behavior was significant. No significant difference in incidence or types of diagnostic or nondiagnostic pathology were found between the nonusers who had had experience with marijuana and the nonusers who had never tried it.

Fifty percent of the users and 40% of their nonuser friends had at some time seen a psychiatrist, psychologist, or other professional counselor. Five of the 100 marijuana users had been psychiatrically hospitalized a total of 13 times; 6 of the 50 controls had had a total of 17 psychiatric hospitalizations. These differences were not statistically signficant. The rather high frequency figures of having at some time sought assistance, or of having been hospitalized psychiatrically, in such young populations, tended to objectively confirm the high lifetime incidence of psychopathology found by the study.

With each subject careful attention was paid to dating the onset of psychiatric symptoms and characterizing the time course of disorders. It was therefore possible for the user group to determine whether the psychiatrically significant episode occurred or began before or after the first use of marijuana. Except for one-quarter of the affective disorders, every diagnosed psychiatric illness began before first marijuana use. Further, in the great majority of instances, psychiatrically significant nondiagnostic experiences of all types occurred before first use of marijuana. The temporal relationship of additional landmarks was also determined. Use of alcohol and tobacco usually preceded marijuana; sexual intercourse nearly always antedated marijuana experience. "Acting out" behaviors—police trouble, arrests, homosexual experience, and heavy drinking—when they occurred, more often preceded marijuana experience than followed it. Utilization of professional help, suicide attempts, and psychiatric hospitalizations, were equally likely to have preceded as followed first marijuana use.

This work was an attempt to systematically study the association of marijuana use and psychiatric illness. The methodological limitations of time, place, legality, sampling biases, and diagnostic controversy are as compelling for this work as for others in the literature. Both populations studied, the regular marijuana users and their nonuser friends, had a high incidence of psychiatric illness. That one group used marijuana and the other did not may have been a reflection of the significantly higher incidence of "acting out" behavior found in the user group. The high incidence of psychopathology found among both groups indicated that at least some regular marijuana users came from a population at high risk for psychiatric problems. As importantly, these psychiatric difficulties almost always preceded use of marijuana. In this group, therefore, regular marijuana use appeared to be a symptom of preexisting significant psychopathology, rather than an etiological factor.

The use of other drugs by these 100 regular marijuana users was also analyzed (Halikas and Rimmer, 1974). Forty-eight subjects were found to have used two or less other drugs, and 52 were found to have used more than two other drugs (mean 7.5). Early antecedent and concomitant behavioral events significantly associated with these "polydrug" users were sought. Childhood discipline contacts, truancy and drop out, earlier age of first illicit drug use, first illicit drug not being marijuana, poor high school socialization, inordinate parental conflicts, poor adolescent adjustment, antisocial behavior, police contacts, homosexual experiences, and self-defeating behavior in adolescence were found to predict later polydrug use from amongst this population. It was felt that these were limit testing events and other problems reflecting internal personality characteristics of the polydrug subgroup of marijuana users. This conclusion was reinforced by the wide variety of deleterious childhood and family life experiences which were found not to be significantly associated with later multiple drug use in this population. Neither social isolation in childhood, a disrupted, or turbulent home life nor parents who served as role models of excessive personal drug use served to distinguish the polydrug group. Events which were significantly associated with multiple drug use, but because of precocious drug involvement by this subgroup were not predictors, included school expulsion or suspension, high school academic problems, earlier age of sexual intercourse, and earlier age of first use of cigarettes and of alcohol. These findings, therefore, tend to support the previously reviewed suggestions that marijuana users may not be a homogeneous group but rather at least two distinct populations whose later drug use reflects earlier life patterns and personality traits.

C. Other Systematic Studies

Beaubrun and Knight (1973) reported on a study of 30 chronic marijuana users and 30 carefully matched controls done in Jamaica. Use of marijuana was daily for at least 7 years. These populations were studied medically as well as psychiatrically. No significant differences in the two groups in incidence of mental illness, alcoholism, abnormal mood, abnormal thought processes, or abnormal behavior were found. The marijuana users had a higher incidence of family history of mental illness and had experienced hallucinations more frequently than controls (which usually occurred during the first occasion of marijuana use). No significant differences were found in neuroticism, extraversion, number of arrests, criminal convictions, use of other drugs, or movement in social or economic position. Furthermore, no medical differences were found.

McGlothlin *et al.* (1970) reported on 29 middle-aged subjects from a larger study who had used marijuana at least two or more times per week for a minimum of 2 years begun in their youth. Two control groups from the larger study were also selected, one of 40 who had never used marijuana and one of 22 who had used it occasionally but never on a regular basis. Both control samples were matched to the marijuana population for demographic and occupational characteristics. The regular marijuana users were found to have been considerably more prone to the use of other drugs, including alcohol, than were the two comparison samples; including for 8 of the 29 development of serious dependence on alcohol, heroin, or amphetamines. A higher proportion of the regular users group were raised in large cities, felt that their parents' marriages were unhappy, and had fathers who used alcohol heavily. Among the user group also, there was a significantly higher incidence of marital discord, job instability, and residence changes. Personality correlates found which distinguished the regular users from the other groups were a belief in the validity of "paranormal" phenomena, involvement in nondrug methods of altering consciousness, and preferences for extremes, risk taking, and the unfamiliar. Though methodologically limited, this work confirmed outcome patterns found by Robins *et al.* (1970) in a different population.

Robins *et al.* (1970) performed a long-term follow-up investigation of 235 Negro boys of normal or better intelligence, selected randomly from elementary school records of the late 1940's and early 1950's with no knowledge of their later behavior. Ninety-five percent were found and interviewed systematically at approximately age 33. Almost half of the group reported having used marijuana at some time. Seventy-six who had first used it in adolescence were compared to 146 subjects who had not used marijuana in adolescence, for long-term outcome status. Of the 76, 32 claimed to have never used any other drug. Significantly more of the adolescent marijuana users on follow-up had failed to graduate from high school, reported marital infidelity, fathered illegitimate children, received financial aid, had adult police records for nondrug offenses, drank heavily enough to create social or medical problems, and reported violent behavior. Marijuana use could not be predicted from variables found on the school records, such as familial disruption, low socioeconomic status, or poor grades, though these variables did predict other later problems. The poorer long-term outcome for adolescent marijuana users found by Robins in this methodologically elegant work merits careful scrutiny.

Such systematic studies provide some clue that perhaps regular marijuana use within the sociological set of the United States during the 1940's, the 1950's, and the 1960's may be related to other risk-taking and dis-social behavior, having common roots in internal personality characteristics indicative of some higher risk for later psychiatric problems; and possibly portending a less than comfortable adjustment to later adult life. As Robins prudently notes in her discussion however, "if marijuana use was responsible for differences in outcome, we were not able to show the mechanism by which the effect occurred . . ."

V. CONCLUSION

The association of marijuana use with psychiatric illness is a complex question which, as presented, currently has no satisfactory answer. Internal controversies within psychiatry limit research in the field. Most anecdotal reports do not present diagnostic criteria used in the investigation. Most reports use descriptive terms which are in large measure interpretative and subject to various definitions. Theoretical formulations modify the perceptions of investigators and affect diagnostic decisions. Valid sample selection is complex and rarely occurs, though crucial toward the development of sound epidemiological prevalence data for psychiatric syndromes. Also, psychiatry of all the medical specialties is the most closely tied to social questions and contemporary societal values. These internal problems have left psychiatric research methodology well behind research in other branches of medicine.

Research into psychiatric aspects of marijuana use is limited by methodological and social complications. Collecting population samples which are epidemiologically representative is impossible where marijuana use is illegal or limited to unrepresentative portions of a society. Cross-cultural problems limit the usefulness of marijuana studies from other societies. Because the physiological and pharmacological effects of marijuana are not clearly defined, clinical studies are limited. The use of other drugs and of illicitly obtained marijuana raises the confounding questions of effects of unknown drugs, dosages, and adulterants in studying populations of users. There are at least two possible acute adverse reactions to marijuana intoxication, the panic anxiety reaction and the toxic acute brain syndrome. Whether from the clinical anecdotal reports linking marijuana with acute and chronic psychopathology will emerge any new diagnostic syndrome, or any clearcut marijuana modified extant psychiatric syndrome, or whether marijuana will indeed be demonstrated as an etiological agent in precipitating a recognized syndrome remains to be proved.

The apparent importance of normal marijuana effects in shaping the quality of adverse reactions is indicated by the predominance of the panic anxiety reaction among untoward syndromes. Weil (1970) has estimated that upwards of 75% of cases in his experience were panic anxiety reactions. Because of the illegal standing of marijuana use, the panic reaction is probably underrepresented in proportion to all marijuana reactions since the milder ones are probably managed by the patient's confreres. What proportion of adverse marijuana reactions in other countries are of the panic anxiety type cannot be estimated because of the many other intercurrent significant variables affecting such a determination. The emotional and psychological set of the user as well as the effect of the setting on precipitation of this reaction appear to be crucial but as yet not clearly elucidated. In the absence of accurate dose-response correlation figures, the significance of unexpected change in dosage must also remain speculative.

The clinical picture of the panic anxiety reaction is dominated by prominent psychological and physiological features of anxiety, in the presence of a clear sensorium, and often with accompanying symptoms of intoxication as well. The content of verbalizations during this panic situation is often determined by the psychological situation of the patient, i.e., ambivalence about the use of the drug causing paranoid or somatic fears, or use of the drug in an abortive therapeutic attempt triggering fears of losing one's mind or worsening of a depressed mood.

The Marijuana Acute Brain Syndrome is apparently quite rare in the United States (Smith and Mehl, 1970). Whether this is a function of the relative weakness of marijuana available as noted by Goodwin (1970) or route of administration (Weil, 1970) or relative safety of the setting (Talbott and Teague, 1969) or because of the absolute rarity of the reaction is unknown. The hallmarks of the clinical picture of this reaction are similar to that of other acute brain syndromes caused by a variety of toxic situations: clouding of mental processes with impairment of orientation, impairment of memory, confusion, impairment of thinking, and impairment of reality testing. Misperceptions, hallucinations, delusions, emotional lability, hyperactivity, and bizarre behavior often occur.

Several traditional psychiatric syndromes have been described in conjunction with marijuana use usually attributing an etiological role to the drug. In some parts of the world, as noted by Grinspoon (1971), this may be administrative shorthand; in the United States this may be accounted for by the heat of controversy and poor psychiatric research methodology.

At least some marijuana users appear to come from a segment of the population at higher risk for a variety of psychiatric disorders. Some do not appear to make as adequate an adjustment to adulthood as comparable nonusing controls. As found in each of the systematic studies of Halikas, Robins, and McGlothlin, antecedents, consequences, and coincidences are complex questions which have yet to adequately parcel out the variable of marijuana use to distinguish its role from that of other associated events in predicting later outcome. The resolution of these questions is necessary before any adequate discussion of the interaction of marijuana use and psychiatric illness can occur without falling into the logical fallacy of *non causa pro causa,* false causes.

Hopefully, the reader will not be deterred by the skepticism of this chapter, but rather will be stimulated to evaluate future work more critically and, possibly, will design methodologically and epidemiologically precise research which will answer some of the questions raised in this review.

ACKNOWLEDGMENTS

The author wishes to acknowledge the vital assistance of Ronald Weller, M.D., in the preparation of this report, particularly noting his help on the study of the literature and his organizational suggestions. This work was supported, in part, by U.S.P.H.S. Grants MH-01110 and DA-00023. The author is the recipient of an NIMH Career Teacher Award in Narcotics, Drug Abuse, and Alcoholism, DA-00023.

REFERENCES

Allentuck, S. (1944). *In* "The Marihuana Problem in the City of New York." Mayor LaGuardia's Committee on Marihuana. As reproduced in Solomon (1966). Jacques Cattell Press, New York.
Allentuck, S., and Bowman, K. M. (1942). *Amer. J. Psychiat.* 99, 248–251.
Anonymous. (1967). *Med. Lett. Drugs Ther.* 9, 73–76.
Anonymous. (1970). *Med. Lett. Drugs Ther.* 12, 33–35.
Baker-Bates, E. T. (1935). *Lancet* 1, 811.
Beaubrun, M. H., and Knight, F. (1973). *Amer. J. Psychiat.* 130, 309–311.
Bernhardson, G., and Gunne, L.-N. (1972). *Inst. J. Addict.* 7, 9–16.
Bey, D. R., and Zecchinelli, V. A. (1971). *Mil. Med.* 136, 21–28.
Bialos, D. S. (1970). *Amer. J. Psychiat.* 127, 819–823.
Bloch, H. S. (1969). *Amer. J. Psychiat.* 126, 289.
Boroffka, A. (1966). *East Afr. Med. J.* 43, 377–384.
Bromberg, W. (1939). *J. Amer. Med. Ass.* 113, 4–12.
Bromberg, W., and Rodgers, T. C. (1946). *Amer. J. Psychiat.* 102, 825–827.
Campbell, D. R. (1971). *Can. Psychiat. Ass. J.* 16, 161–165.
Carlini, E. A. (1968). *Pharmacology* 1, 135–142.
Charen, S., and Perelman, L. (1946). *Amer. J. Psychiat.* 102, 674–682.
Chopra, G. S. (1969). *Int. J. Addict.* 4, 215–247.
Chopra, G. S., and Smith, J. W. (1974). *Arch. Gen. Psychiat.* 30, 24–27.
Chopra, R. N., Chopra, G. S., and Chopra, I. C. (1942). *Indian J. Med. Res.* 30, 155–171.
Clark, L. D., and Nakashima, E. N. (1968). *Amer. J. Psychiat.* 125, 379–384.
Cleckley, H. (1964). "The Mask of Sanity," 4th ed. Mosby, St. Louis, Missouri.
Colbach, E. M., and Crowe, R. R. (1970). *Mil. Med.* 135, 571–573.
Committee on Youth. (1969). *Pediatrics* 44, 131–141.

Davison, K., and Wilson, C. H. (1972). *Brit. J. Addict.* **67**, 225–228.
Feighner, J. P., Robins, E., Guze, S. B., Woodruff, R. A., Winokur, G., and Munoz, R. (1972). *Arch. Gen. Psychiat.* **26**, 57–63.
Fitzgibbons, D. J., and Hokanson, D. T. (1973). *Amer. J. Psychiat.* **130**, 972–975.
Freedman, A. M., and Wilson, E. A. (1964). *Pediatrics* **34**, 283–292.
Gaskill, H. S. (1945). *Amer. J. Psychiat.* **102**, 202–204.
George, H. R. (1970). *Brit. J. Addict.* **65**, 119–121.
Goode, E. (1970). "The Marihuana Smokers." Basic Books, New York.
Goode, E. (1969). *Soc. Probl.* **17**, 48.
Goodwin, D. W. (1970). *Sci. Amer.* **222**, 6.
Grinspoon, L. (1971). "Marihuana Reconsidered." Harvard Univ. Press, Cambridge, Massachusetts.
Grossman, W. (1969). *Ann. Intern. Med.* **70**, 529–533.
Guze, S. B. (1970). *S. Med. J.* **63**, 662.
Halikas, J. A., and Rimmer, J. S. (1974). *Arch. Gen. Psychiat.* **31**, 414–418.
Halikas, J. A., Goodwin, D. W., and Guze, S. B. (1971). *J. Amer. Med. Ass.* **217**, 692–694.
Halikas, J. A., Goodwin, D. W., and Guze, S. B. (1972a). *Comp. Psychiat.* **13**, 161–163.
Halikas, J. A., Goodwin, D. W., and Guze, S. B. (1972b). *Arch. Gen. Psychiat.* **27**, 162–165.
Harding, T., and Knight, F. (1973). *Arch. Gen. Psychiat.* **29**, 635–637.
Harmatz, J. S., Shader, R. I., and Salzman, C. (1972). *Arch. Gen. Psychiat.* **26**, 108–112.
Hogan, R., Mankin, D., Comway, J., and Fox, S. (1970). *J. Consult. Clin. Psychol.* **35**, 58–63.
Jaffe, J. H. (1970). *In* "The Pharmacological Basis of Therapeutics," L. S. Goodman and A. Gilman, eds., 4th ed., p. 276. Macmillan, New York.
Joint Session of Mental Health Association and Orthopsychiatric Association. (1967). *Amer. J. Orthopsychiat.* **37**, 296–299.
Kaplan, H. S. (1971). *N.Y. State J. Med.* **71**, 433–435.
Kaplan, J. (1970). "Marijuna: The New Prohibition." World Publ. Co., Cleveland, Ohio.
Keeler, M. H. (1967). *Amer. J. Psychiat.* **124**, 674–677.
Keeler, M. H. (1968). *Amer. J. Psychiat.* **125**, 386–390.
Keeler, M. H., Reifler, C. B., and Liptzin, M. B. (1968). *Amer. J. Psychiat.* **125**, 384–386.
Kendell, R. E., Cooper, J. E., Gourley, A. J., Copeland, J. R. M., Sharpe, L., and Gurland, B. J. (1971). *Arch. Gen. Psychiat.* **25**, 123–130.
King, F. W. (1970). *J. Amer. Coll. Health Ass.* **18**, 213–217.
Klee, G. D. (1969). *Psychiat. Quart.* **43**, 719–733.
Kolansky, H., and Moore, W. T. (1971). *J. Amer. Med. Ass.* **216**, 486–492.
Kupfer, D. J., Detre, T., Koral, J., and Fajans, P. (1973). *Amer. J. Psychiat.* **130**, 1319–1322.
Liskow, B., Liss, J. L., and Parker, C. W. (1971). *Ann. Intern. Med.* **75**, 571–573.
McAree, C. P., Steffenhagen, R. A., and Zheutlin, L. S. (1969). *Int. J. Soc. Psychiat.* **15**, 102–106.
McGlothlin, W. H., Arnold, D. O., and Rowan, P. K. (1970). *Psychiatry* **33**, 433–443.
McMillan, D. E. (1970). *Science* **169**, 501–503.
McMillan, D. E., Dewey, W. L., and Harris, L. S. (1971). *Ann. N.Y. Acad. Sci.* **191**, 83–99.

Marcovitz, E., and Myers, H. J. (1944). *War Med.* **6,** 382–391.
Marten, G. W. (1969). *Tenn. Med. Ass. J.* **62,** 627.
Milman, D. H. (1969). *J. Pediat.* **74,** 283–290.
Miras, C. J. (1970). *Int. J. Psychiat.* **9,** 533–535.
Norton, W. A. (1968). *Can. Psychiat. Ass. J.* **13,** 163–173.
Panzetta, A. F. (1974). *Arch. Gen. Psychiat.* **30,** 154–161.
Paton, W. D. M., Pertwee, R. G., and Tylden, E. (1973). *In* "Marijuana: Chemistry, Pharmacology, Metabolism and Clinical Effects" (R. Mechoulam, ed.), pp. 335–365. Academic Press, New York.
Perna, D. (1969). *J. Amer. Med. Ass.* **209,** 1085–1086.
Persyko, I. (1970). *J. Amer. Med. Ass.* **212,** 1527.
Robbins, E. S., Robbins, L., Frosch, W. A., and Stern, M. (1970). *Amer. J. Psychiat.* **126,** 1743–1751.
Robins, L. N. (1966). "Deviant Children Grown Up." Waverly Press, Baltimore, Maryland.
Robins, L. N., Darvish, H. S., and Murphy, G. E. (1970). *In* "The Psychopathology of Adolescence" (J. Zubin and A. M. Freedman, eds.), pp. 159–180. Grune & Stratton, New York.
Scher, J. (1970). *J. Amer. Med. Ass.* **214,** 1120.
Siler, J. F., Sheep, W. L., Bates, L. B., Clark, G. F., Cook, G. W., and Smith, W.A.S. (1933). *Mil. Surg.* **73,** 269–280.
Smith, D. E. (1968). *J. Psychedelic Drugs* **2,** 37–47.
Smith, D. E., and Mehl, C. (1970). *Clin. Toxicol.* **3,** 101–115.
Solomon, D., ed. (1966). "The Marihuana Papers," pp. 316–333. Bobbs-Merrill, New York.
Soueif, M. I. (1967). *Bull. Narcotics* **19,** 1–12.
Spencer, D. J. (1970). *Brit. J. Addict.* **65,** 369–372.
Strauss, J. S. (1973). *Arch. Gen. Psychiat.* **29,** 445–449.
Talbott, J. A., and Teague, J. W. (1969). *J. Amer. Med. Ass.* **210,** 299–302.
Tart, C. T. (1970). *Nature (London)* **226,** 701–704.
Thurlow, H. J. (1971). *Can. Psychiat. Ass. J.* **16,** 181–182.
Tylden, E. (1967). *Brit. Med. J.* **3,** 556.
UCLA Interdepartmental Conference. (1969). *Ann. Intern. Med.* **70,** 591–614.
Washow, I. E., Olsson, J. E., Salzman, C., and Katz, M. M. (1970). *Arch. Gen. Psychiat.* **22,** 97–107.
Weil, A. T. (1970). *N. Engl. J. Med.* **282,** 997–1000.
Weil, A. T., Zinberg, N. E., and Nelson, J. M. (1968). *Science* **162,** 1234–1242.
Wikler, A. (1970). *Arch. Gen. Psychiat.* **23,** 320–325.
Williams, E. G., Himmelsbach, C. K., Wikler, A., Ruble, D. C., and Lloyd, B. J. (1946). *Pub. Health Rep.* **61,** 1059–1083.
Wolff, H. G., and Curran, D. (1935). *Arch. Neurol. Psychiat.* **33,** 1175–1215.
Woodruff, R. A., Goodwin, D., and Guze, S. B. (1974). "Psychiatric Diagnosis." Oxford Univ. Press, London and New York.

ADDITIONAL WORK NOT CITED

Anonymous. (1969). *Lancet* **1,** 148.
Anonymous. (1969). *Pub. Health Rep.* **84,** 1084.
Bartolucci, G., Fryer, L., Perris, C., and Shagass, C. (1969). *Can. Psychiat. Ass. J.* **14,** 77–79.

Benabud, A. (1957). *Bull. Narcotics* 9, 1–16.
Bewley, T. H. (1967). *Brit. Med. J.* 3, 603.
Bouquet, R. J. (1944). *J. Amer. Med. Ass.* 124, 1010–1011.
Bromberg, W. (1969). *Amer. J. Psychiat.* 125, 1343–1347.
Casper, E., Janecek, J., and Martinelli, H. (1968). *USARVN Med. Bull.* 40, 60–72.
Chopra, R. N., and Chopra, G. S. (1939). *Indian Med. Res. Mem.* 31, 1–119.
Dally, P. (1967). *Brit. Med. J.* 3, 367.
Goode, E. (1969). *J. Health Soc. Behav.* 10, 83–94.
Harms, E. (1972). *Brit. J. Addict.* 67, 291–296.
Hekimian, L. J., and Gershon, S. (1968). *J. Amer. Med. Ass.* 205, 125–130.
Hogan, R. (1969). *Johns Hopkins J.* 4, 3–4.
Johnson, R. D. (1968). *R.I. Med. J.* 51, 171–178.
Jørgensen, F. (1968). *Acta Psychiat. Scand., Suppl.* 203, 205–216.
Keup, W. (1970). *Dis. Nerv. Syst.* 31, 119–126.
Kornhaber, A. (1971). *J. Amer. Med. Ass.* 215, 1988.
Leonard, B. E. (1969). *Brit. J. Addict.* 64, 121–130.
McGlothlin, W. H., and West, L. J. (1968). *Amer. J. Psychiat.* 125, 370–378.
Medlicott, R. W., Sutherland, D.C., and Medlicott, P.A.W. (1970). *N.Z. Med. J.* 72, 92–95.
Milman, D. H. (1966). *N. Engl. J. Med.* 274, 167.
Murphy, H. B. M. (1963). *Bull. Narcotics* 15, 15–23.
Postal, W. B. (1968). *USARVN Med. Bull.* 10, 56–59.
Roffman, R. A., and Sapol, E. (1970). *Int. J. Addict.* 5, 1–42.
Toker, E. (1966). *Amer. J. Psychiat.* 123, 55–65.
Ungerleider, J. T., Fischer, D. D., Goldsmith, R. S., Fuller, M., and Forgy, E. (1968). *Amer. J. Psychiat.* 125, 352–357.
Wilkins, E. G. (1967). *Brit. Med. J.* 3, 496–497.
Zunin, L. M. (1969). *Mil. Med.* 134, 104–110.

Chapter 12

MARIJUANA USE AND THE PROGRESSION TO DANGEROUS DRUGS *

ERICH GOODE

I. Introduction 303
II. Logical Issues—Descriptive Studies 305
III. Methodological Issues—Descriptive Studies 313
IV. Logical Issues—Causal Mechanisms 320
V. Methodological Issues—Causal Mechanisms 327
References 336

I. INTRODUCTION

The "progression" or "escalation" of marijuana smokers to the use of more potent and dangerous drugs has been the focus of ideological and scientific controversy for well over a generation. Is marijuana a "stepping-stone" drug? Does its use "lead to" heroin, LSD, amphetamine, and/or barbiturate use? Does marijuana "precipitate" or "potentiate" multiple drug use? Does the chronic user of psychedelics, the heroin addict, or the heavy polydrug user start with marijuana? What exactly is marijuana's role in the compulsive use of dangerous drugs?

* This paper is a revision and an updating of the monograph I prepared for the National Commission on Marihuana and Drug Abuse, entitled "Drug Escalation: Marihuana Use as Related to the Use of Dangerous Drugs," and published in *Marihuana: A Signal of Misunderstanding,* The Technical Papers of the First Report of the National Commission on Marihuana and Drug Abuse, U.S. Government Printing Office, Washington, D.C., 1972.

It is precisely in those areas which are most controversial that it becomes necessary for the observer to specify in logical, precise, and empirically testable propositions just what is meant by the questions raised. At the same time, it is in those areas that such questions and issues are least likely to be specified with precision. The sloppier the formulation of a given issue, the lower the probability that one's beliefs will be refuted by empirical evidence and the greater the likelihood that any manner of evidence will appear to confirm it. The question "Does marijuana use lead to the use of more dangerous drugs?" is just such a loose and sloppy formulation. It does not permit either confirmation or disconfirmation. It is entirely possible to answer the question correctly with a "yes" or a "no," given different meanings of the question. Unless we take pains to specify the meaning of the drug progression issue, both the controversy and any attempts to resolve it will be nonsensical. By some definitions of the key variables in question, marijuana does "lead to" the use of more dangerous drugs; by other definitions, it does not. Before we attempt to answer the question, our first job is to find out exactly what the question itself might mean.

It is not altogether clear just how the drug escalation hypothesis could be tested empirically. Claims have been made that the marijuana-to-dangerous drugs progression has been thoroughly documented. Yet, an examination of the data of the available studies reveals that all are seriously flawed and most are fatally flawed. As one observer points out, the "progression hypothesis, as related to marihuana usage, has had a relatively long and undistinguished history" (Meyer, 1972). Two sorts of problems present themselves in assessing the data on this issue: logical and methodological. A *logical* problem would be one whereby the stipulations of a given study preclude any test of the hypothesis in question. A *methodological* problem would be a condition, or a set of conditions, under which a study was conducted which render the data questionable, unreliable, inaccurate, or invalid. Moreover, each of these problems can be subdivided into those which relate to whether a given study attempts to establish the *descriptive* fact of whether or not drug escalation does in fact take place—that is, whether marijuana users actually do "progress" to more dangerous drugs—and those which have to do with the *causal* issue of the specific mechanisms which make for escalation, if and when it does occur. Thus, in assessing the progression thesis, we find ourselves faced with four analytically separate problems, four possible sources of confusion in the commentaries and the studies on the subject: logical issues connected with descriptive studies, methodological issues connected with descriptive studies, logical issues connected with explorations of the causal mechanisms involved, and methodological issues connected with explorations of the causal mechanisms involved.

II. LOGICAL ISSUES—DESCRIPTIVE STUDIES

Probably the most common example of a logical fallacy involved with the presentation of data bearing on the drug progression thesis is the presentation of the proportion of heroin addicts who once smoked marijuana. Such data would be unacceptable on logical grounds because they fail to meet the criterion of relevancy. A study which gathers such data cannot possibly answer the question of whether marijuana smokers do progress to the use of dangerous drugs, specifically heroin, because it is not designed to deal with the issue of drug progression in the first place. In order for such information to be rendered relevant, we would have to know additional facts, facts about other populations which are not included within the scope of a study on heroin addicts. At the very least, we would have to find out: (1) whether the percentage of addicts who once smoked marijuana was substantially greater than that of their peers who did not become addicted; (2) what the percentage of marijuana smokers who did not become addicted to heroin is; (3) what the current heroin addicts' former degree of involvement with marijuana was prior to their addiction; (4) whether nonusers of marijuana became seriously involved in the use of a dangerous drug other than heroin, and what their rate of this involvement is; (5) what the causal links between the two variables, marijuana use and heroin addiction, are; (6) how marijuana progression differs from the use of, and escalation from, other drugs, such as alcohol and tobacco. Thus, on the face of it, the datum that a given proportion of heroin addicts "started with" marijuana does not logically extend to the progression hypothesis. The population of the datum constitutes the end product of a process which we would like to study, but cannot, because we have no other populations with which to compare it.

Nevertheless, studies which take as their principal focus the proportion of heroin addicts who smoked or who "started with" marijuana as evidence of the causal link between the use of these two drugs are conducted (Chapple, 1966; Ball et al., 1968; Chein et al., 1964; Chambers et al., 1968) and frequently cited (Giordano, 1968; Miller, 1968; Gannon, 1972). Probably the most frequently cited study of this genre is a survey conducted among over 2000 narcotic addicts admitted to the federal hospital-prisons in Lexington and Fort Worth in 1965. The research design was devised to answer the following questions: "Given existing social conditions and laws, is the smoking of marijuana associated with the subsequent use of opiate drugs? If so, under what conditions? If not, under what conditions?" (Ball *et al.*, 1968). The authors schematize the issue into a fourfold tabulation (see below), inquiring as to whether cases conform to a "marijuana only," a "narcotics only," or a "marijuana and narcotics" pattern:

	Marijuana use	
	Yes	No
Narcotics use		
Yes	(1)	(2)
No	(3)	(4)

Supposedly, the progression thesis would be confirmed if the bulk of the cases fell into cell (1), where both marijuana and heroin are used. (However, the priority of each drug would be another matter to be investigated.) On the other hand, if a large proportion of the cases fell into cells (2) and (3), then the progression hypothesis would be disconfirmed. However, the relevancy of these data to the questions asked is oblique, since individuals who fall into cell (3) would not appear in the sample at all. The magnitude, or, indeed, the very existence, of "marijuana only" cases would not be known, because they would not come to the attention of officials or researchers located in these federal narcotic institutions. The only thing that we can do with the Lexington data is to compare cells (1) and (2).

Although the report has been widely cited by proponents of the progression hypothesis as strong evidence that marijuana does actually lead to heroin addiction, actually, its data demonstrate almost precisely the opposite contention. The Ball *et al.* (1968) study shows that the issue of whether or not marijuana actually is a precursor to narcotic addiction is totally dependent on the social and cultural setting in which drug use takes place, as well as the nature of the drug market. In other words, any progression that does occur appears not to be a function of the drugs themselves, that is, not "caused by" the use of marijuana itself, but grows out of the nature of the communities in which drug use is embedded. The crucial factor in this study was not the use of marijuana per se, but the existence of an illicit drug subculture. The Ball data demonstrate just how variable and contingent drug progression is.

The majority of the addicts coming from most of the areas of the South

—from Oklahoma in the West, to West Virginia in the North, to Florida in the South—conformed to cell (2), or the "opiates only" pattern. The typical drug history of the addicts coming from 12 states of the South was to have become addicted without the use of marijuana. In other words, in specific social, cultural, and geographical settings, the use of marijuana is not necessary for addiction; marijuana is not a "precursor" to addiction to narcotic drugs. The southern addicts tended to become addicted in isolation from other addicts, without subgroup or subcultural support, and without contact, typically, with "underworld" sources of supply. An extensive pattern of addiction emerged in the South without the accompaniment of extensive marijuana use; the less potent drug was not necessary for precipitating the use of more dangerous drugs.

On the other hand, addicts coming from the North (plus Texas and Louisiana) tended to conform to pattern (1)—marijuana plus narcotics. In these areas, a vigorous drug subculture does exist, and marijuana use tends to precede the use of narcotic drugs. Addicts from the North, especially from metropolitan communities, tended to begin drug use earlier, to also be involved with other criminal activities, to have had an earlier and longer arrest record, to have become addicted specifically to heroin (as opposed to other types of narcotics), to use the intravenous route of administration, *and* to have used marijuana prior to their addiction.

Thus, using drugs, and becoming addicted to narcotics, tends to be the culmination, the most extreme form, of a well-developed highly elaborated way of life, a complex of values and behavior, a "subculture." No single part of the complex "causes" any other. Delinquency or criminal behavior does not necessarily "cause" heroin addiction, although they occur prior in time; they are clearly empirically associated with one another in this type of setting. Each of the elements in the complex is found there as a consequence of these conventions and customary patterns and of market networks established over time. Marijuana use tends to be a part of this complex, but its existence is neither necessary nor inevitable, as the Southern case demonstrates. It is frequently claimed that the relevant statistic from the Ball study is that a clear majority of all addicts used marijuana prior to their addiction; this is often cited as the major finding of the study. In fact, the very authors of this article conclude that marijuana smoking is a "predisposing influence in the etiology of opiate addiction in the United States . . . within the metropolitan host environment." The "incipient addict," they write, "is predisposed to opiate addiction by his use of marihuana" (Ball *et al.*, 1968). Actually, the purpose of the study was to investigate the conditions under which drug progression did occur, as well as conditions under which it did not occur, and thus, to pin-point causes. Demonstrating that marijuana is not necessary for the existence of narcotic addiction, under certain social conditions, shows that marijuana per se has nothing to do with this progression, if and when it does occur, but rather it is the existing of an illicit drug-using subculture that is most crucial in this respect.

It is frequently stated that this tendency for a majority of all narcotics addicts to have once been involved with marijuana is a universal tendency. This is not in fact the case. It is a time-bound, group-bound, and a culture-bound relationship. In fact, prior to the Harrison Act of 1914, designed to curb narcotic addiction in the United States, there were perhaps a million addicts in this country created largely as a consequence of the presence of addicting substances such as morphine and opium in over-the-counter patent medicines. Very few of them had ever smoked marijuana. In summarizing the drug situation in Vancouver prior to 1965, one researcher (Paulus, 1969) writes that "the Narcotic Addiction Foundation had listed approximately 1200 heroin addicts as patients. Very few of these patients had a history of marihuana use previous to the onset of narcotic use. A perusal of the 1200 case files showed that alcohol, barbiturates, or other hard narcotics preceded heroin use, if and when heroin was not the first drug used" (Paulus, 1969). Estimates as to the proportion of narcotic addicts among physicians cluster around 1 or 2 out of 100, far higher than for the population at large (Vaillant et al., 1970; Modlin and Montes, 1964; H. C. Modlin, unpublished observations, 1972). In a study of 98 physicians who were addicted to narcotics, Winick (1961) found that "none of the physicians had ever smoked marijuana." Among the Chinese of Southeast Asia, particularly Hong Kong, heroin and opium use and addiction are of considerable proportions; at the same time, the use of marijuana or hashish is quite rare. What these cases—the "Southern" pattern of narcotic addiction during and before the 1960's, addiction in the United States prior to 1914, addiction to heroin prior to 1965 in Vancouver, narcotic addiction among physicians, and addiction among the Chinese in Southeast Asia—show is that specific social and cultural forces can generate addiction to narcotics on a large scale in the absence of marijuana use. Clearly, then, marijuana is far from a universally necessary condition for addiction.

Another logical problem which necessitates specification is just what is meant by a "dangerous drug." This is not a naturally occurring entity which is possessed of exact properties concerning which all disinterested observers can and do agree. Exactly which substances will be included within the scope of dangerous drugs cannot be decided by nature, but by specific observers with specific opinions on the progression controversy. To indicate the possibility of vastly different answers that might

12. Marijuana Use and Progression to Dangerous Drugs

be obtained according to how the key variable, "dangerous drug," is specified, consider the fact that one observer (Fort, 1968) has constructed a dimension of "hardness" which classifies tobacco and alcohol as hard, or dangerous drugs. Clearly, then, in order to make our analysis meaningful, we would have to specify just which drugs we intend to include within our universe of "dangerous drugs." Our decision to include or exclude certain drugs will in part determine the results of our conclusions.

If we were to examine the total universe of all heavy users of "dangerous drugs" and then check to see if a majority had been involved with marijuana prior to their use of their present drug of choice, the picture would be a great deal more confused than the "progression" advocates portray. Although in most milieux a clear majority of heroin addicts once smoked marijuana, this is not true for the users of most dangerous drugs, nor for most "dangerous drug" users. There are, after all, approximately 10 million alcoholics in the United States. All are heavy and continual users of a decidedly dangerous drug. Many are technically addicted, that is, they would undergo painful and potentially lethal withdrawal symptoms if they discontinued drinking. Yet, only a small minority "started with" the use of cannabis. Likewise, there may be as many as a million American men and women who are literally addicted to one or more of the various sedative-hypnotic prescription drugs, such as one of the barbiturates, methaqualone, and the "minor" tranquilizers. Although these drugs are used on the street for recreational purposes, often in conjunction with other drugs, including marijuana, the typical sedative addict uses them legally, under a physician's guidance (Chambers, 1971; Moffett and Chambers, 1970). Only a tiny minority of these "hidden addicts" was previously involved with marijuana.

In the Narcotic Addiction Control Commission's survey of the drug use patterns of a random sample of 7500 New York State residents in 1970, only 17% of the "regular" (six or more times in the previous month) users of barbiturates were also regular users of marijuana (Chambers, 1971). The comparable figures for regular users of nonbarbiturate sedative-hypnotics was 11%, for users of major tranquilizers it was 14%, and for "relaxants and minor tranquilizers" it was only 8%. The same was not true of users of LSD (100% were also regular users of marijuana), of users of cocaine (the figure was also 100%), or methedrine (91%). Heroin was between these two sets of figures; just over half, or 53%, of all regular users of heroin were also regular users of marijuana. Clearly, then, marijuana is used differentially by regular users of different dangerous drugs. Marijuana is closely associated with the use of some dangerous drugs, but not others. Thus, if our universe is the regular or the heavy users of all dangerous drugs, and we were to examine their use of marijuana prior to, or in conjunction with, the dangerous drug they are currently using, we would find that a small minority uses, or once used, cannabis. For the typical dangerous drug user, marijuana was not a facilitative escalation drug; in fact, it was not in his or her drug history at all. It is specifically among those dangerous drugs, the legal prescription drugs, whose users are numerically greatest that marijuana use figures least heavily. What we would have to find out is why is marijuana more prominent in the drug progression patterns of users of certain dangerous drugs than others. The progression thesis is refuted if we examine the undifferentiated mass of all regular and heavy users of all dangerous drugs, because most are users of alcohol and many are users of prescription drugs; relatively few are narcotic addicts. It is only by logically excluding users of specific drugs from our consideration of who is a user of dangerous drugs that we are able to confirm the progression hypothesis. *In general,* the thesis does not hold up, because most present users of dangerous drugs did not "start with" the use of marijuana. But it is confirmed if we examine specific drugs and ignore others. We would have to find out what produces this distinct and curious pattern if we are to make any headway on this issue. The importance of spelling out logical problems before investigating an issue becomes clear at this point.

In fact, the logical implication of the progression thesis is that marijuana is the first of a series of illegal and dangerous drugs, a series that eventually terminates in heroin addiction. This pattern turns out to be markedly atypical, even for the heroin addict. When it is stated that a given addict "started with" marijuana, it is usually forgotten that the first dangerous, psychoactive, and for them, illegal, substance that adolescents experiment with and use regularly is either alcohol or nicotine in tobacco. Adolescent drinkers and smokers are significantly more likely to use dangerous drugs than is true of their nondrinking and nonsmoking peers. A survey conducted in the late 1960's among a cross-section of Michigan high school students showed that the strongest statistical relationships that were found were between tobacco and alcohol use and the use of marijuana. The authors state: "Such relationships suggest that there are several overall similarities in the way these substances are regarded by adolescents." Not only were adolescent smokers and drinkers more likely to experiment with marijuana, but they were also markedly more likely to think of marijuana as harmless. In general, these researchers state: "it is possible that drinking leads to an increased confidence in the safety of drugs. On the other hand, drinkers may be a select group to begin with, a group without a deep suspicion of drugs" (Bogg *et al.*, 1968).

12. Marijuana Use and Progression to Dangerous Drugs

In a study of my own among the students in an undergraduate course on "deviance and delinquency," I found that smokers of ordinary tobacco cigarettes were roughly twice as likely to experiment with all dangerous drugs, from marijuana to heroin (Goode, 1972a). The same pattern held for all illegal drugs and for all levels of cigarette smoking. A clear case could be made, then, for a progression from tobacco and alcohol to dangerous drugs. Instead of the dangerous drug user "starting with" marijuana, typically, he or she starts with ordinary household substances. Again, it is an arbitrary mental exercise to exclude this process from consideration in examining the escalation hypothesis. If we wish to understand the "progression" from marijuana to dangerous drugs, if and when it occurs, we would be remiss if we were not to understand an earlier and even more basic process. When the statement "marijuana leads to the use of dangerous drugs" is made, it is assumed that no other process can adequately explain the progression that obtains—that cannabis is unique in this regard. It is only by logically blocking out the cigarettes and alcohol "escalation" issue that one is able to take seriously marijuana's role in this process. The data indicate that there may be a kind of *general drug-taking disposition*. Marijuana users appear to be *selectively recruited* out of the general population. Even before smoking marijuana for the first time, the young potential drug user is already different from his or her peer who does not and never will use illegal drugs (Goode, 1973). This makes the specific role of any given drug problematic. I will return to this crucial issue when I deal with the theories on the mechanisms which make for drug escalation.

Another logical problem which never receives attention in discussions of the progression hypothesis is what level of dangerous drug use should be included within our concept. Does marijuana use lead to *experimentation* with dangerous drugs, that is, at least one-time "use"? Or does it lead to an actual physiological addiction? Even before we examine the data on this issue, we have to decide beforehand what our concepts mean, logically, and what manner of data fall within the ambit of our definitions. Otherwise our efforts will be futile and meaningless. Many observers assume that there is an automatic polarization between the heavy user, or addict, and the complete abstainer—that once someone initiates the use of a given dangerous drug, he or she is basically similar in all important respects to someone else who also uses the same drug. This dichotomy is fallacious. What we actually see is a *continuum* encompassing all shades and degrees of dangerous drug use. Moreover, the patterns of use associated with different drugs are quite distinct from one another. Drugs differ in regard to the rates of *persistence* typically attached to their use (M. J. Hindelang, unpublished observations, 1971);

that is, out of the total universe of at least once users, what proportion are currently and regularly using the drug? Caffeine and nicotine are two drugs with extremely high rates of persistence; of all those who have ever taken these drugs at least once, an extremely high proportion are not only using them currently, but also regularly, even heavily. Alcohol, likewise, has a high rate of persistence; the proportion of those who have ever drunk liquor and who are presently drinking is higher than the proportion who has quit for good. Many drugs are typically used on a much more experimental and episodic basis. Cocaine, for instance, partly because of its cost, partly because of the great difficulty in obtaining it, is used in the United States on an extremely infrequent basis. (In other milieux, such as among the Indians of South America, it is typically used on a much more regular basis.) In the Narcotic Addiction Control Commission study cited earlier, only 27% of all at least once users of cocaine had used it at all in the 30 days prior to the survey, and only 6% of all current users were regular users, that is, had taken it six or more times in the previous 30 days (Chambers, 1971). LSD was also used episodically in the usual case; only a quarter of all current users took it regularly. On the American college campuses, opium is an esoteric luxury drug; only 2% of the opium smokers in a survey I conducted said that they had used it weekly or more in the 6 months prior to the survey (Goode, 1972b).*

In contrast, marijuana is a drug with far higher persistence than most dangerous drugs. In two college surveys I did, the median point of use for marijuana was almost exactly once per week (Goode, 1972b); for no other illegal drug was the frequency even half that high. A survey at York University in Toronto found that while only a quarter (or 26%) of the marijuana users had taken the drug less than ten times, this was true of 57% of the at least once users of psychedelics, 45% of the users of amphetamine, and 71% of the users of opiates (Kohn and Mercer, 1971). In a study of almost 1000 residents of three large cities in the Netherlands, Cohen (1972) found the persistence patterns of hashish and alcohol to be almost identical: 21 vs. 23%, respectively, were daily users, and 16 vs. 14% were monthly or less users. But not one user of LSD took it daily, only 2% took it several times weekly, and 69% took it once every 2 months. Opium was used more frequently than LSD, but far less frequently than hashish or alcohol. After reviewing the data from his survey of school children in Toronto, Smart comments on the persistence of

* As with cocaine, opium is used in other settings with much greater average frequency; these facts should direct our attention away from the intrinsic properties of a given drug in predicting patterns of use and toward how it fits in with the society and culture in which its use takes place.

12. Marijuana Use and Progression to Dangerous Drugs

marijuana in comparison with that of other drugs: "It is only for marihuana that regular users outnumber experimenters" (Smart, 1971).

Thus, if we were to conclude that in the typical case marijuana use is a "stepping stone" to serious, intense, and chronic dangerous drug involvement merely because a certain proportion of users had tried the drug, we would be very much in error. Dangerous drug use for the average at least once user is experimental and episodic rather than frequent and regular and is most often discontinued. Even experimentation with a given dangerous drug does not typically "lead to" serious daily use of that drug; it typically leads to a discontinuation of the use of that drug.

III. METHODOLOGICAL ISSUES—DESCRIPTIVE STUDIES

The methodological problems associated with testing the existence of the progression process are far more numerous, and yet they are at the same time less fatal than the logical ones. A study may be conducted in such a fashion that its data may be questionable on one of a number of grounds, but its findings may still be suggestive, informative, and useful; they may indicate the tendency that more adequate data will assume. On the other hand, there are many methodological flaws which will render a study's conclusions altogether invalid. How serious a methodological problem is has to be decided on a study-by-study basis. Of all such flaws, perhaps drawing a biased sample of subjects is the most common.

An escalation study exemplifying the problems associated with sampling was sponsored by the Narcotic Addiction Control Commission. A 5 and 10 year follow-up survey was conducted with about 700 males who were, in 1957 and 1962, referred to the New York City Youth Counsel Bureau, "an agency established for handling juvenile and youthful persons alleged to be delinquent or criminal and not deemed sufficiently advanced in their misbehavior to be adjudicated by the courts" (Glaser et al., 1969). Three groups of youths were compared: those who had committed marijuana, heroin, and nondrug offenses, all of whom had come to the attention of the Youth Counsel Bureau. The study then checked the appearance of the names of the members of these three groups on the Narcotics Register, supposedly "the most complete file of its type available anywhere in the United States."

The data appear to confirm the progression hypothesis. Only 12% of youths who committed nondrug offenses in 1957 and 15% in 1962 appeared 5 to 10 years later (1963–1967) on the Narcotics Register. But this was true of 40% of the young men who committed marijuana offenses in 1957 and 41% in 1962. The figures for those involved in heroin offenses who, 5 to 10 years later, appeared on the Narcotics Register were 49 and 53%. The authors of this report summarize these findings by stating that: *"we can conclude that among New York City male adolescents apprehended for relatively unadvanced delinquency, marijuana use is almost as portentous of adult heroin use as is actual use of heroin as an adolescent"* (Glaser et al., 1969; the emphasis is theirs).

Although these researchers do strongly qualify the applicability of their findings to groups other than juvenile delinquents, it must be pointed out that methodological problems inherent in their data render the study's findings even more narrowly applicable than this qualification would have it. The marijuana smoker whose use of the drug is so conspicuous as to come to the attention of authorities cannot be said to represent marijuana users as a whole. To come to the attention of any agency of law enforcement of any kind is to be part of a highly special and unrepresentative social group. Such users are far more likely to be more heavily involved with marijuana, to be implicated in the more heavily sanctioned marijuana-related activities, such as selling, and to be incautious about their marijuana use. A nonstatistical participant–observation study of drug use in the predominantly Black and Chicano working-class neighborhoods of Oakland, California (Blumer et al., 1967) emphasized the importance of different "styles" of drug use. The most common style of marijuana use, the so-called "cool" style, emphasized using marijuana inconspicuously, weaving it into hedonistic, recreational activities, avoiding illegal activities other than marijuana use, avoiding drugs other than marijuana, and avoiding official notice, particularly arrest.

The kind of marijuana use style which was most likely to attract attention, and to result in arrest was the so-called "rowdy" style. "Rowdy" marijuana users were very likely to attract official attention, to commit a variety of crimes, often violent ones, to become arrested, to become placed on a record such as the Youth Counsel Bureau's, and, in addition, to move on to the use of more dangerous drugs such as heroin, and, therefore, to appear eventually on the Narcotics Register. The "rowdy" marijuana user, therefore, was specifically that type of user who was most likely to get into the Narcotic Addiction Control Commission's study sample. The more cautious user was both unlikely to be studied as well as unlikely to later use heroin. The NACC probably selected the segment of marijuana users which has the very highest likelihood of later heroin use. The progression hypothesis holds up best in the very group wherein the Commission gathered its data.

12. Marijuana Use and Progression to Dangerous Drugs

In addition, lower-class adolescent slum dwellers are far more likely to come to the attention of formal agencies of legal control than is true of the middle-class suburban or college youth. For the latter, informal, nonrecord, nonarrest implementation is more likely than with the former. Again, it is a certainty that the progression to heroin is most likely among the former; middle-class young people and college youth are both less likely to come to official notice and to use heroin. The process of officially recording an individual's illegal behavior is contingent on social class, neighborhood, race, and education. Official notice is, therefore, immersed in the very process the NACC authors are trying to explain. The problem is not with degrees of official notice, as the authors state—that is, appearing on Youth Counsel Bureau's list, in contrast with appearing before the courts—but with official involvement at all as opposed to no involvement at all.

Thus, what the NACC drug progression study shows is that young marijuana smokers in New York City whose use is so conspicuous as to attract the attention of authorities have almost as high a likelihood of becoming seriously involved with heroin as adults as do young heroin users whose use of their drug is similarly conspicuous. Youths unfortunate or incautious enough to become apprehended for nondrug offenses had a much lower likelihood. "Being apprehended for marijuana crimes" and "being apprehended for heroin crimes" clearly were indicators of a similar behavioral syndrome, while "being apprehended for nondrug crimes" tapped into a distinctly different type of behavior. However, what this study says for the progression hypothesis cannot be said for sure. Its applicability does not extend beyond individuals who are arrested. Nearly all heavily involved users of heroin become arrested in their drug careers; on the other hand, a tiny minority of all marijuana smokers are ever arrested. So that if we compare marijuana arrestees with heroin arrestees, we are comparing a small segment of a very large group with the full spectrum of a smaller group. To reason about the characteristics of marijuana users *in general* from the characteristics of marijuana *arrestees* is clearly invalid.

Perhaps the most consistently documented generalizations in the drug use literature are ones which bear directly on the escalation hypothesis: (1) Marijuana smokers are significantly more likely, on a statistical basis, to try and use any and all dangerous drugs than is true of abstainers from marijuana; and (2) the greater the frequency of smoking marijuana, the greater the likelihood of experimenting with and using regularly all dangerous drugs. No investigator exploring relationships between these variables has failed to find a powerful and unambiguous correlation between them. This has been true for college and for slum populations, as well as for a random sample of the general population. It has been found to be true for men and for women, for adults and for high school adolescents, for Blacks and whites, for the entire range of the social class spectrum, for the populations of the United States, Canada, and Great Britain, in fact, for every segment of these groups and populations that has ever been studied. The greater tendency of marijuana users, and especially regular and heavy users, to also use dangerous drugs may be taken as an established fact.

In the survey conducted by the Narcotic Addiction Control Commission of 7500 New York State residents in 1970, regular marijuana smokers (those who had used the drug six times or more in the 30 days prior to the study) stood a significantly higher statistical likelihood of being regular users of *all* drugs, from minor tranquilizers taken via prescription, to heroin, always used illegally (Chambers, 1971). However, the magnitude of this relationship was strikingly greater for illegal than for prescription drugs. Smoking marijuana only doubled a person's actuarial chances of being a regular user of minor tranquilizers, tripled one's chances of taking nonbarbiturate sedatives regularly, multiplied by almost five times the chance of taking barbiturates regularly; all these drugs were secured by legal prescription far more than illegally. On the other hand, marijuana users stood 17 times the likelihood of also being regular heroin users, 22 times the likelihood of being regular users of methedrine, 12 times of taking cocaine regularly, and almost 31 times the chance of using LSD on a regular basis. Thus, although using marijuana increases one's statistical chances of using any drug, it increases them far more for illegal drugs than for legal drugs.

Also, frequency of marijuana smoking is powerfully correlated with the use of other drugs. The more that a given individual uses cannabis, the greater are his or her chances of using one or any of a wide range of psychoactive drugs. As one looks from experimenters through regular users to heavy, daily, "chronic" marijuana smokers, the percentage trying all dangerous drugs increases. This is an unambiguous relationship, and it occurs almost without exception. In an exploratory study of my own (Goode, 1969, 1970) of a nonrandom sample of New York City marijuana smokers, I found that infrequent, or less than monthly, users were extremely unlikely to have tried three or more drugs aside from and in addition to marijuana (9%), slightly more frequent users were a bit more likely to have done so (19%), more regular users even more likely (29%), frequent smokers even more likely (69%), and daily smokers the most likely of all (92%). The same pattern of a stepwise relationship was true of all drugs. For instance, only 22% of the less than monthly smokers had tried LSD, but 82% of the daily users had done so. All in-between levels of marijuana use were also in-between with regard to the use of LSD. When I repeated the same correlation on an undergraduate population several years later, exactly the same relationship obtained (Goode, 1971). In Table I, I present the percentage of marijuana users of two different levels of use who have tried one representative drug, LSD and/or the psychedelics, from a dozen or so studies; in addition, the likelihood of marijuana abstainers trying LSD is also presented. Table II shows the percentages of a sample trying a number of different drugs, also arranged

TABLE I

Marijuana Use and the Use of LSD and/or Psychedelics (Hallucinogens)

Reference	Marijuana nonusers	Lowest marijuana use category	Highest marijuana use category
Wolk (1968)	0	—	22
King (1969)	0	—	18
Goode (1969, 1970)	—	22	82
Russell (1970)	1	34	67
Whitehead (1970); Whitehead et al. (1972)	1	—	31
Mirin et al. (1971)	—	17	100
Goode (1971)	1	7	65
Josephson et al. (1972)	1	0	55
Hochman (1972); Hochman and Brill (1973)	1	29	57
Fisher and Brickman (1973)	0	15	95
Smart and Fejer (1973)	0	—	31
Johnson (1973)	0	8	68

TABLE II

Percent Trying Various Drugs By Marijuana Use in Past Six Months[a]

Marijuana use	Amphetamines	LSD	Barbiturates	Opium	Cocaine	Heroin	Methedrine
3 times per week or more	61	65	44	28	29	14	28
3 times per month to 2 times per week	46	32	15	12	4	3	8
At least once	19	7	4	2	3	1	6
Never	5	1	2	1	0	0	0

[a] From Goode (1971).

by frequency of marijuana use. It would be difficult to argue away the existence of this relationship, although the strength of it, or the amplitude of the figures, will no doubt vary.

Even data so unambiguous as these should be examined with care. The methodological flaws in these studies should at least be mentioned. We do not know from these self-report studies of drug use that the substance which was asked about or mentioned was in fact the substance which was actually smoked, ingested, or injected. Samples of drugs sold illicitly on the street are quite often not as advertised; purported, alleged drugs are frequently something altogether different. Hence, we may receive a distorted picture of what specific drugs were taken by our subjects or respondents by relying solely on what they tell us they take. However, this warning does not apply equally to all drugs. Easily obtainable or manufactured drugs, or those whose identity can be readily detected visually, are far less likely to be bogus than those which are difficult or expensive to synthesize or obtain. Mescaline, peyote, psilocybin, and THC are never, or almost never, as advertised; they are almost always bogus (Cheek et al., 1970; Marshman and Gibbins, 1970; Tennant et al., 1973). LSD is usually genuine although often impure. Cocaine and heroin are also usually as advertised, but they contain far more adulterant, by bulk, than the active drug. Cannabis is typically genuine. (Incidentally, marijuana distributed and sold in the United States is almost never treated, or "laced," with more potent substances such as opium or mescaline. Although such samples may be found from time to time, they are extremely rare; the explanation is simple: The cost is prohibitive.) However, the special problem that marijuana poses is the enormous variability in *potency*. In a study of the chemical composition of a variety of strains of *Cannabis sativa*, it was demonstrated that different plants contain several hundred times more Δ^9-THC, the principal psychoactive agent in cannabis, than others do, from less than one-fiftieth of 1% to about 5% (Doorenbos et al., 1971; Fetterman et al., 1971). This makes it impossible to fully understand the pharmacological process of habituation to the chemicals in cannabis from self-reports of use. When a respondent reports having smoked marijuana daily for the past year, the researcher does not know for sure whether his THC intake is similar to or very different from someone else who has also smoked daily, or similar to or very different from another respondent who has smoked marijuana weekly. This potential source of error assumes prominence when the possible sources of the mechanism behind cannabis escalation is considered, and this applies particularly to tolerance. If we make use of such self-report data, as we all have to for the present, we have to assume that by looking at large numbers of cases these possible errors cancel

12. Marijuana Use and Progression to Dangerous Drugs 319

each other out. From what we know, this is a reasonable assumption, but making it represents a far from ideal solution to the problem.

Another methodological problem involved with studies showing greater rates of dangerous drug use among marijuana users, particularly chronic users, is that they almost never specify the chronological time sequence of the progression. We very rarely know in any of these studies precisely when a given subject uses marijuana for the first time, begins using it regularly, and then when he or she initiates heroin use. From the bulk of the studies now available, all we know is that respondents who use marijuana tend to also be those who use heroin. Both could have been initiated at the same time, or either before the other. In order to get a clearer picture of the process of the progression from cannabis to dangerous drugs, we would have to have a detailed picture of the natural history, or the drug "career" of large numbers of users; the drug "biography," in time sequence, should be on the agenda of any researcher exploring this question. *Longitudinal* data are needed.

However, as with the THC content of cannabis, this is a troublesome, but not fatal problem. Drug sequences have been established empirically. In the typical case, alcohol and cigarettes do tend to be used prior to marijuana, and marijuana is most often used prior to the use of dangerous drugs such as barbiturates, LSD, amphetamines, and heroin (Goldstein and Gleason, 1973; M. J. Hindelang, unpublished observations, 1971; Cohen, 1972; Steffenhagen *et al.*, 1972). We know, in short, what a modal sequence of use looks like, but this is still, at present, lacking in sufficient detail. We have not established at risk figures for specific lengths of marijuana use relating to probabilities of trying and becoming seriously involved with each dangerous drug. Ideally, we would like to know the likelihood that a cross-section of marijuana users will try a number of dangerous drugs *given* daily use for one year, given daily use for two years, and so on. Without these data, we have to take guesses as to the role marijuana plays in drug progression.

Another problem longitudinal data would solve is our present reliance on cross-sectional nonpanel studies. That is, we can, with the data presently at hand, compare different individuals with different levels of marijuana use in regard to their rates of dangerous drug use. We do not have the information on different marijuana use levels of the same individuals at different points in time. We have to assume that other variables are equal when we compare groups of individuals with various levels of marijuana use, but of course other things are never equal; if we are lucky, errors do cancel each other out, but this is a haphazard fashion of conducting research. Fortunately, panel studies on drug progression have been undertaken and are underway at this writing.

IV. LOGICAL ISSUES—CAUSAL MECHANISMS

It is always difficult to interpret relationships between social variables. A correlation, even a strong and unambiguous one, is not a demonstration of causality; it is a fallacy to automatically equate correlation with cause. Suggesting a theory to explain why a given relationship prevails is only a first step, a step which entails the search for more detailed correlations, in other words, the search for further information. In order to render observed correlations meaningful, we should propose a model, an explanation, a specification of the mechanism by which outcomes should be expected to obtain. It might be possible to agree on what the facts say, but the question of why they say what they say is a different and far more complex matter.

Explanations for the phenomenon of drug escalation can be divided into those which invoke factors *intrinsic* to marijuana use and those which are *extrinsic* to it. The question of whether marijuana use, in and of itself, causes the use of more dangerous drugs, or whether it has to do with factors which happen to be, but which are not necessarily, associated with marijuana use, is central. The issue is whether dangerous drug use is a necessary or an artificial feature of continued marijuana use.

"Intrinsic" explanations for drug progression can be divided into pharmacological and "pseudo-pharmacological" (Meyer, 1972). The pseudo-pharmacological explanation posits that it is the marijuana *experience*—getting high on marijuana—that predisposes one to further adventures in drug intoxication. A team of sociologists opine that "the incipient addict is predisposed to opiate addiction by his use of marihuana," because, among other things, "marihuana is taken for its euphoric effect—produces a high" (Ball *et al.*, 1968). One problem with this supposed explanation is that it does not specify any *variables*. It attributes causal power to an experience which is shared by everyone who smokes marijuana, and yet not all who smoke marijuana escalate to heroin addiction, or even to the experimentation with dangerous drugs. It is a well-known axiom in science that a constant cannot explain a variable outcome. We are still left with the question of why it is that a certain proportion of marijuana users (the vast majority) do not progress to heroin and another proportion (a tiny minority) do use and become addicted to heroin. The pseudo-pharmacological "experience" mechanism, getting high, has no explanatory power. Moreover, this theory does not explain what is substantially different between the marijuana and the alcohol intoxication experience.

Alcohol, like marijuana, is taken among adolescents principally for its intoxicating properties, for "euphoric" purposes. Therefore, both should, other things being equal, be equivalent in their potency to produce heroin addicts. If other factors are not equal, we should look to these other factors to explain the escalation, if and when it occurs.

The same stricture applies to another supposed explanation for cannabis progression; it is that "a youngster who, despite warnings to the contrary, has started to smoke hash and has found it harmless, may then feel that heroin and cocaine . . . may be equally harmless and try them too with disastrous results" (Glatt, 1969). As with the pseudo-pharmacological explanation, no variables are specified, only the speculation that all marijuana users share the same basic experience which would incline them toward the use of more dangerous drugs. But clearly, this process cannot explain progression, because all marijuana users do not use heroin (Triesman, 1973). This explanation turns out to explain nothing.

Intrinsic explanations also face a snag in interpreting the near-ubiquity of marijuana in various drug scenes. (Although, as I pointed out earlier, there are many patterns of dangerous drug use where marijuana is not used at all.) Marijuana is, as Jordan Scher points out, a *vade mecum* of the drug world; it "cuts across all categories of preferential adult drug use" (Scher, 1967). This is not quite true; it is, however, found very frequently in illegal, street drug scenes. It also tends quite often to be discontinued specifically among heroin addicts, but not among regular users of cocaine, LSD, and methedrine (Chambers, 1971). Thus, marijuana is almost always, but not quite always, implicated in the use of a number of dangerous drugs. The logical problem here is attributing a common, even typical, temporal sequence with causal power. Is A the cause of B, or does B often follow A because of factors external to them both, on which they are both causally dependent? Using drugs is simultaneously participating in a certain social group. In order for the progression hypothesis to make sense, it is necessary to nullify the causality of social interaction and learning in this process. A simple example will illustrate. Learning to drive an automobile almost always occurs before learning to fly an airplane. The first is implicated in the behavioral system of the second. Yet they are not causally linked, in the usual meaning of cause and effect. A tiny proportion of automobile drivers "go on" to become pilots, and no one could possibly argue that it is necessary to have driven to fly. That the two are connected *in some way* is clear, but it is specifically *how* and *why* that we wish to understand. Thus, we must move away from saying that marijuana and dangerous drug use are a "common sequence" toward saying that they occur in some specific fashion together causally.

The intrinsic explanation par excellence is the *biochemical* explanation; here, tolerance to the effects of the drug THC explains why someone should escalate to more potent drugs. By smoking more, one enjoys it less; eventually one becomes immune to the effects of cannabis, and in order to reach the same level of euphoria that one did early in one's contact with marijuana, it becomes necessary to use increasingly stronger drugs. Nahas (1973) argues this position by writing that "tolerance to *Cannabis* gives a physiological basis to the necessity for the frequent smoker to increase dosage, or to use more potent psychotropic drugs such as other hallucinogens or the opiates. . . . The demand for the pleasureable sensations caused by *Cannabis* will require in time larger and larger amounts of the drug. A biological urge will develop to substitute more potent drugs for *Cannabis,* in order to reach a similar feeling of detachment from the world."

Nahas and those who invoke biochemical processes as the key mechanism in the etiology of drug progression make a number of logical and empirical assumptions which merit scrutiny. If any one of them is invalid, then the biochemical argument as a whole is invalid.

First, that tolerance to marijuana's subjective effects does in fact occur among humans at a certain level of frequency, chronicity, and dosage.

Second, that this level of cannabis use is, in fact, actually attained by users in significant numbers, that is, that cannabis tolerance is not merely a potentiality at some abstract level of use, but it actually occurs at a level which is empirically common among current users.

Third, that this tolerance action substantially and irretrievably reduces the level of euphoria attainable by the use of marijuana over time, i.e., that the same prior level cannot be reached by increasing the dosages of cannabis.

Fourth, that the use of marijuana is, in fact, abandoned on the inception of use of one or another dangerous drug.

Fifth, that the motivation of large numbers of users to attain a state of euphoria (and/or oblivion) is sufficiently great as to actually impel them to the use of, and eventually the heavy and chronic use of, one or another of the dangerous drugs.

Sixth, that these dangerous drugs will be available in a given society or community and specifically available to marijuana smokers.

Seventh, that the effects of these dangerous drugs will actually be experienced by users as sufficiently similar to those of cannabis, and sufficiently euphoric (and/or oblivion-producing) as to merit continued use subsequent to abandoning cannabis.

Physiological and behavioral tolerance has been exhibited with the continued administration of THC to a variety of species of animals (Mc-

Millan, 1970; Dewey et al., 1972; Domino, 1972; Lomax, 1971). However, the connection of these findings to our inquiry is tangential at best. First, it may not be safe to assume that the physiological and pharmacological actions of a drug can automatically be translated across animal species, and from animals to humans. This is an empirical question which should be proposed for testing, not assumed. Such precise comparable data for human beings are not yet available. Second, the doses administered in these animal experiments are often massive, hundreds of times greater than doses human beings actually take. For instance, one study (Ford and McMillan, 1972) administered a dose of 1.8 gm of THC per kilogram of body weight to pigeons. An average dose of cannabis consumed by man in a real-life setting would be one cigarette weighing 1 gm which is 1% THC. Third, tolerance is not a unitary phenomenon; properly discussed, it always refers to specific actions. A drug which produces tolerance in one organ or in one function may not in others. Certainly physiological tolerance in any of its many manifestations cannot be equated with behavioral tolerance, and neither can it be equated with tolerance to marijuana's subjective effects. Clearly, we are interested in the marijuana *experience,* that is, how the drug's effects are apprehended subjectively, in exploring the progression hypothesis, and not simply the "objective" actions of chemical substances on the human body. For instance, at least one observer speculates that behavioral tolerance may be, to a major degree, a function of learning to cope under the influence—a condition of state-dependent learning—rather than to diminishing effects of the drug (Ferraro, 1972).

Clearly "compensatory behavior" which acts "to attenuate initially adverse behavioral effects of the drugs" and diminishing effects at the cellular level are two radically different phenomena. To further underscore the importance of differences in effects among different species, the researcher who proposed this theory of behavioral compensation did most of his experimental work with chimpanzees (Ferraro and Grilly, 1973; Grilly *et al.,* 1973), the animal species closest to man, while those who propose cellular tolerance as the crucial mechanism in diminishing behavioral effects did their work with lower animal species (McMillan and Dewey, 1972).

Lastly, tolerance may occur to specific subjective effects but not to others. This is especially important when considering a drug so complex as cannabis. For instance, it may be that the contradictory stimulation and depression effects act in opposite directions with regard to tolerance. No researcher can afford to dismiss such a proposal out of hand.

In an experiment which allowed 20 human subjects, half of whom were heavy, chronic marijuana smokers, the other half occasional users, free access to cannabis over a 21-day period, it was found that there was no significant relationship between the day of smoking and the ratings of degree of subjective intoxication, although, oddly enough, cigarettes smoked late in the day, on any given day, tended to be judged significantly more potent than those smoked early in the day. Also, the scores on a "subjective drug effects" questionnaire did not change over the course of the experiment. However, the quantity smoked was higher for the last 5-day period than for the first 5-day period, both for the casual users (4.1 cigarettes per day vs. 2.8) and the heavy users (7.8 vs. 5.7). The authors suggest that "no tolerance to subjective effects occurred as the smoking period progressed for most experienced users" (Mendelson and Meyer, 1972).

Moreover, questionnaire and interview studies have shown that, interestingly enough, it is not the infrequent, short-term user that expresses the most pleasure and the most agreement that specific effects occur, but the frequent, long-term chronic user. This is a finding which has been confirmed in a number of different studies (Tart, 1970, 1971; Goode, 1970; Hochman, 1972; Hochman and Brill, 1973). For instance, in one survey of a 10% random sample of UCLA students, the subjective effect "increased sexual pleasure" was checked by 23% of the occasional users as occurring always, and 27% said that it happened to them often. But 39% of the chronics said always, and 44% said often. Sixty-five percent of the occasionals said that marijuana intensified their sense of taste often or always; 80% of the chronics agreed (Hochman, 1972). In my own interview study of 200 New York marijuana smokers, it was the more frequent users that were more likely to answer "yes" to questions of sexual arousal. Of the frequent, or three times a week or more, marijuana smokers, over half (52%) said that marijuana stimulates their sexual desire, and three-quarters said that it increased their sexual enjoyment; the figures for less than weekly users were 30% and 49% (Goode, 1970). It would be difficult to argue that the data show diminishing subjective effects as users increase their frequency of use. As to how we might explain these findings may be a different matter, but the findings themselves would be difficult to dismiss.

A basic problem with this version of the progression thesis, which might be called the *tolerance-disillusionment* model, is that it is specifically the chronic user who enjoys marijuana most, and it is the user who most enjoys marijuana that is most likely to progress to the use of more dangerous drugs. The tolerance-disillusionment model proposes an *abandonment* of cannabis with the onset of the use of dangerous drugs. As we have seen, this does not occur. It is the heavy user of dangerous drugs that is *most* likely to use cannabis. If we were to take the bio-

12. Marijuana Use and Progression to Dangerous Drugs

chemical explanation seriously, we would be at a loss to explain these hard facts. If we were to ask what sorts of patterns would we expect given a biochemical mechanism for drug progression, we would have to propose precisely the opposite predictions from the pattern which actually prevails. Even before an empirical test of the direct action of chronic marijuana use has been set up, the logical and empirical preconditions for such a theory have been found to be invalid. The "Nahas thesis" on drug escalation seems to be without any foundation whatsoever. The facts suggest that it has been disproven.

Once we abandon the biochemical thesis, at least three hypotheses for drug progression remain. These are termed by sociologist Bruce Johnson (1973) the *disturbed personality* theory, the *sophisticated stepping-stone* theory, and the *subculture* theory. The disturbed personality theory, when scrutinized closely, turns out to be more of a *denial* that marijuana "causes" dangerous drug use than an affirmation, although its proponents do not realize it. "An individual who feels inadequate or perhaps perverted sees in drugs a way out of himself and into a totally new body and mind" writes physician Graham Blaine (1966). "Often this search for a new self is what leads to escalation and a frantic search for new drugs which lead to addiction." In other words, marijuana use is the first step in a kind of supermarket-like search for oblivion. It clearly does not have the power of "solving" the desperate problem, and so it is abandoned for drugs which are more capable of blotting out the pain of the real world. Eventually, the search ends in addiction. The problem with this theory is that logically it means something quite different from what it seems to imply. In an effort to show that marijuana use is "bad," it is necessary to demonstrate its connection with other "bad" phenomena, mental disturbance and heroin addiction. But in this case, the link is magical, because marijuana use itself has nothing to do with experimentation with dangerous drugs. In fact, it turns out to be a *dead-end;* far from "causing" dangerous drug use, it *delays* it. This model views marijuana use as one stop along an inevitable trek. It is the "disturbed personality" that turns first to marijuana and then to addicting drugs; it is not marijuana use that "causes" the later, and, ultimately, successful search for oblivion.

The "sophisticated stepping-stone" theory (Johnson, 1973) admits the influence of factors outside the intrinsic action of cannabis itself, but holds that extrinsic factors alone cannot account for the process of drug progression. This approach toward the phenomenon insists that there is a significant unexplained effect that cannot be ruled out; the effects of cannabis itself are, along with other factors, an independent influence in turning users toward dangerous drugs. This is a polygenetic theory. Certainly social and cultural factors provide impetus in escalation. Certainly disturbed personalities are more attracted to both heavy marijuana use and dangerous drugs. Certainly availability has to be considered. But the intrinsic effects of the drug marijuana should not be ruled out. The precise mechanism is rarely spelled out, but in all probability it is specifically marijuana which is to blame for a significant portion of drug progression that obtains.

In a classic early study of over 200 black males between the age of 30 and 35 who had attended elementary school in St. Louis beginning 25 years prior to the survey, Robins and Murphy (1967) found a strong correlation between marijuana use and the use of all dangerous drugs, including heroin. Of the 109 subjects who had tried at least one drug, 103 had taken marijuana at least once; 27 of the marijuana users had also tried heroin and 22 had become addicted to it. This same pattern held for other drugs as well. "Virtually everyone who used any drug used marijuana. . . . It served as the introduction to drugs for most of those who went on to other drug use" (Robins and Murphy, 1967). Although the authors remind the reader that "half of the marijuana users never used any other drug," they suggest that their data are "in keeping with the commonly held belief that marijuana is a stepping stone to heroin." In addition, the use of marijuana, especially when initiated in adolescence, correlated with a wide range of other forms of behavior which the authors feel are harmful and "deviant": dropping out of high school, being sexually unfaithful in one's marriage, reporting violent behavior, fathering illegitimate children, drinking heavily, and so on. The authors suggest that they "cannot rule out the possibility that the use of marijuana itself was in part responsible" for the "poorer outcome" of the subjects who used marijuana, in comparison with those who abstained; "every attempt to *rule out* a direct harmful effect of marijuana use has failed" (Robins *et al.*, 1970). Thus, the effects of cannabis *may* independently contribute to socially and personally harmful behavior, including experimentation with, and ultimately, addiction to, dangerous drugs.

The sophisticated stepping-stone theory is basically a *residue* explanation. Even after all the important sociological and psychological variables have been controlled, some unexplained influence which appears to be traceable to the effects of marijuana remains. Thus, the intrinsic independent effect of cannabis is more a supposition than a datum. What unexplained variance that remains is attributed to the action of cannabis rather than empirically traced to it.

Actually, the Robins and Murphy data show that drug progression is an outcome which is highly *contingent* on extrapharmacological, sociological variables: "More than one-third of the high school dropouts who used marijuana also used heroin. But among graduates, only one in eight who tried marijuana then tried heroin" (Robins and Murphy, 1967). In fact, if we adopted an actuarial approach and asked which adolescent variables gave us the greatest power in predicting adult heroin use, dropping out of school was just such a variable, as one observer points out (Meyer, 1972). The fact that pharmacological processes (drug progression, heroin use, and heroin addiction) are dependent on social variables (school performance) should make us suspicious of the power of pharmacological processes as explanatory variables.*

V. METHODOLOGICAL ISSUES—CAUSAL MECHANISMS

The subcultural theory of drug progression denies the validity of all "intrinsic" explanations and emphasizes the overwhelming importance of social and cultural forces in determining drug use in general and drug progression specifically. It is social interaction, social and cultural definitions, and social settings which determine the forms drug-related behavior will take, and not the chemistry of the drug or the interaction between the chemical and the organism into which it is introduced. People do not escalate from the use of marijuana to more dangerous drugs, if and when they do, because of any intrinsic property resting with cannabis itself; rather, it is totally a function of the kinds of people who use the drugs, their attitudes and values, their friendship and interaction networks, activities routinely associated with the use of specific drugs, and so on. All the variation in rates of progression from group to group, from culture to culture, from one historical era to another, and from one society to another can be accounted for by the social and cultural characteristics of the group, the culture, the era, the society, in short, by nonpharmacological factors. The use of marijuana per se, that is, in the sense of a biochemical phenomenon, cannot account for any of the variation in the use of dangerous drugs. The biochemical explanation is com-

* In an analysis of data collected for the National Commission on Marihuana and Drug Abuse which I conducted (Goode, 1972c), the Robins *et al.* thesis on the persistence of the effect of marijuana after sociological variables have been controlled was not confirmed. Although users were more likely to commit criminal offenses than nonusers, and regular users more than occasional users, this relationship disappeared when factors such as the use of drugs other than marijuana, the drug use of one's friends, race, age, and education were held constant. In this study, the "harmful outcomes" suggested by the Robins team as a possible effect of marijuana use are only indirectly related; the independent contribution of marijuana use itself was almost exactly nil.

pletely spurious as a mechanism accounting for the progression from marijuana to more dangerous drugs.

Clearly, involvement with the drug subculture is a variable, just as the use of marijuana varies from user to user; there are varying degrees of involvement with the drug subculture. This does not mean simply close relationships with others who use drugs. Not all drugs are *sociogenic*, that is, the use of some drugs does not form the basis for the creation and the maintenance of a sociological group. Some drug-related activities are conducted in relative isolation, without group support. For instance, the use of meperidine by physician narcotic addicts does not lend itself to a feeling of identity or friendships among users: There is no "subculture" of physician narcotic addicts. The same can be said of users of prescription drugs. Housewives who routinely use tranquilizers or antidepressants on the advice of their physician do not form a community, do not believe things which are similar to one another, but distinctly different from nonusers, do not relate to one another more intimately because of their drug use, and do not think of themselves as belonging to a group with a name. The use of prescription drugs does not entail participation within a specific social group.

The same cannot be said for the use of marijuana, LSD, heroin, or for the illegal street usage of prescription drugs; there are subcultures of illegal drug users. This does not mean that users are part of a world apart from nonusers, participate in, and identify with a social community with boundaries as distinct as occupation (physicians, lawyers, and policemen), gender, race, or religion. But it does mean that users maintain some degree of difference from nonusers, that the community at large thinks of users as forming something of a group, that users have somewhat different beliefs and practices, that using does form the basis of some measure of identity, and that users are more likely to interact, especially frequently and closely, with users than with nonusers. Clearly, some drug users form a more distinct group or subculture than others. The use of marijuana entails far less of a commitment to a distinct and special subculture than the use of heroin. "Subcultureness" must be seen as a matter of degree; it forms a continuum, not a dichotomy.

Moreover, different individuals are involved to a differential degree in each of the various drug subcultures. I found that *frequency of use* of one's drug of choice is closely correlated with group involvement. I asked the daily marijuana smokers in a sample of users the following question: "When you meet a person for the first time, is the fact that he smokes marijuana one of the first half-dozen things you think about?" The great majority (81%) said yes. But among infrequent, or less than monthly marijuana users, a small minority (16%) agreed. The same

12. Marijuana Use and Progression to Dangerous Drugs

pattern held up regardless of which indicator of subcultural or group involvement I chose. Frequent users were also far more likely to have friends who also smoked marijuana regularly. When I asked what proportion of their friends smoked marijuana weekly or more, between half and two-thirds (62%) of the daily smokers said that over 60% of their friends did, but this was true of only one less than monthly user in ten (9%). Heavy users were also far more likely to participate in marijuana-related activity than sporadic users. Nearly all (96%) daily users said that they had bought marijuana at least once; but between a third and a quarter (29%) of the less than monthly users had done so. The figures for selling marijuana at least once were 92% for the daily users and 11% for the less than monthly users (Goode, 1969).

It was also true, as I pointed out earlier, that heavy marijuana users were significantly, even strikingly, more likely to use drugs other than and in addition to marijuana than was true of infrequent users. This is a massive, linear, stepwise relationship.

> The more that one smokes the greater the *salience* that marijuana has in one's life, and the greater the likelihood that it is involved in one's evaluation of others. Heavy marijuana use . . . (1) implicates the individual in intense and extensive social interaction with other marijuana users, (2) involves him with numerous marijuana users, (3) involves him with numerous marijuana-related activities, (4) alters the role of marijuana as a relevant criterion in his conceptions of others, (5) changes his conception of himself as a drug user (Goode, 1969).

And moreover

> it increases the likelihood of taking drugs in addition to marijuana *which the subculture approves of*. (Even daily use of marijuana will not involve the individual in heroin use if it is absent from the group in which he interacts.) The more that the individual smokes marijuana, the greater is the likelihood that he will have taken drugs other than marijuana. The more that he smokes, the more *extensive* his drug experience is likely to be. Moreover, the greater the proportion of one's friends who are also regular marijuana smokers, the greater is the likelihood that one has taken drugs other than marijuana, and the more extensive one's experience with other drugs is likely to be (Goode, 1969).

In short, I saw a remarkable "concatenance of many factors relating to marijuana use"; frequency of marijuana use was an excellent index of involvement with the drug-using subculture. The obvious question then arises: Do heavy users try more dangerous drugs because of the action of cannabis itself, as the biochemical model proposes? My data suggest, but do not demonstrate, that the social and cultural variables dominate this relationship. But since frequency of use and involvement with the subculture are so tightly bound up with one another, separating them in order to test their independent contribution would be a difficult task.

Kandel has shown that the single most powerful predictor of adolescent marijuana use is friends' use. "Involvement with other drug-using adolescents is the most important correlate of adolescent marihuana use," she writes.

> The proportion of adolescents who report having used marihuana 60 times or more increases from 2 percent among those whose friends have never used marihuana to 48 percent among those whose friends have themselves used the drug 60 times or more. . . . Indeed, we find that use of marihuana and of other illegal drugs is what friends have most in common. With the exception of certain demographic characteristics (such as age, sex, and race), on no other activity or attitude . . . is similarity between friends as great as on illegal drug use (Kandel, 1973).

Again, these data suggest that drug progression is a function of the nature of social relationships, and not of a biochemical reaction. How might we test the subcultural hypothesis?

These relationships were explored by Johnson (1973); in 1970 he conducted a questionnaire study of 3500 students attending colleges in and near the New York metropolitan area. Johnson divided his sample into four levels of marijuana use: (1) nonusers, or abstainers; (2) experimental users (less than monthly in the past six months); (3) moderate users (monthly or more, but less than weekly); (4) regular users, who said that they smoked marijuana weekly or more in the six months prior to the survey. What we are interested in as the dependent variable is, of course, the use of dangerous drugs, particularly heroin.

Johnson found, as do all researchers, a positive, significant, linear relationship between the frequency of marijuana use and the use of all dangerous drugs, heroin included. Almost no abstainers from marijuana (or less than 1%) had tried heroin at least once. This was 1% among experimental users, 5% among moderate users, and 17% among regular, or weekly or more, users. The same basic pattern was replicated for all dangerous drugs. For instance, less than one-half of 1% of the marijuana abstainers had tried a psychedelic drug, 8% of the experimenters had done so, 32% of the moderate users, and 68% of the regular users had tried one or more of the hallucinogenic drugs.

Johnson then set out to determine what variables influenced the relationship between marijuana use and the use of dangerous drugs. A crucial explanatory variable was differential exposure to and interaction with drug-using friends. There is, of course, a positive correlation be-

12. Marijuana Use and Progression to Dangerous Drugs

tween the use of marijuana and having at least one friend who used one or more dangerous drugs. Over nine-tenths of the marijuana abstainers said that they had no heroin-using friends (91%); this was true of only half (49%) of the weekly marijuana users. Only 2% of the abstainers said that they had an *intimate* friend who used heroin, but a quarter (24%) of the regular marijuana smokers did. The same held for all the dangerous drugs. Three-quarters (75%) of the marijuana abstainers had no friends at all who used a psychedelic drug, but only one in ten (9%) of the weekly users said this. But one abstainer in ten (8%) had an intimate friend who used hallucinogens, and three-quarters of the regular marijuana users were this close with a user of LSD-type drugs (74%). The crucial question, then, is the relative contribution of these two variables, frequency of marijuana use and having dangerous drug-using friends, to our dependent variable, the use of dangerous drugs, especially heroin. By holding frequency of use constant, this question can be tested.

In one sense, the various versions of the stepping-stone theory are correct: Almost none of the marijuana abstainers had tried heroin, whether or not they had heroin-using friends. Among experimental marijuana users with no heroin-using friends, only one-half of 1% had tried heroin. This rose to 5% of the marijuana experimenters who had at least one heroin-using friend. And another 5% of the *regular* users without any heroin-using friends had tried heroin themselves. But almost half, or 45%, of the regular marijuana users with at least one heroin-using friend had tried heroin. As one moved from experimental to regular use of marijuana, the concomitant use of heroin rose only slightly when heroin use by one's friends is held constant. But as one moved from not having to having heroin-using friends, with marijuana use controlled, the likelihood of trying heroin rises markedly. It is obvious that having heroin-using friends is far more potent in influencing heroin experimentation than is one's level of marijuana use. Even the regular use of marijuana does not "lead to" the use of heroin in the absence of having heroin-using friends.

Earlier work (Carey, 1968; Goode, 1969) pointed to the importance of buying and selling both marijuana and other dangerous drugs in this process. For instance, I found that marijuana users who had also bought the drug were significantly more likely to have tried LSD (59%) than users who had never bought marijuana (23%). The same held for selling marijuana; 72% of those who had sold marijuana at least once had tried LSD, but this was true of only 30% of those who had never sold it (Goode, 1969). Johnson therefore explored the role of buying and selling drugs in gaining heroin-using friends. Among respondents who have bought marijuana but never sold it, 4% of the experimental users and 8% of the regular users had at least one intimate heroin-using friend, clearly a very small increase, indicating a negligible impact of using marijuana as the independent variable. Among users who had both bought and sold marijuana, as well as one or more other dangerous drugs, a quarter (25%) of the experimental users and a third (36%) of the regular users had one or more intimate friends, again, a small increase. The increases from 4 to 8% and from 25 to 36% (that is, the independent impact of frequency of marijuana use on acquiring heroin-using friends) are fairly small. But the jumps from 4 to 25 and from 8 to 36% (that is, the independent impact of involvement with buying and selling on acquiring heroin-using friends, with use controlled) are obviously far more marked. It becomes clear, then, that involvement in selling drugs is considerably more potent and influential in having heroin-using friends and, hence, in eventually using heroin oneself, than is the factor of one's own frequency of using marijuana. The original correlation between frequency of use and the use of dangerous drugs does not appear to be the result of use at all, but the result of interaction and involvement with others who use—of one's own integration into the drug-using subculture. The causal link between marijuana use and the use of dangerous drugs can be traced not to a biochemical reaction, but to social relations. The use of marijuana is merely an external manifestation of something far more basic that underlies it: involvement with and in a drug-using subculture.

Two cultural and subcultural factors appear to account for the reason why marijuana users, and particularly frequent and regular users, are more likely to try and use dangerous drugs than is true of abstainers. The first is a *selective recruitment* process, and the second is a *selective interaction and socialization* process.

The selective recruitment process explains why young drinkers of alcohol and smokers of ordinary tobacco cigarettes are more likely to "go on" to the use of marijuana and dangerous drugs. This is the same reason why marijuana users are more likely to engage in premarital sex (Goode, 1972d, Johnson, 1973), to become active in liberal politics (Hochman, 1972), and so on. It also explains why such a peculiar fact that coffee drinkers should be more likely to use marijuana and dangerous drugs than is true of those who do not drink coffee (Blum et al., 1969). Or why people who take aspirin stand a higher likelihood of using illegal dangerous drugs (Estes and Johnson, 1971). It is simply because no social group or category, almost no participants in any activity, form a random selection of the general population. It is not because marijuana use "causes" sexual excitation, or a liberal ideology, it is not because drinking coffee "causes" one to "go on" to dangerous drug use, or taking aspirin stimulates the need for stronger drugs, but because those who use marijuana, drink coffee, and take aspirin are statistically a bit different from those who do not; they are already inclined in a number of different directions even before they partake of the various activities in question. Almost nothing is equally participated in by all social groups. We will observe differences between participants vs. nonparticipants of any activity in a wide range of different ways—not because that activity necessarily has anything to do with these differences, but because the people who take part in them are already a bit different in a number of ways. Knowing this basic fact will insulate us from making absurd causal inferences.

It seems to be the case that users of *any* psychoactive drug stand a higher statistical chance of using any other. The Narcotic Addiction Control Commission's survey of New York State residents confirms this generalization (Chambers, 1971). Using barbiturates regularly (six or more times in the month prior to the survey) increased by approximately 10 times the likelihood of using "pep pills," heroin, methedrine, and LSD, and increased by about 5 times using marijuana regularly. Using diet pills (almost all purchased via a legal prescription) increased by 2 times the chance of using barbiturates regularly, 15 times using pep pills, 5 times using heroin, and about 15 times using LSD and methedrine. Blum's data (Blum *et al.*, 1969) also show clearly that the correlation between marijuana use and the use of dangerous drugs is matched by a similar correlation between legal household substances like tobacco and alcohol, and dangerous drug use. The statistical correlation between marijuana and the opiates, for example, was significant and fairly strong ($r = 0.24$). But the correlation between tobacco and marijuana was higher ($r = 0.31$) and that between the sedatives and the opiates was also higher ($r = 0.25$), and between alcohol and marijuana was almost as high ($r = 0.22$). Correlation between alcohol and the amphetamines was slightly below that for marijuana and alcohol ($r = 0.19$), and that between tobacco and the amphetamines only slightly below that ($r = 0.17$). The highest correlation of all was between marijuana and the use of the hallucinogens ($r = 0.55$), which are, typically, drugs of extremely episodic use.

These patterns obtain not because becoming intoxicated on this or that drug "leads to" a bigger and better "kick" or "thrill," but because individuals who use drugs tend to be selectively recruited from segments of the populace which are to some degree different from individuals who do not use drugs, even before drug use even takes place. There is to some degree a drug-taking disposition and orientation, just as there is something of a drug-abstention orientation. Thus, many of the relationships we observe between the use of marijuana and the use of dangerous drugs—or the use of marijuana and just about anything else—can be accounted for in part simply by virtue of the fact that marijuana users are statistically somewhat different from abstainers, with or without marijuana use. We have to hold these differences constant before making any generalizations about the "effects" of the drug.

The second process, selective social interaction and socialization, also operates here as well. Not only are marijuana users already different even before they smoke their first marijuana cigarette, but they also become different as a result of the distinctive social relations and activities they engage in during the course of their marijuana-related activity. Two such factors have been mentioned: making dangerous drug-using friends and engaging in the buying and selling of marijuana and other dangerous drugs. It is entirely possible that marijuana's illegal status adds a dimension not shared by the legal drugs. Its subterranean status makes its use not simply a question of the selective recruitment into a certain activity by a segment of society which is somewhat different from the population at large. Something else is occurring as well. Its criminal character gives its use, possession, and sale an added socializing and subcultural power not evidenced by the possession and use of the legal drugs.

Many of the same methodological strictures which have been directed against descriptive studies also apply to explanatory studies. Some apply with even greater force, however. Kandel's research (1973) indicates that drug users are often inaccurate in their assessment of the drug use of others whom they know; in her study, they significantly overestimate the use of alcohol, tobacco, and prescription drugs by their own parents. Thus, studies which use crucial variables which rely on the respondent's *perception* of a given condition, for instance, friends' use of drugs, parents' use of drugs, and the extent of drug use in their school, should instead seek out the primary source of information. Of course, perceptual data may be sought out, but they are not the same thing as direct information, and often they are very different from one another.

Establishing the time order of our explanatory variables should emerge as a central task in this investigation. Studies conducted in the past (including my own) have been surprisingly casual about which drugs were used and how frequently and in what specific sequence. Instead of empirically establishing the precise connection between the time order of drug taking and drug progression, we have relied too long on questions about at least one time experimentation of certain drugs taken at some time or another in the respondent's life prior to the survey. For example, stepping-stone advocates would predict that the young person who escalates from marijuana to heroin will make a more likely candidate for a committed addict than the one who experiments with heroin before ever getting the chance to become disillusioned with marijuana, because marijuana has "potentiated" him into chronic drug use. The subculture theory would predict the opposite, because the fact that someone has been presented with the opportunity to try heroin, and who does in fact try it, is a rough although accurate measure of that individual's integration into the drug-using subculture, and hence on that ground alone would be more likely to become addicted to heroin. Time-order data would answer questions such as these. Time information on when crucial events occurred in a respondent's life need not apply only to the use of specific drugs. For instance, if making drug-using friends is of great explanatory power, we would want to find out information about whether one first makes friends who use drugs and then trys the drugs or whether experimentation took place first, or whether the order is more subtle, dialectical, more complex. At what point in a marijuana user's "career" does he begin selling marijuana? At what point does he sell dangerous drugs? Our present information is patchy on these questions. More sophisticated and detailed information is clearly called for.

The possible importance of the role of the precise chemical composition of black market drugs was illustrated a few years ago in the study of the connection between the ingestion of LSD and chromosomal aberrations. Early research indicated that LSD might contain mutagenic properties. After more careful studies were conducted, it was realized that subjects who had ingested pure LSD demonstrated no increases in chromosomal breakages, but that those who had taken "illicit, alleged" LSD, purchased on the street, exhibited about triple the rate of breaks found normally. This indicates that the early findings resulted not from the LSD ingested, but from the impurities found in black market LSD (Dishotsky *et al.*, 1971). At the same time, we must also be careful to make a clear distinction between laboratory conditions and real-life conditions. If the substance sold on the street and advertised as LSD does, in fact, cause damage to the human body, it is not absolutely crucial exactly what element in it really causes the damage; anyone who ingests it runs a risk of bodily damage. If heavy doses of THC injected into animals do produce behavioral and physiological tolerance, this datum may be irrelevant for real-life human use of small doses of self-administered natural cannabis, smoked every other night. Laboratory conditions are not street conditions, and we must always be aware that findings from one cannot automatically translate into the other. The assumptions that have to be made to do so have to be critically examined at each step of the reasoning process.

REFERENCES

Ball, J. C., Chambers, C. D., and Ball, M. J. (1968). *J. Crim. Law, Criminol. Police Sci.* **59,** 171–182.
Blaine, G. B., Jr. (1966). "Youth and the Hazards of Affluence." Harper Colophon, New York.
Blum, R. H., *et al.* (1969). "Students and Drugs." Jossey-Bass, San Francisco, California.
Blumer, H., Sutter, A., Ahmed, S., and Smith, R. (1967). "The World of Youthful Drug Use." School of Criminology, University of California, Berkeley.
Bogg, R. A., Smith, R. G., and Russell, S. (1968). "Drugs and Michigan High School Students." House of Representatives, Lansing.
Carey, J. T. (1968). "The College Drug Scene." Prentice-Hall, Englewood Cliffs, New Jersey.
Chambers, C. D. (1971). "An Assessment of Drug Use in the General Population." Narcotic Addiction Control Commission, New York.
Chambers, C. D., Moffett, A. D., and Jones, J. P. (1968). *Int. J. Addict.* **3,** 329–342.
Chapple, P. A. L. (1966). *Brit. J. Addict.* **61,** 269–282.
Cheek, F. E., Newell, S., and Joffe, M. (1970). *Science* **167,** 1276.
Chein, I., Gerard, D. L., Lee, R. S., and Rosenfeld, E. (1964). "The Road to H." Basic Books, New York.
Cohen, H. (1972). *Int. J. Addict.* **7,** 27–55.
Dishotsky, N. I., Loughman, W. D., Mogar, R. E., and Lipscomb, W. R. (1971). *Science* **172,** 431–440.
Domino, E. F. (1972). *Ann. N.Y. Acad. Sci.* **191,** 166–191.
Doorenbos, N. J., Fetterman, P. S., Quimby, M. W., and Turner, C. E. (1971). *Ann. N.Y. Acad. Sci.* **191,** 3–12.
Estes, J. W., and Johnson, M. (1971). *Clin. Pharmacol. Ther.* **12,** 883–888.
Ferraro, D. P. (1972). *In* "Current Research in Marijuana" (M. F. Lewis, ed.), pp. 49–95. Academic Press, New York.
Ferraro, D. P., and Grilly, D. M. (1973). *Science* **179,** 490–492.
Fetterman, P. S., Keith, E. S., Waller, C. W., Guerrero, O., Doorenbos, N. J., and Quimby, M. W. (1971). *J. Pharm. Sci.* **60,** 1246–1249.
Fisher, G., and Brickman, H. R. (1973). *Dis. Nerv. Syst.* **34,** 40–43.
Ford, R. D., and McMillan, D. E. (1972). *Fed. Proc., Fed. Amer. Soc. Exp. Biol.* **31,** 506.
Fort, J. (1968). *J. Psychedelic Drugs* **2,** 1–14.
Gannon, F. (1972). "Drugs." Warner, New York.
Giordano, H. L. (1968). *FBI Law Enforce. Bull.* **37,** 2–5 and 16.
Glaser, D., Inciardi, J. A., and Babst, D. V. (1969). *Int. J. Addict.* **4,** 145–155.
Glatt, M. M. (1969). *Brit. J. Addict.* **64,** 109–114.
Goldstein, J. W., and Gleason, T. C. (1973). *Proc. 81st Annu. Conv. Amer. Psychol. Ass.*, pp. 305–306.
Goode, E. (1969). *Soc. Probl.* **17,** 48–64.
Goode, E. (1970). "The Marijuana Smokers." Basic Books, New York.
Goode, E. (1971). *Brit. J. Addict.* **66,** 335–336.

Goode, E. (1972a). *Int. J. Addict.* **7**, 133–140.
Goode, E. (1972b). In "Student Drug Surveys" (S. Einstein and S. Allen, eds.), pp. 123–127. Baywood Publ. Co., Farmingdale, New York.
Goode, E. (1972c). In "Marihuana: A Signal of Misunderstanding," Vol. I, pp. 447–469. US Gov't. Printing Office, Washington, D.C.
Goode, E. (1972d). *Amer. J. Psychiat.* **128**, 1272–1276.
Goode, E. (1973). "The Drug Phenomenon." Bobbs-Merrill, Indianapolis, Indiana.
Grilly, D. M., Ferraro, D. P., and Marriott, R. G. (1973). *Nature (London)* **242**, 119–120.
Hochman, J. S. (1972). "Marijuana and Social Evolution." Prentice-Hall, Englewood Cliffs, New Jersey.
Hochman, J. S., and Brill, N. Q. (1973). *Amer. J. Psychiat.* **130**, 132–139.
Johnson, B. D. (1973). "Marihuana Users and Drug Subcultures." Wiley, New York.
Josephson, E., Haberman, P., Zanes, A., and Elinson, J. (1972). In "Student Drug Surveys" (S. Einstein and S. Allen, eds.), pp. 1–8. Baywood Publ. Co., Farmingdale, New York.
Kandel, D. (1973). *Science* **181**, 1067–1070.
King, F. W. (1969). *Psychiatry* **32**, 265–276.
Kohn, P. M., and Mercer, G. W. (1971). *J. Health Soc. Behav.* **12**, 125–131.
Lomax, P. (1971). *Res. Commun. Clin. Pathol. Pharmacol.* **2**, 159–167.
McMillan, D. E. (1970). *Science* **169**, 501–503.
McMillan, D. E., and Dewey, W. L. (1972). In "Current Research in Marijuana" (M. F. Lewis, ed.), pp. 97–114. Academic Press, New York.
McMillan, D. E., Dewey, W. L., and Harris, L. S. (1971). *Ann. N.Y. Acad. Sci.* **191**, 83–99.
Marshman, J. A., and Gibbins, R. J. (1970). *Ont. Med. Rev.* **37**, 1–3.
Mendelson, J. H., and Meyer, R. E. (1972). In "Marihuana: A Signal of Misunderstanding," Vol. II, pp. 69–246. U.S. Gov't. Printing Office, Washington, D.C.
Meyer, R. E. (1972). In "Biochemical and Pharmacological Aspects of Dependence and Reports on Marihuana Research" (H. M. Van Proog, ed.), pp. 205–213. Bohn, Haarlem, Netherlands.
Miller, D. E. (1968). *Suffolk Univ. Law Rev.* **3**, 81–96.
Mirin, S. M., Shapiro, L. M., and Meyer, R. E. (1971). *Amer. J. Psychiat.* **127**, 1134–1140.
Moffett, A. D., and Chambers, C. D. (1970). *Soc. Work* **15**, 54–59.
Nahas, G. G. (1973). "Marihuana—Deceptive Weed." Raven Press, New York.
Paulus, I. (1969). *Int. J. Addict.* **4**, 77–88.
Robins, L. N., and Murphy, G. E. (1967). *Amer. J. Pub. Health* **57**, 1580–1596.
Robins, L. N., Darvish, H. S., and Murphy, G. E. (1970). In "The Psychopathology of Adolescence" (J. Zubin and A. Freedman, eds.), pp. 159–178. Grune & Stratton, New York.
Russell, J. (1970). "Survey of Drug Use in Selected British Columbia Schools." Narcotic Addiction Foundation of British Columbia, Vancouver.
Scher, J. (1967). *Int. J. Addict.* **2**, 171–190.
Smart, R. G. (1971). In "Drug Dependence and Abuse Resource Book" (P. F. Healy and J. P. Manak, eds.), pp. 295–306. National District Attorneys Association, Chicago, Illinois.
Smart, R. G., and Fejer, D. (1973). *Brit. J. Addict.* **68**, 117–128.
Steffenhagen, R. A., McAree, C. P., and Nixon, H. L., II. (1972). *Int. J. Addict.* **7**, 285–303.

Tart, C. T. (1970). *Nature (London)* **226**, 701–704.
Tart, C. T. (1971). "On Being Stoned." Science and Behavior Books, Palo Alto, California.
Tennant, F. S., Jr., Glasser, M., McMillan, C., and Shannon, J. (1973). *Med. Dig.*, pp. 49–52.
Triesman, D. (1973). *Int. J. Addict.* **8**, 667–682.
Vaillant, G. E., Brighton, J. R., and McArthur, C. (1970). *N. Engl. J. Med.* **282**, 365–370.
Whitehead, P. C. (1970). "Drug Use Among Adolescent Students in Halifax." Youth Agency, Province of Nova Scotia, Halifax.
Whitehead, P. C., Smart, R. G., and Laforest, L. (1972). *Int. J. Addict.* **7**, 179–190.
Winick, C. (1961). *Soc. Probl.* **9**, 174–186.
Wolk, D. J. (1968). *J. Amer. Coll. Health Ass.* **17**, 144–149.

Chapter 13

MARIJUANA AND HUMAN AGGRESSION

JARED R. TINKLENBERG

I. Introduction 339
II. Basic Considerations 340
   A. Pharmacological Properties 340
   B. Dose-Response Characteristics 340
   C. Time-Action Characteristics 341
   D. Drug–Drug Interaction 341
   E. Cumulative Effects and Tolerance 341
   F. Psychological and Environmental Influences 342
   G. Individual Variation 342
   H. Predrug Personality Characteristics 343
   I. Aggression Process Factors 343
III. Sources and Limitations 344
IV. Laboratory Data 345
V. Field Studies of Marijuana and Human Aggression 347
   References 354

I. INTRODUCTION

The relationship of marijuana to human aggression has been a controversial question for many years. Observations and reports from diverse sources have resulted in a serious and persistent conflict of opinion. The aim of this chapter is to (1) outline fundamental factors that influence drug effects on behavior; (2) describe the sources and limitations of the available data; and (3) review the salient studies that have been used in assessments of the relationship between marijuana and aggression. For the purposes of this chapter, aggression is simply defined as intentional behavior that results in physical injury to the victim.

II. BASIC CONSIDERATIONS

Any assessment of the relationship of marijuana or other drugs to aggressive behavior should include consideration of the following fundamental factors: pharmacological properties of the drug, dose-response and time-action characteristics, drug–drug interactions, cumulative effects and tolerance, psychological and environmental variables, individual variation, predrug personality, and aggression process factors.

A. Pharmacological Properties

Marijuana is a crude preparation of *cannabis sativa*, a plant found in most parts of the world either growing wild or under cultivation. The principal active chemicals in cannabis are the tetrahydrocannabinols (THC) and their metabolites. Heredity and environment of the individual plant have an important influence on drug content. In addition, the parts of the plant vary in THC content; few active ingredients are found in the roots, stems, and seeds while more is found in the resinous top leaves and flowers. The variability in drug content of marijuana available in the United States usually ranges from no THC to 5% or more.

The pharmacological properties of marijuana do not fit clearly into any of the usual categories of drug classification. Depending on the dose, time-action considerations, and set and setting, marijuana exerts a mixture of euphoric, sedating, and hallucinogenic effects (Hollister, 1971).

The basic pharmacological effects of marijuana are described in other chapters in this treatise. However, one effect especially relevant to the consideration of human aggression is that in tasks requiring sustained effort, marijuana appears to reduce physical strength or at least the inclination toward strenuous exertion (Hollister *et al.*, 1968; Hollister, 1971).

B. Dose-Response Characteristics

Investigations over a wide range of doses of marijuana have established dose-dependent effects on many physiological and psychological variables. At lower doses, behavioral responses to marijuana are likely to correlate with psychological and environmental variables quite independently of pharmacological properties (Jones, 1971). However, as with other drugs, when dosage is increased psychological and environmental variables become less potent and pharmacological effects assume dominance. Low, moderate, and high doses and the related euphoric, sedating, or hallucinogenic effects may necessarily exert varied influences on the several components of human aggression.

C. Time-Action Characteristics

The effects of marijuana change during the course of the drug action. Behavioral effects are usually most pronounced when tissue concentrations of the drug are rapidly changing, especially at the onset of drug effect. When smoked, the onset of drug effect is almost immediate and peak effects are noted in 10–30 minutes; when ingested, the onset is at about ½ to ¾ hour and peak effects are noted from 1 to 2 hours. Any marijuana influence on aggressive behavior is likely to be modified as drug effects wax and wane with the time-action curve.

D. Drug–Drug Interaction

Various psychoactive agents are sometimes used either intentionally or inadvertently with marijuana; additives have ranged from the opiates to various hallucinogens. Tart (1971) reported that some users deliberately combine alcohol or amphetamines with marijuana to potentiate drug effects. Although users may be unaware of adulterants, the behavioral effects of the added chemicals may be considerable since drug–drug interaction can be greater than the effects expected from each drug used separately (Bressler, 1968). (For a review of drug–drug interaction see Davis *et al.*, 1973.) Adulteration and multiple drug use seriously complicate field studies on the behavioral effects of a specific drug; aggressive behavior erroneously attributed to marijuana may actually derive from adulterants or from drug–drug interactions.

E. Cumulative Effects and Tolerance

There is increasing evidence that chronic cannabis users respond to a given dose differently than casual users (Lemberger *et al.*, 1971; Mendelson and Meyer, 1972; Meyer *et al.*, 1971; Smith and Mehl, 1970). Although tolerance to most of the effects of cannabis has been noted in chronic users, the mechanisms are unknown. Paradoxically, some observers have also reported increased sensitivity to certain subjective effects with the recurrent use of marijuana (Weil et al., 1968). In any event, the important consideration for marijuana–aggression interactions is that the amount of previous exposure to marijuana influences the behavioral response to a given dose. A heavy pattern of previous marijuana consumption can also become important if use is suddenly discontinued. Withdrawal reactions following the chronic use of marijuana do occur, although they are not as severe as with many other psychoactive agents and seldom linked with aggressive behavior (Mendelson and Meyer, 1972).

F. Psychological and Environmental Influences

Personal and group expectations are derived from the personalities and experiences of the individuals involved in a drug-taking situation. The physical and social milieu interact with these expectations to create a "set and setting" which contribute variable but often powerful determinants of behavior. Jones (1971) conducted a series of experiments suggesting subjective highs from marijuana at low doses are more a result of set and setting than of drug properties. Many users familiar with marijuana contend that they can control drug effects and "come down" if necessary (Tart, 1971). Low dose intoxication may be directly related to set and setting reinforcements. However, while it is possible that regular users may learn to control certain behavioral effects at low doses, there is no evidence that at higher doses experienced users have volitional control over the total range of drug effects.

The Jones experiments identified another set and setting factor of special significance in assessing the relevance of laboratory studies to human behavior in natural settings: Subjects tested alone behaved differently from those studied in a group. Subjects were quiet, relaxed, and slightly drowsy when tested alone; however, when tested in a group situation, they became elated, euphoric, and exhibited uncontrolled laughter and a marked lack of sedation. Therefore, in assessing marijuana's contribution to behavior it is important to note the circumstances under which the drug was taken.

G. Individual Variation

Individual response to the same drug, dosage, and setting may differ dramatically. Most laboratory subjects characterize the marijuana experience as pleasant. However, several investigators, including our group, have observed paradoxical reactions ranging from dysphoria and agitation to psychotic disorder. Unusual reactions in laboratory settings are rare; sampling techniques and screening procedures directed toward the selection of "normal" subjects serve to reduce the possibility, but individual variation remains an important factor in evaluating field studies.

H. Predrug Personality Characteristics

Certain individuals demonstrate characteristic and relatively enduring behavioral patterns that repeatedly result in assaultive or other criminal behavior regardless of drug use. These individuals, variously described as antisocial, dyssocial, sociopathic, or psychopathic, typically manifest tendencies toward various forms of deviancy that may include both aggressive behavior and drug use (Goodwin et al., 1971; Hare, 1970; Robins, 1970; Schuckit, 1973). Attempts to establish a cause and effect relationship between drug use and criminal behavior have produced mixed results; some field studies have found sociopathic behavior antedated drug use while others have found the opposite. In any event, deviant individuals who have incorporated aggression into their repertoire of usual coping behaviors may use aggressive responses regardless of concomitant drug use. Indeed, this group of sociopaths may contribute to a large part of the statistical correlation found between drugs and crime. It appears reasonable to assume that both forms of deviancy, drug use and aggression, may not proceed one from the other, but may share a common matrix. One must not infer, however, that drug use has no influence on the behavior of these individuals. Any drug, including marijuana, may induce alterations in perception and reinforcement that enhance or reduce the possibility of violence.

I. Aggression Process Factors

Human violence is usually the culmination of a series of interactions between two or more individuals. Age, sex, race, location of the encounter, the availability of weapons, and other variables may all influence behavior at any stage of the aggression process. Throughout the entire process, the presence of drugs in the assailant, the victim, or both may alter perceptions or responses and contribute to the final outcome.

The relative contributions of the basic factors listed above vary in each case and are extremely difficult to determine precisely; nevertheless, they must be considered in a meaningful analysis of the evidence used to assess the interactions between marijuana and human aggression (Tinklenberg and Murphy, 1972).

III. SOURCES AND LIMITATIONS

In general, two types of data are available for assessment: (1) data collected from laboratory studies in which calibrated amounts of tetrahydrocannabinol, the active ingredient in marijuana, are administered to selected individuals under controlled conditions so that specific physiological and behavioral effects can be measured; and (2) field survey information from investigations of the behavior of admitted marijuana users gathered from self-reports or official sources. Both of these approaches have limitations. Considered alone, each approach leaves the investigator with the uneasy knowledge that he is not completely describing the complex interaction of marijuana intoxication and aggressive behavior.

The controlled setting of a laboratory study is essential for obtaining basic pharmacological data and related behavioral changes. Drug administration can be controlled for potency and purity thereby eliminating variables of dose as well as drug–drug interaction. In addition, both dose-response and time-action functions can be closely observed. At the same time, however, important psychological and environmental variables that also influence behavioral responses to marijuana are omitted. Sampling techniques also limit inferences from clinical studies since selection of subjects is usually confined to "normals." Certain deviant, disturbed, or otherwise abnormal individuals who extensively use drugs in social settings are generally excluded from observation. As a result, idiosyncratic reactions are minimized and unusual effects that occur in the general population may be less frequently observed in the laboratory.

Similarly, it is difficult to study the full aggression process in the laboratory. Although measurements may be made of certain components of human aggression such as hostility, frustration, impulsivity, or willingness to inflict pain on another individual, the total complex series of events leading to human aggressive attack cannot practically or ethically be replicated (Bandura, 1973). In addition, since powerful causal conditions as well as important social variables are omitted in human laboratory studies, the responses of individuals in such controlled settings are incomplete indicators of responses in other situations.

On the other hand, field studies are limited by lack of controls for personality predisposition, drug dosage, and purity. Populations in field studies tend to be biased since most investigations are confined to accessible groups such as prisoners or students. Extrapolation from these special groups to the total population of marijuana users is necessarily limited. Field studies are further complicated by differences in drug potency in natural settings that permit wide variation in the relative influences of psychological and pharmacological effects on behavior. Finally, lack of controls for drug purity seriously complicates assessments of marijuana use and aggression. Marijuana may be deliberately or inadvertently adulterated with other psychoactive substances that may exert important behavioral effects erroneously attributed to marijuana.

Although the two major sources of available data, laboratory and field studies, have inherent limitations, when cautiously and skillfully combined they provide useful information for the investigation of possible relationships between marijuana and aggressive behavior.

IV. LABORATORY DATA

Ethically, the totality of human aggression cannot be studied in a controlled laboratory setting; however, certain components of aggression have been investigated. In a study involving the effects of tetrahydrocannabinol (THC), Clyde Mood Scale ratings indicated that 1 hour after an oral dose of 30 to 70 mg of THC subjects' self-ratings of moods showed an elevation of "friendly" and a decrease in aggressive feelings; but 5 hours after the drug was ingested self-ratings indicated they were substantially less "friendly" than during baseline conditions (Hollister et al., 1968). An obvious limitation to these findings is that the apparent decrease in friendliness toward the end of the study may be related to the tedium of a long experiment rather than any pharmacological effects of marijuana.

Other investigators have observed a marijuana-associated reduction in social interaction among subjects studied in groups. In two separate studies, Babor (1973) investigated the relationship between marijuana and social behavior among 10 casual and 10 heavy users during a 21-day smoking period. Although marijuana smoking tended to be a group-centered activity, subjects did not always engage in social interaction during and after smoking. Verbal interactions in task-oriented discussions decreased markedly for both casual and heavy users during the first quarter of the smoking period, returned to baseline for heavy users thereafter, but continued to decrease for casual users. Babor interpreted his findings as suggesting that the pharmacological effects of marijuana may suppress social interaction by making subjective experience more salient.

A study designed to measure the effects of marijuana on hostile behavior compared intoxicated and nonintoxicated states for two groups of 5 subjects each, one casual and the other chronic users (Salzman *et al.,* 1973). Buss-Durkee self-report measurements indicated that total hostility as an affective state was significantly decreased following group session intoxication for both casual and chronic marijuana users. During intoxication, as compared to baseline, subjects were seen by their colleagues as consistently more friendly, receptive, understanding, and cooperative (Hostility Interpersonal Perception Scale). However, when audio tapes of the group interactions were later rated according to a Verbal Interpersonal Hostility Scale, the experimenters found that the overall amount of verbal hostility did not change but shifted from overt criticism in the nondrug state to indirect sarcasm in the drug state.

Changes in mood were also measured by Mendelson and Meyer (1972) as part of an operant free choice marijuana consumption study of two groups of subjects, 10 heavy (2–5 year history of daily use) and 10 casual users (used for 1 year, one to two times per month). Although both groups of subjects generally reported positive mood changes after smoking marijuana (e.g., less hostility and anxiety and more friendliness and carefreeness), paradoxically they also reported feeling more depressed at the same time. The authors could not explain this finding from the data available. As the 31-day experiment (5-day predrug, 21-day drug, and 5-day postdrug) progressed, casual users generally reported an overall relative increase in negative mood states and a decrease in positive mood states. Heavy users did not show an overall trend toward dysphoria during the 21-day drug taking, but did describe an increase in negative feelings during the postdrug period. These findings are difficult to interpret in terms of actual human aggression; however, there were no reports of any direct aggressive behavior during this study. When a measurement of risky and conservative betting strategies was made for heavy users, fewer risky bets were chosen during the marijuana period than during the nondrug period. The authors suggest that, at least for one type of risk-taking strategy, marijuana induced more conservative behavior.

In another study, the levels of aggression in 15 experienced marijuana users during conditions of 0, 25, and 100 μg/kg of smoked THC were tested by measuring the intensity of electric shock that they thought they were using to negatively reinforce another human subject who was apparently performing a learning task (Bloom, 1972). In reality, no shocks were delivered. Analysis indicated a statistically nonsignificant *decrease* in overall aggression with increased dosage of marijuana and a significant increase in shock level over blocks of trials (an order effect in which there is a tendency to increase intensity of the shock with each successive trial). The highest level of aggression occurred with the placebo dose while the lowest level of aggression correlated with the most potent dose of THC.

In summary, relatively few laboratory studies have directly investigated the relationship of marijuana to human aggression. The few measures that have been made of certain components of aggression have produced no evidence that acute or chronic marijuana intoxication incites or enhances aggressiveness in controlled settings. To the contrary, laboratory investigations indicate that marijuana generally induces a reduction in physical interaction, an increase in positive mood states, and a reduction in hostility and certain components of aggressive behavior.

V. FIELD STUDIES OF MARIJUANA AND HUMAN AGGRESSION

The first of several large scale investigations of the social impact of marijuana use was conducted in 1893–1894 when the Indian Hemp Drugs Commission (1969) held a lengthy series of hearings on cannabis cultivation and use in India. The Commission concluded that, rarely, excessive use of hemp drugs may lead to violent crime, "But for all practical purposes, it may be laid down that there is little or no connection between the use of hemp drugs and crime."

During the succeeding years, seven separate investigations conducted by the governments of Canada, Great Britain, and the United States have taken up the question of marijuana and its possible contributions to aggressive behavior (Advisory Committee on Drug Dependence, 1968; Commission of Inquiry into the Non-Medical Use of Drugs, 1970, 1972; Mayor's Committee on Marijuana, 1944; National Commission on the Causes and Prevention of Violence, 1970; National Commission on Marijuana and Drug Abuse, 1972; President's Commission on Law Enforcement and Administration of Justice, 1967; White House Conference on Narcotic and Drug Abuse, 1963). None of these investigative groups reached a conclusion substantially different from that of the Indian Hemp Drugs Commission.

The latest and most comprehensive marijuana report was completed by the United States National Commission on Marijuana and Drug Abuse in March of 1972. The reader is referred to that excellent two-volume report for a detailed review of the data. The following is a summary of the more salient studies reviewed by the Commission as well as subsequent research studies on marijuana and human aggression.

Various types of field studies have been used to investigate the possible contributions of marijuana to violent crime. One common approach entails retrospective case analyses of crimes committed by alleged marijuana users, although such case reports usually are limited by inherent methodological constraints and inadequate attention to the basic considerations previously outlined (Section II). They do, however, indicate that as with all psychoactive drugs, a few individuals demonstrate peculiar, abnormal susceptibility to the effects of marijuana intoxication. These adverse reactions, which may be partially analogous to the poorly defined entity of "pathological intoxication" with alcohol or "bad trips" with LSD, are characterized by irrational, frenzied, poorly controlled behavior which may entail aggressive actions (George, 1970). Since adverse reactions do not occur with most individuals who use the same dose of marijuana in the same setting, these unusual effects are often termed idiosyncratic reactions. Predisposing personality disorders seem to be an important influence in these cases (Ausubel, 1964; Bloomquist, 1971; Bromberg, 1934, 1939; Charen and Perelman, 1946; Grinspoon, 1971; Kaplan, 1970; Malmquist, 1971; National Institute of Mental Health, 1972).

The behavior of the individual who demonstrates an adverse reaction to marijuana intoxication or withdrawal from marijuana in some instances resembles that of a schizophrenic patient, even after all effects of the drug have dissipated (Fraser, 1949; Grossman, 1969; Kaplan, 1971; Tennant and Groesbeck, 1972). Although appropriate systematic data are not available, idiosyncratic reactions with marijuana seem to be infrequent and generally occur in individuals with prior psychiatric disturbance or when other drugs are concomitantly used (Gaskill, 1945; Keeler, 1967; Keup, 1970; Smith, 1968; Tennant and Groesbeck, 1972; Weil, 1970). These reactions probably account for most of the case reports of human aggression which are directly linked to the use of marijuana (Allentuck and Bowman, 1942; Asuni, 1964; Klee, 1969; Talbott and Teague, 1969).

Case reports most often indicate that marijuana usually sedates the user rather than incites him to violence (Blum, 1969a; Chopra, 1940; Chopra and Chopra, 1939; Freedman and Rockmore, 1946a, b; Maurer and Vogel, 1967; Mayor's Committee on Marijuana, 1944; National Institute of Mental Health, 1970, 1972; White House Conference on Narcotic and Drug Abuse, 1963). Similarly, large-scale studies of marijuana users in the general population have not shown them to be more likely than nonusers to commit violence or aggressive acts (Goode, 1970). When Blumer et al. (1967) assessed drug use among a large group of lower-class minority youth, they found that marijuana was the drug of preference for those youths who sought to affect a "cool" rather than "rowdy" image. Although some marijuana users were rowdy, these individuals formed a small subgroup who generally preferred alcohol and had been reared in aggressive circumstances. The authors noted that a shift from a "rowdy" to a "cool" nonviolent life style involved the smoking of marijuana, which the youths felt had a socializing effect.

Another study which assessed aggression among marijuana users included a large group of people known to have increased marijuana use for signs of an increase in violence. Blum (Blum et al., 1969) found in his survey of 1300 students at a large university that 1% of all marijuana users (19% of the total sample) reported fights or other criminal behavior which they attributed to the drug, whereas 8% of all alcohol users (94% had used alcohol) reported fights and 2% reported other offenses while under the influence of alcohol. Blum's survey is supported by Kaplan's observation that despite a marked increase in marijuana use by students in recent years, there is no evidence to indicate a concomitant increase in assaultive crimes on the University of California campuses (Kaplan, 1970).

Subsequently, Goode (1972) analyzed a large interview study that compared 559 young male marijuana users and nonusers in West Philadelphia for significant differences in criminal behavior attributable to marijuana use per se. Respondents denied any criminogenic effects from marijuana and nearly all reported no aggressive behavior during marijuana intoxication. When six representative crimes were specifically studied for marijuana or alcohol use 24 hours or less before commission of the crime, analysis showed that most crimes were committed in a drug-free state. In terms of absolute numbers, alcohol was considerably more often involved in the commission of crimes than was marijuana. However, no relative assessment could be made since the interview data did not include the frequency of use of alcohol. A comparison of the offense rates of users and nonusers yielded a simple positive relationship between marijuana use, frequency of use, and offense rate. But the application of several sociological variables (race, education, age, the use of other drugs, and having drug-using friends) either reduced or eliminated the relationship. When all six variables were applied simultaneously, less than 1% of the variance in committing offenses could be attributed to the use of marijuana per se. On the basis of the data, the author argues that the relationship between marijuana and crime is spurious, since a definite relationship between the psychopharmacological properties of marijuana and crime would not be so substantially reduced with the application of sociological variables.

Certain methodological limitations noted by the author of this study merit mentioning. So few individuals admitted to serious crimes that it was necessary to base the analysis on more "trivial" offenses. It is not clear whether this is consistent with the rate of serious crime in the general population or reflects an appropriate hesitancy to admit to more serious crimes. In any event, despite the experience of researchers that drug users tend to be frank about their drug use and behavior, self-report studies must always be interpreted with caution. Further, it should be remembered that the data did not necessarily reflect behavior during drug intoxication since dose and time action information were not obtained. And finally, without data on the relative frequencies of use of marijuana and alcohol, no inferences can be made as to whether a given number of hours of intoxication with either drug puts the individual at greater risk of criminal behavior. Indeed, the higher incidence of alcohol-related crime may simply reflect a greater frequency of alcohol use. As marijuana use increases, the number of crimes committed under the influence of marijuana may also increase, but in Goode's words: "... marijuana's *direct* contribution to the commission of crimes, especially aggressive crimes, is an independent issue, and one in need of exploration."

Another type of field study entails the use of incarcerated prisoners to determine the percentages of violent crimes purported to be committed by marijuana users. In some investigations a high percentage of individuals convicted for violent crimes has been marijuana users (Committee on Ways and Means, 1937; Lambo, 1965) and in others the percentage is low (Andrade, 1964; Bromberg, 1939). No valid inferences can be made from percentages of crimes committed by users as a result of the lack of precise evidence of use before or at the time of the crime, the failure to use adequate comparison groups, and other deficiencies in the basic considerations previously discussed in Section II.

Studies assessing the criminality of persons arrested for marijuana use show that, as one would expect, some users do have prior and subsequent criminal records that may include violent offenses (Gardikas, 1950). However, most investigations that have compared the rates of violence for convicted criminals who were marijuana users with appropriate control groups of non-marijuana-using criminals, have indicated that marijuana users were apprehended for fewer violent or other crimes than non-users (Blum, 1969; Bromberg and Rodgers, 1946; Maurer and Vogel, 1967; Soueif, 1971).

Another method of investigating interactions between marijuana use and criminal activity involves the large scale assessment of individuals arrested for but not necessarily convicted of criminal activity (Eckerman *et al.*, 1971). Interviews, urine analyses, and record reviews were conducted on a systematic sample of 1889 individuals arrested during 1971 in six metropolitan areas of the United States: Brooklyn, Chicago, Los Angeles, San Antonio, New Orleans, and St. Louis.

13. Marijuana and Human Aggression 351

The aim of the study was to discern possible correlations between arrest charges and drug use patterns based on the assumption that if no difference in arrest charges exists between users and nonusers, drug use is probably not an important variable in arrest charges. Out of the total sample, 979 (51.8%) men admitted to using marijuana at least once during their life, but not necessarily at the time of the crime. They were categorized as "Ever Users" of marijuana. The marijuana "Ever Users" when compared with the 677 "Non-Drug Users" who claimed they did not use any of the ten drugs studied (marijuana, heroin, cocaine, barbiturates, amphetamines, methadone, hashish, psychedelics, tranquilizers, and special substances) did not produce positive urine specimens and were not listed on official records as drug users. Although the marijuana "Ever Users" were more often charged with robbery and buglary, they were less frequently arrested for criminal homicide, forcible rape, aggravated assaults, and other assaults. Thus, the marijuana users were less likely to be charged with crimes involving definite aggression as defined earlier (Section I) than were subjects categorized as "Non-Drug Users." A similiar distribution of arrest charges was found for hashish users.

Arrestees in the "Ever Used" marijuana category were also compared with the 223 "Other Drug Users" who did not admit to using marijuana but claimed they did use at least one of the other nine drugs studied. Again, the marijuana group was more frequently charged with robbery, but less often arrested for aggravated assaults and other assaults. This study indicates while marijuana or hashish users were proportionately more often arrested for robbery than arrestees claiming they did not use these drugs, they were less frequently arrested for aggressive crimes. It should be emphasized that this study was necessarily limited by the fact that the "Ever Used" category did not reflect the number of individuals under the influence of the drug at the time of the crime or arrest, but only that at some time in their lives they had used marijuana.

We are conducting interview and record studies of incarcerated adolescent delinquents in California to assess possible interactions between drug use and aggressive behavior (Tinklenberg and Woodrow, 1974). Since these young males, who are generally from lower socioeconomic minority urban backgrounds, constitute a high risk group for both aggressive crime and the use of psychoactive drugs, we thought an intensive study of overall drug use might identify any special relationship of marijuana to violence as compared to other drugs. An assaultive group of 50 subjects convicted of crimes involving actual tissue damage was compared for patterns of drug use with a matched group of 80 incarcerated subjects never charged or convicted of violent crimes. We found that the assaultive group used marijuana significantly less often than the nonassaultive subjects. Therefore, overall extent of marijuana use was not a positive predictor of assaultive crime.

Fifty-six assaults committed by the 50 assaultive subjects were examined for specific drug involvement. As shown in Table I, 6 (17%) of the 36

TABLE I

Comparison of Drug and Non-drug Assaults

	n	Total assaults (%)	Drug assaults (%)
Alcohol	17	30	47
Secobarbital	8	14	22
Alcohol + secobarbital + marijuana	3	5	8
Alcohol + secobarbital	2	4	6
Marijuana	2	4	6
Amphetamine	1	2	3
Alcohol + amphetamine + marijuana	1	2	3
Glue	1	2	3
Dextromethrophan	1	2	3
	36	65	101
Non-drug	20	36	—
	56	101	—

drug-related assaults involved marijuana alone or combined with other drugs; whereas 31 (86%) of the drug-related assaults involved alcohol or secobarbital alone, together, or in combination with other drugs. The comparatively low incidence of marijuana involvement in criminal aggression among these subjects is emphasized by the fact that median lifetime usage of marijuana for these subjects was greater than that of either alcohol or secobarbital. In contrast, the relatively high incidence of secobarbital involvement was particularly striking since the median lifetime usage of secobarbital for the assaultive group was approximately one-fifth that of alcohol and one-sixth that of marijuana (Tinklenberg et al., 1974).

The drug-related criminal assaults committed by this group of young male delinquents tended to support behavioral expectations based on their personal experience of drug effects. When asked to identify the single drug of all those they had used that was most likely to enhance aggressive behavior, none of the assaultive or nonassaultive subjects identified marijuana, but 78% of the assaultive and 56% of the nonassaultive subjects selected secobarbital. When second choices were obtained, there

13. Marijuana and Human Aggression

was a definite tendency to identify alcohol as the drug next most likely to enhance aggressiveness.

As shown in Fig. 1, marijuana was identified as the single drug most

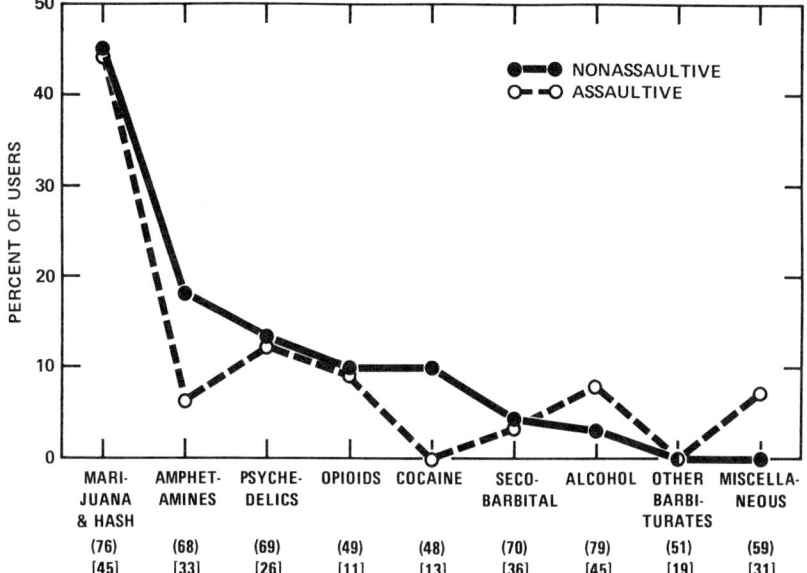

Fig. 1. Drug selected in response to the question: "Of all the drugs you've used was there one drug that helped you 'cool it' when you got angry or mad, so you didn't get into a fight?" In order to ensure an informal comparison, the number shown includes only subjects who had used at least one other drug in addition to the drug selected. Number in parentheses, nonassaultive; number in brackets, assaultive. Reprinted with permission from the Association for Research in Nervous and Mental Disease.

likely to *decrease* the possibility of violence by a large proportion of nonassaultive and assaultive subjects who had used marijuana and at least one other drug. We wanted to know in what way their behavior was different during marijuana intoxication. In response to our inquiry the following comments were offered:

> It just made me relax. I didn't forget the trouble but I saw it from a different viewpoint and saw it wasn't worth fighting over.
>
> Made me feel good and warm toward others . . . friendly and overwhelmed with life.
>
> I just gave the peace sign and said 'cool it man.' I think I put out a lot of good vibes cus I didn't get into a hassle.

> When I was smoking marijuana I didn't want to fight anybody. I just felt lazy.
>
> You know, it lets you think, 'maybe I should bust him alongside the head.' You say, 'Why should I do that, that's what he wants me to do. Why satisfy him.' I just walk away.
>
> A couple of joints, man, relaxed me. I started being more aware. I wouldn't mess up. I'd give the dude a chance.

These comments are of interest in reference to observations that when drugs are used repeatedly they are taken primarily for the drug effect per se (Schoolar and Idanpaan-Heikkila, 1970). Based on interviews with chronic LSD users, Allen and West (1968) concluded that psychedelics appear to be used by certain individuals in an "escape from violence." Results from our studies suggest that there may be a subgroup among these incarcerated young men who are using marijuana in part for what they perceive to be the drug's aggression-reducing effects.

In conclusion, there is no convincing evidence that the pharmacological properties of marijuana incite or enhance human aggression. Field and laboratory studies suggest that set and setting, personality predispositions, and sociological variables account for most of the associations observed between marijuana and violence. Indeed, marijuana may be a useful tool for future research in models of aggression; contrary to many central nervous system depressants, marijuana may exert influences that tend to inhibit brain mechanisms subserving assaultiveness. There is suggestive evidence, at any rate, that the use of marijuana facilitates acquiescence in some individuals and hence reduces the possibilities for human aggression.

ACKNOWLEDGMENTS

The author wishes to thank Patricia Murphy and Peggy Murphy for their research and editorial assistance. The author's research reported in this chapter was supported in part by the van Ameringen Foundation and the Commonwealth Foundation.

REFERENCES

Advisory Committee on Drug Dependence. (1968). "Cannabis." HM Stationery Office, London.
Allen, J. R., and West, L. J. (1968). *Amer. J. Psychiat.* **125**, 364–370.

13. Marijuana and Human Aggression

Allentuck, S., and Bowman, K. (1942). *Amer. J. Psychiat.* **99**, 248–251.
Andrade, O. M. (1964). *Bull. Narcotics*, **16**, 23–28.
Asuni, T. (1964). *Bull. Narcotics* **16**, 17–28.
Ausubel, D. P. (1964). "Drug Addiction: Physiological, Psychological and Sociological Aspects." Random House, New York.
Babor, T. F. (1973). *Psychopharmacol. Bull.* **9**, 51–52.
Bandura, A. (1973). "Aggression: A Social Learning Analysis." Prentice-Hall, Englewood Cliffs, New Jersey.
Bloom, R. (1972). "The Effects of Tetrahydrocannabinol on Aggression in Humans." University Microfilms, Ann Arbor, Michigan.
Bloomquist, E. R. (1971). "Marijuana, The Second Trip." Glencoe Press, Beverly Hills, California.
Blum, R. H. (1969). *In* "Crimes of Violence" (A Staff Report to the National Commission on the Causes and Prevention of Violence, Prepared by D. J. Mulivihill and M. M. Tumin), Vol. 13, pp. 1461–1523. US Gov't. Printing Office, Washington, D.C.
Blum, R. H. and Associates. (1969). "Students and Drugs. Drugs II." Jossey-Bass, San Francisco, California.
Blumer, H., Sutter, A., Ahmed, S., and Smith, R. (1967). "ADD Center Project Final Report: The World of Youthful Drug Use." Univ. of California Press, Berkeley.
Bressler, R. R. (1968). *Amer. J. Med. Sci.* **225**, 89–93.
Bromberg, W. (1934). *Amer. J. Psychiat.* **91**, 303–330.
Bromberg, W. (1939). *J. Amer. Med. Ass.* **113**, 4–9.
Bromberg, W., and Rodgers, T. C. (1946). *Amer. J. Psychiat.* **102**, 825–827.
Charen, S., and Perelman, L. (1946). *Amer. J. Psychiat.* **102**, 674–682.
Chopra, R. N. (1940). *Indian Med. Gaz.* **75**, 356–367.
Chopra, R. N., and Chopra, G. S. (1939). *Indian J. Med. Res. Mem.* **31**, 1–119.
Commission of Inquiry into the Non-Medical Use of Drugs. (1970). "Interim Report of the Commission of Inquiry into the Non-Medical Use of Drugs." Queen's Printer, Ottawa.
Commission of Inquiry into the Non-Medical Use of Drugs. (1972). "Cannabis." Queen's Printer, Ottawa.
Committee on Ways and Means. (1937). "Taxation on Marihuana" (U.S. Congress, House of Representatives). US Gov't. Printing Office, Washington, D.C.
Davis, J. M., Sekerke, H. J., and Janowsky, D. S. (1973). *In* "Drug Use in America: Problem in Perspective. The Technical Papers of the Final Report of the National Commission on Marihuana and Drug Abuse," Appendix, Vol. 1, pp. 181–208. US Gov't. Printing Office, Washington, D.C.
Eckerman, W. C., Bates, J. D., Rachel, J. V., and Poole, W. K. (1971). "Drug Usage and Arrest Charges among Arrestees in Six Metropolitan Areas of the United States" (U.S. Dept. of Justice, Bureau of Narcotics and Dangerous Drugs). US Gov't. Printing Office, Washington, D.C.
Fraser, J. D. (1949). *Lancet* **2**, 747–748.
Freedman, H. L., and Rockmore, M. J. (1946a). *J. Clin. Psychopathol.* **7**, 765–782.
Freedman, H. L., and Rockmore, M. J. (1946b). *J. Clin. Psychopathol.* **8**, 221–236.
Gardikas, C. G. (1950). *Enkephalos* **1**, 201–211.
Gaskill, H. S. (1945). *Amer. J. Psychiat.* **102**, 202–204.
George, H. R. (1970). *Brit. J. Addict*, **65**, 119–121.
Goode, E. (1970). "The Marijuana Smokers." Basic Books, New York.
Goode, E. (1972). *In* "Marihuana: A Signal of Misunderstanding. The Technical

Papers of the First Report of the National Commission on Marihuana and Drug Abuse," Appendix, Vol. 1, pp. 446–469. US Gov't. Printing Office, Washington, D.C.
Goodwin, D. W., Crane, J. B., and Guze, S. B. (1971). *Quart. J. Stud. Alc.* 32, 136–147.
Grinspoon, L. (1971). "Marihuana Reconsidered." Harvard Univ. Press, Cambridge, Massachusetts.
Grossman, W. (1969). *Ann. Intern. Med.* 70, 529–533.
Hare, R. D. (1970). "Psychopathy: Theory and Research." Wiley, New York.
Hollister, L. E. (1971). *Science* 172, 21–28.
Hollister, L. E., Richards, R. K., and Gillespie, H. K. (1968). *Clin. Pharmacol. Ther.* 9, 383–391.
Indian Hemp Drugs Commission (1969). "Report of the Indian Hemp Drugs Commission, 1893–1894." Waverly Press, Baltimore, Maryland.
Jones, R. T. (1971). *Pharmacol. Rev.* 23, 359–369.
Kaplan, H. S. (1971). *N.Y. J. Med.* 71, 433–435.
Kaplan, J. (1970). "Marijuana—The New Prohibition." World Publ. Co., Cleveland, Ohio.
Keeler, M. (1967). *Amer. J. Psychiat.* 124, 674–677.
Keup, W. (1970). *Dis. Nerv. Sys.*, 31, 119–126.
Klee, G. D. (1969). *Psychiat. Quart.* 43, 719–733.
Lambo, T. A. (1965). *Bull. Narcotics* 17, 3–13.
Lemberger, L., Axelrod, J., and Kopin, I. J. (1971). *Ann. N.Y. Acad. Sci.* 191, 142–154.
Malmquist, C. P. (1971). *Amer. J. Psychiat.* 128, 461–465.
Maurer, D. W., and Vogel, V. H. (1967). "Narcotics and Drug Addiction." Thomas, Springfield, Illinois.
Mayor's Committee on Marihuana. (1944). "The Marihuana Problem in the City of New York: Sociological, Medical, Psychological and Pharmacological Studies." Jacques Cattell Press, Lancaster, Pennsylvania.
Mendelson, J. H., and Meyer, R. E. (1972). *In* "Marihuana: A Signal of Misunderstanding. The Technical Papers of the First Report of the National Commission on Marihuana and Drug Abuse," Appendix, Vol. 1, pp. 68–246. US Gov't. Printing Office, Washington, D.C.
Meyer, R. E., Dillard, R. C., Sapiro, L. M., and Mirin, S. M. (1971). *Amer. J. Psychiat.* 128, 198–204.
National Commission on the Causes and Prevention of Violence. (1970). "To Establish Justice, to Insure Domestic Tranquility." US Gov't. Printing Office, Washington, D.C.
National Commission on Marihuana and Drug Abuse. (1972). "Marihuana: A Signal of Misunderstanding." US Gov't. Printing Office, Washington, D.C.
National Commission on Marihuana and Drug Abuse. (1973). "Drug Use in America: Problem in Perspective." US Gov't. Printing Office, Washington, D.C.
National Insitute of Mental Health. (1970). "Marijuana" (U.S. Congress, House of Representatives, Statement to the Select Committee on Crime). US Gov't. Printing Office, Washington, D.C.
National Institute of Mental Health. (1972). "Marihuana and Health" (U.S. Department of Health, Education and Welfare). US Gov't. Printing Office, Washington, D.C.
President's Commission on Law Enforcement and Administration of Justice. (1967). "Task Force Report: Narcotics and Drug Abuse." US Gov't. Printing Office, Washington, D.C.

Robins, L. N. (1970). *Semin. Psychiat.* **2**, 420–434.
Salzman, C., Kochansky, G. E., and Porrino, L. J. (1973). *Psychopharmacol. Bull.* **9**, 54–55.
Schoolar, J. C., and Idanpaan-Heikkila, P. (1970). *In* "Drug Dependence" (R. T. Harris, W. A. McIsaac, and C. R. Schuster, Jr., eds.), pp. 268–279. Univ. of Texas Press, Austin.
Schuckit, M. A. (1973). *Quart. J. Stud. Alc.* **34**, 157–164.
Smith, D. E. (1968). *J. Psychedelic Drugs* **2**, 37–47.
Smith, D. E., and Mehl, C. (1970). *Clin. Toxicol.* **3**, 101–115.
Soueif, M. I. (1971). *Bull. Narcotics* **23**, 17–28.
Talbott, J. A., and Teague, J. W. (1969). *J. Amer. Med. Ass.* **210**, 299–302.
Tart, C. T. (1971). "On Being Stoned." Science and Behavior Books, Palo Alto, California.
Tennant, F. S., and Groesbeck, C. J. (1972). *Arch. Gen. Psychiat.* **27**, 133–136.
Tinklenberg, J. R., and Murphy, P. (1972). *J. Psychedelic Drugs* **5**, 183–191.
Tinklenberg, J. R., and Woodrow, K. M. (1974). *In* "Aggression: Proceedings of the 1972 Annual Meeting of the Association for Research in Nervous and Mental Disorders" (S. H. Frazier, ed). Williams & Wilkins, Baltimore, Maryland.
Tinklenberg, J. R., Murphy, P. L., Murphy, P., Darley, C. F., Roth, W. T., and Kopell, B. S. (1974). *Arch. Gen. Psychiat.* **30**, 685–689.
Weil, A. T. (1970). *N. Engl. J. Med.* **282**, 997–1000.
Weil, A. T., Zinberg, N. E., and Nelson, J. M. (1968). *Science* **162**, 1234–1242.
White House Conference on Narcotic and Drug Abuse. (1963). "Proceedings of the White House Conference on Narcotic and Drug Abuse." US Gov't. Printing Office, Washington, D.C.

Chapter 14

EFFECTS OF MARIJUANA ON DRIVING IN A RESTRICTED AREA AND ON CITY STREETS: DRIVING PERFORMANCE AND PHYSIOLOGICAL CHANGES*

HARRY KLONOFF

I. Introduction ... 359
II. Methods ... 362
   A. General Procedure ... 362
   B. Experimental Procedure ... 364
III. Results ... 372
   A. Course—Driving Skills Measures ... 372
   B. Street—Driving Skills Measures ... 375
   C. Course and Street Comparisons ... 377
   D. Course and Street—Physiological Measures ... 380
   E. Postdriving Interview ... 385
   F. Driving Questionnaire ... 386
IV. Discussion ... 388
V. Conclusion ... 394
   References ... 396

I. INTRODUCTION

One of the first comprehensive reviews of the effects of drugs on driving was published by Nichols (1971). Le Dain (1972) was the first to report a study of the effects of two levels of smoked marijuana (1.4 mg Δ^9-THC and 5.9 mg Δ^9-THC) and a single dose of alcohol (average blood alcohol

*An abbreviated version of this chapter was published in *Science* 186, pp. 317-324, 25 October 1974 (copyright 1974 by the American Association for the Advancement of Science).

level was 0.07%) on 16 subjects who drove a vehicle in a restricted traffic-free area. Le Dain concluded: "The low marijuana dose and placebo conditions were not different in terms of the number of poles or road cones hit. Both the higher marijuana dose and the alcohol condition produced small increases in hits, which were reliably different from placebo, but not significantly different from each other. The higher cannabis dose resulted in a slight (7%) but consistent decrease in driving speed." No other study has been uncovered to date which has dealt with the effects of marijuana on driving in a real life situation. One other study that may well be a landmark is that of Coldwell et al. (1958), and this dealt with the effects of alcohol on driving in a restricted area.

All the published studies relevant to marijuana and driving have employed a psychomotor model or some type of laboratory driving simulator. Crancer et al. (1969) investigated the effects of marijuana and alcohol on simulated driving with 36 subjects and in part concluded: "Subjects experiencing a social marijuana high accumulated significantly more speedometer errors than when under control conditions, whereas there were no significant differences in accelerator, brake, signal, steering, and total errors. Impairment in simulated driving performance does not seem to be a function of increased marijuana dosage or inexperience with the drug." Crancer's methodology has been questioned and in particular the potency of the marijuana he used (Le Dain, 1972).

Dott (1972) used a simulated risk paradigm and found that a potentially hazardous passing situation resulted in heightened cautiousness and accurate judgment of risk for the marijuana subjects, but more aggression and less adequate judgment of risk for the subjects under the influence of alcohol. Whereas decision reaction time was prolonged during non-emergency trials for both marijuana and alcohol subjects, response to emergency signals was impaired by alcohol but not by marijuana. Bech et al. (1973) and Rafaelsen et al. (1973) also used a simulator to determine the effects of oral doses of marijuana and alcohol on driving. They found that marijuana had a much stronger effect than alcohol on the estimation of time and distance; both marijuana and alcohol increased brake time and start time; alcohol increased while marijuana decreased the number of gear changes; and mean speed was not changed with either drug but variation of speed was affected by both marijuana and alcohol. Ellingstad et al. (1973) reported a simulator study in which marijuana influenced the accuracy of passing-time judgments but did not adversely affect risk-taking/decision-making capabilities, while alcohol affected the latter but not the former. Moskowitz et al. (1973), using the UCLA driving simulator, found a marijuana dose-related impairment in response to a subsidiary task (increase in errors of recognition and delay in response to the visual recognition task) and to an auditory signal detection task in conditions of both concentrated and divided attention. Other studies, such as Binder (1971) and Kielholz et al. (1972), imply that they are engaged in investigating cannabis and simulated car driving, but this does not turn out to be so.

Another area of the literature that is relevant to the present study is that of physiological monitoring during driving. There are few relevant published studies and even fewer dealing with actual driving situations. The most comprehensive review in this area is that of Wilde and Curry (1970). Taggart and Gibbons (1967) reported preliminary results of electrocardiogram (ECG) studies in normal London traffic and in competitive motor-racing. Simonson et al. (1968) reviewed cardiovascular changes reported during automobile driving and point out that heart rate responds instantaneously to critical situations during driving, the increase of heart rate of 20 to 40% being directly related to traffic density and critical traffic situations. Whereas more speed did not affect heart rate, some effect was noted with driving experience. In their monitoring of five subjects during 30 minutes of city driving, they found that heart rate increased on the average from 70 to 95 beats per minute.

Hulbert (1957) analyzed the galvanic skin response (GSR) in traffic on 21 subjects in terms of idealized path, driver actions, clarity of the GSR record, and amount of traffic activity along the route. A trend was noted regarding drivers' GSRs and changes in the traffic situation. Michaels (1960) continuously monitored the GSR in terms of frequency and magnitude in 10 subjects in urban test routes during five traffic periods. During the continuous test run, events per minute were 2.42 and 1.71 for the two routes taken, while average GSR magnitude was 2.28 and 2.23 for the respective routes. Of the measurable responses, 95% were caused by eight types of traffic interference, the most frequent being other vehicles in the traffic stream. Taylor (1964) measured the rate of occurrence of GSR in 20 drivers during a range of road conditions. Taylor found significantly different rates between his subjects, but some of the differences between subjects could be accounted for by length of experience as drivers and age. There was, however, no variation in the GSR rate for the variety of road and traffic and lighting conditions sampled. He concluded that: "Driving is a self-paced task governed by the level of emotional tension or anxiety which the driver wishes to tolerate."

The final area in the literature that is relevant to the present study is that of physiological monitoring during marijuana smoking in a laboratory setting. Le Dain (1972) provided a most comprehensive review of the literature on the cardiovascular system. Researchers on marijuana have, however, paid less attention to autonomic measures such as GSR and respiration. One exception is Gale and Guenther (1971) who found the basal level conductance to be significantly lower during the drug sessions and they relate this to a state of relaxation or sedative effect. Low et al. (1973) also found that GSR reactivity decreased for the marijuana conditions compared with baseline and placebo condition.

Domino (1972) reported a minor decrease in respiratory rate with smoked marijuana. Low et al. (1973), however, reported a slight drop in respiration rate with smoked marijuana for their placebo condition and slight increases for low- and high-drug doses, respectively. Tashkin et al. (1973) found no differences in respiration rate with oral Δ^9-THC for their placebo and drug conditions. Gostomzyk et al. (1973), on the other hand, found that respiratory rate was 20% higher under the influence of hashish.

The logistics of planning research on the effects of marijuana on driving were covered in Chapter 1 of this volume. The purposes of the present study were to determine: (1) the effects of low and high doses of marijuana on driving performance in a restricted, traffic-free area, i.e., driving course, and on the streets of Vancouver, including the downtown area, during peak hours of traffic flow; (2) physiological responses (heart rate, GSR, and respiration) during these driving experiences; (3) the relationships between physiological measures on the course and the street; and (4) the nature of the relationships between driving performance measures and physiological parameters on the course and the street.

II. METHODS

A. General Procedure

1. CRITERIA FOR VOLUNTEERS AND SCREENING PROCEDURE

All subjects were volunteers who met the following criteria: (1) age between 19 and 31; (2) light and restricted use of psychoative drugs (33 of the 64 subjects had experimented with psychoactive drugs other than marijuana or hashish at some time, but not during the past year); (3) not on any form of prescribed drug regimen; (4) good physical health; and (5) no signs of serious personality disorder. There was no advertising for volunteers and interested individuals became aware of the project through the grapevine.

Prospective subjects were initially interviewed by the project coordinator, informed about the general nature of the experiment, given an opportunity to ask relevant questions regarding the project, and were then given the opportunity of volunteering for the study. Those volunteers who

14. Effects of Marijuana on Driving

satisfied all the above criteria were then interviewed by a psychiatrist and provided informed consent (signed release and consent form).

Volunteers were asked to refrain from using psychoactive drugs for one week prior to the experimental session and during the course of the experiment.

2. BACKGROUND CHARACTERISTICS OF SUBJECTS

The project population for the course portion of the study consisted of 64 volunteers (43 men and 21 women) assigned to experimental conditions as follows: low-dose drug, 13 men and 8 women; high-dose drug, 14 men and 8 women; and placebo, 16 men and 5 women. Of these, 38 volunteers (25 men and 13 women) also participated in the street-driving portion of the study and were assigned to experimental conditions as follows: low-dose drug then placebo, 5 men and 4 women; placebo then low-dose drug, 7 men and 3 women; high-dose drug then placebo, 6 men and 2 women; and placebo then high-dose drug, 7 men and 4 women. Mean age of the study population was 23.89 years (SD 2.99, range 19 to 31). Educational level of the population was as follows: high school, 22%; 1 year of university, 12%; 2 to 4 years of university, 30%; bachelor's degree, 30%; master's degree, 3%; and doctorate, 3%. This is a highly educated group, the large majority being university trained and 36% having university degrees. Occupation was classified into the following six categories: postsecondary students, 38%; professional, 20%; semiprofessional, 3%; service, technical, and clerical, 20%; skilled and semiskilled, 11%; and housewife, 8%. The majority of the volunteers were postsecondary students. Of the group, 62% were single, 32% married, and 6% divorced, separated, or living common-law.

All the subjects had prior experience driving, mean years of driving experience was 6.92 (SD 3.14 years).

3. MARIJUANA AND PLACEBO

Low dose was defined as standardized *Cannabis sativa* labeled as containing 0.70% Δ^9-THC, and high-dose as containing 1.2% Δ^9-THC. The physical characteristics of the placebo were identical to those of the *Cannabis sativa* plant material, but free of cannabinols. The placebo, when smoked, smelled and tasted like the marijuana cigarettes made from the unextracted plant material.

Marijuana and placebo were administered in the form of cigarettes of standard size and weight (0.70 gm)—low-dose 4.90 mg Δ^9-THC and high-dose 8.40 mg Δ^9-THC—and the smoking was standardized (Klonoff, 1973).

4. DRIVING QUESTIONNAIRE AND POSTDRIVING INTERVIEW

A driving questionnaire was completed by the volunteers and the items dealt with past driving history, the use of drugs and alcohol in a context of driving, and reported effects of marijuana on driving.

For the course portion of the study, subjective evaluation of marijuana and placebo was obtained at the conclusion of the second session. In addition, a statement regarding change of performance in driving after smoking was obtained from each subject. For the street portion of the study, a dictated account of reactions to the driving experience was obtained.

B. Experimental Procedure

1. DESCRIPTION OF PHYSIOLOGICAL SYSTEM

Physiological data were obtained from a portable FM/FM battery powered telemetry system using FM subcarrier multiplexing (with a maximum transmission range of 100 feet—EKEG Electronics). The system carried in the automobiles consisted of the following: (1) ECG, 2 Beckman bio-potential electrodes* were placed on the subject's chest, one on the sternum and the other on the fourth intercostal space (left side), and the signal was increased by means of an integrated circuit differential instrumentation amplifier; (2) respiration, a nasal thermistor probe was placed under the subject's clearest nostril and respiration was measured by a Whetstone bridge configuration; and (3) GSR, 2 Grass silver chloride electrodes were placed on the subject's first and third fingers of the right hand and GSR was measured by means of skin resistance changes. Each of the amplified signals was then used to drive an FM subcarrier oscillator multiplexed on to a main FM carrier in the standard FM band. The received FM signal was then converted back by means of demodulators and recorded on a Hewlett Packard 3960, 4 channel FM Instrumentation Tape Recorder powered by a 12 V car battery. The fourth channel of the tape recorder was used as a stimulus marker. A portable battery-powered oscilloscope was used to confirm the operation of the system. The tape was subsequently played back using the same tape recorder onto an 8 channel Beckman Type R dynograph to produce visual write-outs of the physiological data.

2. DESCRIPTION, OPERATION, AND SCORING OF DRIVING COURSE

The driving course was made up of eight practical road tests arranged in sequence on a T-shaped paved area of about 50,000 ft². The course, in

* One reference electrode was placed on the right side of the chest.

terms of tasks, distances, and cones, is shown in Fig. 1. The eight driving tasks were as follows: (1) Slalom, consisted of cones placed in a straight line. The subject was instructed to swing back and forth between the cones. (2) and (3) Tunnels of varying length, the two tunnels each consisted of two rows of cones. The subject was instructed to drive between the rows of cones. (4) Funnel, the funnel consisted of two rows of cones and the distance between the cones diminished from start to finish. The subject was instructed to drive between the two rows. (5) Risk, the task consisted of two rows of cones whose distance apart was either 6 ft 2 in. or 5 ft 6 in. The smaller gap was not passable because the outside width of the wheelbase of the vehicle was 5 ft 8 in. The subject was instructed to stop 20 ft from the cones and decide whether the gap was passable or not. If the subject decided it was passable, he had to drive through the gap, otherwise to drive around it. (6) Back-up, the back-up consisted of driving in reverse, making a right angle turn and then backing through two rows of cones. (7) Corner, the subject was instructed to accelerate to 20 mph on a straight away, then slow to 10 mph and go through a right curve made up of two rows of cones. (8) Braking, the braking apparatus was attached to the front bumper of the car and triggered by the driving observer. The emergency braking situation was cued by the firing of a 22 calibre paint cartridge. The shot provided the cue to stop as quickly as possible and the paint on the pavement served as a reference point for measuring braking distance. This test was done only when the subject was between tasks and his speed was 15 mph (the speed he was asked to maintain between tasks).

Points of entry into the course (slalom, back-up, and corner) and order of tasks (slalom, tunnel I, tunnel II, funnel, risk, back-up, and corner) were kept constant between blocks for all subjects. Once the subject had begun a trial, he followed the same order of tasks noted above to the task preceding the point of entry. The braking was done on a random basis within blocks but between tasks.

In the scoring for all the tasks except the slalom and risk, each cone hit was recorded as one. For slalom, the scoring was as follows: 1 point for touching cone; 2 points for direct hit and knockdown of cone; and 2 points for backing up to avoid hitting cone. For risk, the scoring was as follows: impassable option, 0 points for refusing and 4 points for accepting; passable option, 4 points for refusing and 0, 2, or 4 points depending on number of side hits. The scoring was done by four persons who were able to count the cones contacted by the vehicle as it traversed the course.

A Chevrolet Nova compact equipped with automatic transmission, power brakes, and power steering was used for the course portion of

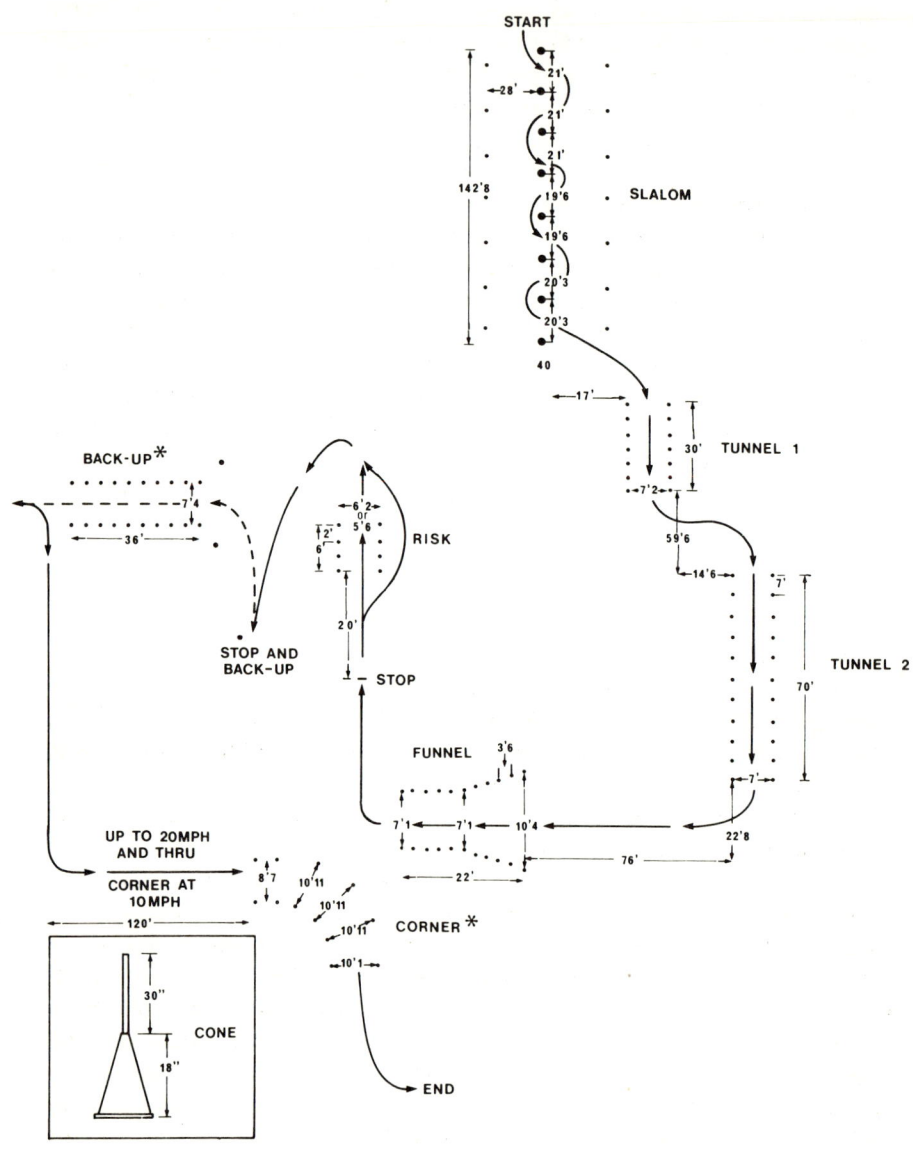

Fig. 1. Description of course. →, Route followed from start position of slalom; *, alternate start position; ●, represents one cone; — — →, backing up.

the study. Safety features installed were dual brakes and an auxilliary ignition. A Chevelle Malibu intermediate equipped with automatic transmission, standard brakes, and power steering was used for the city streets portion of the study. Safety features installed were a dual steering wheel, dual brakes, and an auxilliary ignition.

3. COURSE DRIVING PROCEDURE

The first session began with the placement of the electrodes on the subject. The subject and apparatus were then taken into the Nova and driven to the course. The subject, with the driving observer in the front seat, drove around the course twice to learn about order of tasks, scoring of tasks, and braking procedure. During the five trials of block I, the subject was told to drive the course while the driving observer provided cues for improving performance and feedback regarding errors, clearance of cones, and handling of the vehicle. A minimum of two practice braking sequences was carried out to shape the response. There was an interval of five minutes between blocks to enable the subject to relax. During the five trials of block II, the only instructions given to the subject were concerned with points of entry into the course sequence. There was no feedback. Two braking tests were done and measured. There was an interval on the average of one week between sessions.

For session II, the electrode procedure and driving on the course were identical to that of session I. At the start of the second session, the subject was told to run through the course five times (block III), to become refamiliarized with the tasks and the course. A minimum of one braking test was also done during block III to reestablish the response. After the car was parked, the subject smoked a marijuana or placebo cigarette. After a 3 minute postsmoking period to obtain baseline physiological data, the five trials of block IV and the two braking tests were completed. The interval between blocks III and IV was on the average 15 minutes.

Blocks I to III were accordingly practice and block IV was experimental. Neither the subjects nor the research staff were aware of condition assignment, experimental sequence (which of the 3 blocks was the baseline), or the final scoring system.

4. PHYSIOLOGICAL DATA ACQUISITION ON COURSE

a. Recording Time. Before each of the two driving sessions, heart rate and respiration baselines were recorded for 4 minutes in a laboratory. Baseline measures of skin resistance for the GSR were established prior to each block of five trials. Recording of all three measures in the automobile for the first session was done during the five trials of block II. Recording in the automobile for the second session was done during the five practice trials of block III, for a 3 minutes period following the smoking with the automobile parked (postsmoking baseline), and during the five experimental trials of block IV. The approximate recording time for each block of trials was 20 minutes.

b. Scoring of Physiological Measures. i. HEART RATE. Sampling of time intervals approximated task lengths and was as follows: 10 seconds per trial for tunnel I, tunnel II, funnel, risk, corner, and braking; 20 seconds per trial for back-up; and 30 seconds per trial for slalom. A score was derived by summing each task over five trials and then converting to beats per minute for blocks II and/or III and then compared with IV.

ii. GSR. Sampling of time intervals was as per heart rate. Scoring was in terms of fluctuations (any movement from baseline greater than one-quarter of the largest response) and amplitude (the highest fluctuation of each task for each trial as a fraction of the maximal fluctuation). The fluctuations and amplitudes were then summed over five trials and means obtained for blocks II and/or III and then compared with IV. The fluctuations were then converted to frequency per minute. The rationale for this procedure was that although stimulus onset cannot be readily identified, random feedback occurs because of cone hits, and habituation can still be defined.

iii. RESPIRATION. Sampling of 2 minute time intervals was included for each trial of the three blocks. A score was the summed rate of five trials for each of the three blocks, converted to rate per minute.

Thus heart rate and GSR measures enable comparisons to be made between tasks and blocks, while respiration permits comparisons only between blocks.

5. CITY STREETS DRIVING PROCEDURE

The first session began with the subject driving the Chevelle dual-control car around the campus for 10 minutes in order to become familiarized with the vehicle. The subject then returned to the hospital and the electrodes were placed on the subject. A marijuana or placebo cigarette was then smoked by the subject. As a result of placing of the subject and apparatus in the vehicle and calibration of apparatus, there was on the average a 6 minute interval before driving. The subject was told that he would be responsible for observing all traffic regulations and should drive as if being examined for a driver's license. The subject was then instructed to drive to a designated intersection in the center of the downtown area, and after arriving at this point was instructed to drive to another designated intersection in a residential area, and after arriving there was instructed to drive back to the University hospital. The approximate distance was 16.8 miles and driving time was on the average 46 minutes. With the exception of the familiarization period, the procedure was repeated during the second session, on the average one week later.

During the pilot phase of the study, two trained driving observers (who had been employed as examiners by the British Columbia Motor Vehicle Department) were in the vehicle to ensure reliability of the scoring system. But during the study proper, only one (same) driving observer was present in the front seat of the car.

Driving took place on the streets of Vancouver during daylight hours, between 12:00 noon and 8:30 PM from Monday through Friday. As time of day of the two sessions for each subject was standardized, traffic conditions encountered by individual subjects was more or less controlled. Traffic conditions were categorized and the distribution of the group among these categories was as follows: light, 25%; moderate, 47%; and heavy, 28%. The modal traffic encountered was therefore moderate. Road conditions were categorized and the distribution of the group among these categories was as follows: dry, 67%; damp, 18%; and wet, 15%. The modal road condition encountered was therefore dry.

On the course, only the final block (IV) was preceded by smoking (placebo or drug high or drug low). On the street, each session was preceded by smoking (low- or high-doses and placebo counterbalanced for each subject for each session). The double-blind procedure was maintained on the street-driving portion of the study as well, in terms of experimental conditions and scoring procedure.

6. SCORING PROCEDURE FOR CITY STREETS

The British Columbia Department of Motor Vehicles driver examination format served as the basis for measuring driving skills on city streets. Eleven behavioral components involved in driving were selected and quantified. The components reflecting driving skills and their respective raw score ranges were as follows: (1) general driving habits, including (a) posture (0–5), (b) starting–stopping (0–5), (c) carelessness with driving regulations (0–10), (d) turning (0–10), (e) lane changing (0–10), (f) regard for traffic signals (0–10), (g) poor driving habits, e.g., turning head while talking (0–10); (2) cooperation (0–5); (3) attitude (0–5); (4) irritability (0–5); (5) judgment (0–5); (6) speed, (a) too fast (0–5) or (b) too slow (0–5); (7) care while driving, (a) careless (0–5) or (b) overcautious (0–5); (8) confident, (a) overconfidence (0–5) or (b) lack of confidence (0–5); (9) tension, (a) tense (0–5) or (b) lethargic (0–5); (10) aggression, (a) aggressive (0–5) or (b) passive (0–5); and (11) concentration, (a) fixation (0–5) or (b) attention wanders (0–5). The driving observer assigned a raw score to each category at the end of the respective sessions. In order to reflect change between the two sessions and to relate the change between sessions to experimental conditions (drug/placebo and placebo/drug paradigms), the difference scores for each category were always derived from drug minus placebo conditions.

In order to compare categories and to provide a meaningful composite (total) score, the raw scores were transformed to an arithmetically weighted scoring system of 1 to 7. The transformed score rationale derived from a pilot study and the format was decided on before the study proper began. The driving observer was unaware of the transformed score procedure.

TABLE I

Raw and Transformed Scores for Behavioral Components of Driving

Transformed difference scores	Raw difference scores		
	General driving habits	Speed	Remainder of categories
1	−11 or less	−4 or less	−3 or less
2	−7 to −10	−3	−2
3	−3 to −6	−2	−1
4	±2	±1	0
5	3 to 6	2	1
6	7 to 10	3	2
7	11 or more	4 or more	3 or more

Table I indicates the basis for assigning transformed scores (1 to 7) for general driving habits, speed, and then the remaining 9 categories. For each of the 11 categories a transformed score of 4 indicates no change, transformed scores 1–3 reflect improvement, and transformed scores 5–7 decline. The total transformed score range is accordingly 11–77; 44 indicates no overall change, less than 44 reflects overall improvement, and more than 44 indicates overall decline.

As driving on city streets results in the encountering of emergent events on a random basis, the number of emergent events was recorded by the driving observer for each session regardless of experimental condition. Each event was scored by the driving observer on a scale from 0 to 20, according to his assessment of the dangerous nature of the event. For the

14. Effects of Marijuana on Driving

population under investigation, the number of events between sessions and between experimental conditions should be equivalent. Significant differences in the incidence of emergent events between experimental conditions would accordingly be related to that experimental condition.

7. PHYSIOLOGICAL DATA ACQUISITION ON STREETS

a. Recording Time. Before each of the two driving sessions, heart rate and respiration baseline measures were recorded for 5 minutes in a laboratory. After being seated in the automobile, a baseline resistance was established for the GSR prior to continuous recording. Subsequent to the smoking (approximately 10 minutes) and seating of the subject in the automobile (approximately 6 minutes), a continuous recording was obtained for the two driving sessions (approximately 46 minutes per session).

b. Scoring of Physiological Measures. i. TRAFFIC PATTERNS. In all three measures, recording was continuous during the two driving sessions. Five types of traffic conditions or areas were defined in advance; namely, residential through streets (light traffic and regular traffic flow); residential side streets (light traffic, right-of-way undefined, and school and playground areas); local commercial area (medium traffic and fluctuations in speed); downtown area (heavy traffic conditions and restrictions); and higher speed areas with multiple lanes (medium to heavy traffic and tightness in maneuvering). Scoring was derived from time spent in each of the five areas and an area was included only if time spent in that area was greater than 3 minutes. The scoring was as follows: heart rate, beats per minute for each of the five areas; GSR, fluctuations per minute for each of the five areas, analysis of amplitude was not done; and respiration, rate per minute for each of the five areas.

The rationale for all measures was to provide an index of stress for various traffic conditions. The premise was made that the large sample size and the lengthy recording period for each subject would randomize stress-inducing events among the five traffic conditions or areas and would thus permit probability statements of stress related to traffic condition.

ii. EVENTS. Events were defined in terms of: turns, through major intersections, and for heart rate only, parking. The total time of the event was scored. The scoring was as follows: heart rate, beats per minute for each of the three types of events; GSR, the average number of fluctuations per minute for each of the two types of events; and respiration, rate per minute for each of the two types of events. Thus, different traffic condition effects on all measures can be compared as well as the effects of specific events.

III. RESULTS

A. Course—Driving Skills Measures

1. DATA ANALYSIS

For the data analysis and reporting of results on driving skills, each of the five trials for the four blocks was scored as outlined above. Because the nature of the tasks followed a learning model, block III was used as the baseline measure and block IV as the experimental measure. In order to control for warmup effect, boredom, and fatigue, only the middle trials (2–4) for each of the respective blocks were used in the data analysis.

2. LEARNING BETWEEN BLOCKS OF TRIALS

The initial analysis of the data was by linear regression. Using the baseline scores for trials 2 to 4 of blocks I, II, and III, a line was fitted through this data. For each of the seven tasks as well as the total score, a predicted value for block IV was then calculated along with the 95% confidence interval about the predicted point. Finally, the means for placebo, drug low, and drug high conditions were checked to see if they were within that confidence interval.

The results of Table II lend themselves to a learning model interpretation. First, the actual scores for each of the tasks as well as the total score decrease (performance improves) from blocks I through III. Second, learning (slope of line column) occurs at a significant rate for three of the tasks (slalom, tunnel I, and tunnel II) and for total score. A further examination of Table II reveals that only actual scores of the drug conditions for block IV were beyond the upper limits of the confidence interval. Specifically, with the low-dose group there was a drug effect on learning with two of the tasks and the total score and with the high-dose group five of the tasks and the total score.

3. EFFECTS OF MARIJUANA AND PLACEBO ON DRIVING SKILLS

Turning now to the performance scores within and between groups, difference scores were used to enable each subject to be his own control in terms of change between the baseline and experimental blocks (trials

TABLE II

Linear Regression for Course Scores ($N = 64$)

Task	Actual scores for blocks I	II	III	Predicted score for block IV	95% Confidence interval for predicted score block IV	Slope of line	Actual scores for block IV for conditions Placebo	Low	High
Slalom	10.5	9.8	9.0	8.3	±1.6 (6.7– 9.9)	−0.7[a]	8.9	8.8	10.4[b]
Tunnel I	3.9	2.7	1.5	0.3	±1.2 (−0.9– 1.5)	−1.2[c]	1.0	2.6[b]	3.0[b]
Tunnel II	8.1	6.6	5.1	3.5	±1.9 (1.6– 5.4)	−1.5[c]	2.8	5.0	6.9[b]
Funnel	2.1	1.9	1.7	1.4	±1.0 (0.4– 2.4)	−0.2	1.2	1.7	2.9[b]
Back-up	8.1	7.1	6.1	5.0	±2.6 (3.4– 7.6)	−1.0	6.0	6.0	7.0
Corner	3.5	3.4	3.4	3.3	±0.7 (2.6– 4.0)	−0.1	2.9	4.1[b]	3.1
Risk	4.4	3.9	3.4	2.9	±1.2 (1.7– 4.1)	−0.5	4.0	3.8	4.7[b]
Total	40.7	35.4	30.1	24.8	±5.4 (19.4–30.2)	−5.3[c]	26.8	31.9[b]	38.1[b]

[a] $p < 0.05$.
[b] Beyond upper limits of confidence interval.
[c] $p < 0.001$.

2–4 of blocks III and IV). Table III shows that the driving skills of the placebo group improved significantly between blocks III and IV, the low-dose group skills declined somewhat but not significantly, whereas the skills of the high-dose group declined extensively and significantly. In comparing the low- and high-dose groups with each other and each, in turn, with the placebo group, the differences were significant in all

TABLE III

Mean Difference (d) Scores, t Tests, and Duncan's Multiple Range Test for Course Scores ($N = 64$)

Experimental condition	N	Mean d score	t	Duncan's multiple range
Placebo	21	−5.5	−2.41[a]	
Low	21	+1.0	0.54	
High	22	+8.2	2.85[b]	
				($F = 11.99, p < 0.001$)
Low vs. high	—	—	−2.10[c]	$p < 0.05$
Placebo vs. low	—	—	−2.21[c]	$p < 0.05$
Placebo vs. high	—	—	−3.71[d]	$p < 0.01$

[a] $p < 0.02$.
[b] $p < 0.01$.
[c] $p < 0.05$.
[d] $p < 0.001$.

analyses. Specifically, the driving skills of both drug groups are adversely affected when compared with the placebo group.*

Braking distance was analyzed separately within and between experimental conditions. Braking distance decreased between the baseline and the experimental condition for the placebo ($t = -2.41$, $p < 0.05$), low-dose drug ($t = -1.33$), and high dose drug ($t = -0.65$) groups. The only significant change (decrease in braking distance), however, occurred with the placebo group. In comparing the braking distance of the placebo group with the low-dose drug group and then with the high-dose drug group, neither difference was significant (placebo vs. low-dose drug, $t = 0.68$; placebo vs. high-dose drug, $t = 1.09$).

Statistical tests permit inferences about differences between groups, and in this study differences between the placebo and drug groups. But this is a generalization that requires qualification in terms of the number within each experimental condition that changed, the direction of their change, and the extent of change.

Table IV provides information regarding absolute change in perform-

TABLE IV

Frequency and Percentage of Decline, No Change, Improvement, Significant Decline (+6 or More for Course and 47 or Higher for Street), No Change (+5 to −5 for Course and 42 to 46 for Street), and Improvement (−6 or Less for Course and 41 or Lower for Street) by Experimental Condition—Course and Street

	Course ($N = 64$)					Street ($N = 38$)			
	Placebo		Low		High		Low		High
	Freq.	%	Freq.	%	Freq.	%	Freq.	%	Freq.	%
Decline (+)	5	24	12	57	16	73	10	53	15	79
No change (0)	1	5	1	5	1	4	1	5	1	5
Improvement (−)	15	71	8	38	5	23	8	42	3	16
Significant decline	3	14	7	33	12	55	8	42	12	63
No change	10	48	9	43	7	31	5	26	4	21
Significant improvement	8	38	5	24	3	14	6	32	3	16

ance in terms of decline, no change, and improvement of driving skills. Although there was variability within experimental conditions, the differences between the placebo group and the drug groups, and in par-

* Duncan's multiple range test revealed significant differences for placebo vs. high-drug for trial 1 ($p < 0.01$) and trial 5 ($p < 0.05$), as well as for low- vs. high-drug for trial 1 ($p < 0.05$).

ticular the high-dose drug group, are very striking, e.g., 71% of the placebo group improved their performance while 73% of the high-dose drug group declined in their performance.

Absolute scores overstate the nature of change, and a criterion measure was accordingly used to determine significant change in performance. From the linear regression analysis (Table II), it may be noted that the confidence interval for total score was ±5.4, and ±5 was accordingly used as a cutoff for determining significant decline and improvement. No change therefore means that the subject was permitted to decline or improve five points in either direction. Significant decline was defined in terms of a gain of six or more points between the baseline and experimental blocks, whereas significant improvement was defined in terms of a loss of at least six points between the baseline and experimental blocks. The findings regarding significant change (Table IV) can accordingly be summarized as follows: of the placebo group, 14% showed a significant decline in their driving skills, 48% showed no change in performance, and 38% improved their driving skills significantly; of the low-dose drug group, 33% declined significantly, 43% showed no change, and 24% improved significantly; and of the high-dose drug group, 55% declined significantly, 31% showed no change, and 14% improved significantly.

B. Street—Driving Skills Measures

1. DIFFERENTIAL EFFECTS OF MARIJUANA AND PLACEBO ON DRIVING SKILLS

In the analysis of data, the counterbalanced drug/placebo and placebo/drug sessions were combined for the respective low-dose and high-dose drug groups. The mean score for the low-dose group was 45.1 and for the high-dose group 47.5. An analysis of the scores as they differ from the cutoff point of 44 revealed significant findings for the high-dose group ($t = 2.33$, $p < .05$) but not for the low-dose group ($t = 0.56$). The scores were then categorized in terms of: decline, above the cutoff score of 44; no change, score of 44; and improvement, below the cutoff score of 44. Table IV also summarizes the distribution by experimental condition.* Although there was variability within the low- and high-dose

---

* Two females who were initially assigned to placebo/high-dose drug refused to drive during the second session and were accordingly brought in subsequently for their second session and given low-dose drug. The two subjects were then assigned to the high-dose group regarding driving performance and the low-dose group for the assessment of behavioral components of driving.

drug groups, both groups declined in their performance, i.e., 53% for the low-dose group and 79% for the high-dose group.

As was pointed out with the course data, absolute scores overstate the nature of change and here again the 95% confidence interval was used as a basis for inferring significant change. The 95% confidence interval was ±1.99 for the scores of all subjects, and this interval was related to the cutoff score of 44 in order to determine categories of significant change. Decline was accordingly defined as scores of 47 or higher, no change as scores between 42 and 46, and improvement as scores of 41 or lower. The findings regarding significant change (Table IV) can accordingly be summarized as follows: 42% and 63% of the respective low- and high-dose groups showed a significant decline in their driving performance; 26% and 21% of the respective groups showed no change; and 32% and 16% of the respective dose groups improved significantly.

2. BEHAVIORAL COMPONENTS OF DRIVING

In addition to a global estimate of driving performance, the behavioral components of driving were also analyzed. Table V presents a comparison of the 11 behavioral components of driving for those subjects whose driving did not change significantly or in fact improved significantly with those subjects whose driving declined significantly. Of the 11 categories, there was no appreciable difference between the subjects below and above the cutoff point for cooperation and attitude. There was some difference (of the order of 5 to 15%) in the comparison of those subjects above and below the cutoff point in general driving skills, irritability, speed, confidence, tension, and aggression. The greatest difference (of the order of 16% to 29%) in the comparison of subjects above and below the cutoff point occurred in judgment, care while driving, and concentration.

3. EMERGENT EVENTS

Emergent events were scored separately in terms of frequency of occurrence and the degree of hazard involved (magnitude) was rated from 0 to 20. For the group as a whole, the number of emergent events recorded for the placebo session was 8, and for the drug session (unrelated to dose) 18. The probability of occurrence of events for the drug session, using the placebo session as the criterion, was highly significant ($p < .001$). Whereas there was a significant difference between the placebo and drug conditions regarding frequency of emergent events, the mean magnitude of events for the drug condition was slightly but not significantly higher, i.e., 5.5 for the drug condition compared with 5.2 for the placebo condition.

TABLE V

Behavioral Components of Driving Performance for No Change and Significant Improvement Subgroup (Below Cutoff Point) Compared with the Significant Decline Subgroup (Above Cutoff Point)

Driving categories	Direction of change	Change[a]	Subjects below cutoff point ($N = 19$)[b]		Subjects above cutoff point ($N = 19$)[b]	
			Freq.	%	Freq.	%
General driving		+	17	45	12	32
		−	2	5	7	18
Cooperation		+	18	47	19	50
		−	1	3	0	0
Attitude		+	19	50	18	47
		−	0	0	1	3
Judgment		+	13	34	5	13
		−	6	16	14	37
Irritability	Less	+	14	37	12	32
	More	−	5	13	7	18
Speed	Closer to speed limit	+	17	45	12	32
	Unduly slow or fast	−	2	5	7	18
Care	Appropriately careful or cautious	+	16	42	5	13
	More careless, hypercautious	−	3	8	14	37
Confidence	Appropriately confident	+	15	39	9	24
	Overconfident, lacks confidence	−	4	11	10	26
Tension	Less tense, less lethargic	+	15	39	9	24
	More tense, more lethargic	−	4	11	10	26
Aggression	Less aggressive, less passive	+	15	39	11	29
	Unduly aggressive or passive	−	4	11	8	21
Concentration	More attention, less fixation	+	9	24	3	8
	More fixation, less attention	−	10	26	16	42

[a] (+) Improved/no change; (−) declined.
[b] Frequencies different than for Table IV.

C. Course and Street Comparisons

1. RELATIONSHIPS BETWEEN SUBJECTIVE RATING OF MARIJUANA "HIGH" ON THE COURSE AND SUBJECTIVE EVALUATION OF PERFORMANCE

When subjects were asked to rate the "high" experienced during the driving session on a scale from 0 to 10 (0, no effect; 1–2, minimal "high"; 3–6, moderate "high"; 7–10, very "high"), the ratings of the experimental groups were distributed as follows: placebo group, no effect or minimal effect (48%) and moderate effect (52%); low-dose group, minimal effect (5%), moderate effect (33%), and extensive effect (62%); and high-dose group, minimal effect (5%), moderate effect (41%), and extensive effect (54%). For the placebo group, the moderate effect of 52% noted was somewhat above the 44% reported in another study by Klonoff (Chapter 1, this volume), but the inference is the same, namely, about half of the number of subjects misidentify placebo as a psychoactive agent and these subjects may accordingly be viewed as placebo reactors. The phenomenon of placebo reaction may have particular relevance in this study in helping to explain variability of findings among the placebo condition subjects.

In comparing the placebo group subjects' ratings of "high" experienced during the driving sessions with their respective scores on the course, the following emerged: all 10 of those subjects who reported no or minimal effect improved significantly or showed no change in their performance, in terms of cutoff points established. Of the 11 subjects whose subjective ratings were in the moderate range, 8 improved significantly or showed no change while 3 declined significantly. One might accordingly infer that these 3 subjects were placebo reactors and that these subjects more or less accounted for the variability within the placebo group. Whereas subjective ratings did bear a relationship to course scores for the placebo group, no such relationship is evident for either the low- or high-dose drug groups; the two drug conditions cutoff scores were proportionately distributed between categories of subjective rating of "high."

What is the relationship between assessment of performance after the fact and actual performance? Of those 34 subjects who reported their performance had improved in the experimental block compared with the practice blocks, only the subjects of the placebo group were realistic in their appraisal (100% level of accuracy), whereas 56% and 58% of the respective low- and high-dose groups were accurate in their post hoc appraisals. The trend in accuracy of prediction was, however, different for the 30 subjects who reported their performance had worsened. In this instance, the highest accuracy of assessment was registered for the high-dose group (70%), with significantly lesser levels for the placebo group (37%) and for the low-dose group (25%). It may be more than coincidental that the 3 subjects in the placebo group who accurately assessed their performance as having declined were the identified placebo reactors, and we might surmise that they were engaging in a self-fulfilling prophesy. The high-dose group accuracy of assessment might, on the other hand, be explained in terms of threshold of drug effect.

2. COURSE AND STREET SCORES AS RELATED TO SEX AND PRIOR DRIVING EXPERIENCE

A number of variables which may produce differential effects on driving were also included in the data analysis. For the course, difference scores for trials 2–4 between blocks III and IV were again used as the basis for comparison. The first variable considered was sex and there were no significant differences for the experimental conditions: placebo, $t = 0.50$; low dose, $t = 1.17$; and high dose, $t = 1.68$. The second variable analyzed was driving experience, and this was defined in terms of: at least 5 years of driving and on a more or less daily basis; less than 5 years of driving. There were no significant differences for any of the experimental conditions: placebo, $t = 1.77$; low dose, $t = 0.61$; and high dose, $t = 1.35$. The third variable examined was previous driving while under the influence of marijuana and this was defined in terms of: never or infrequent and frequent (more than 50 times). The findings were as follows for the experimental conditions: placebo, $t = 0.36$; low dose, $t = -0.53$; and high dose, $t = -0.42$.

These same variables were analyzed with respect to scores obtained by those subjects who drove on the street. Regarding sex, here again there were no significant differences for the low-dose group ($t = 0.67$) or the high-dose group ($t = 1.37$). Regarding driving experience, no significant differences were obtained for the low-dose group ($t = 0.04$) or the high-dose group ($t = 1.90$). Regarding previous driving while under the influence of marijuana, here as well no significant differences emerged for the low-dose group ($t = 0.03$) or for the high-dose group ($t = 0.65$).

3. DESCRIPTION OF UNUSUAL BEHAVIOR ON THE COURSE AND EMERGENT EVENTS ON THE ROAD

Observations by the driving observer who was in the car while the course was being driven by subjects may illustrate some of the more unusual examples of behavior noted during the drug condition. Transient episodes of preoccupation and possibly confusion were noted regarding the order of tasks to be followed as well as with respect to the internal and external course markers. Behavior that was more characteristic of confusion involved loss of set where a subject had to be redirected after continuing off the course. Another example was a momentary forgetting to change into the appropriate gear during the back-up task, i.e., from forward drive to reverse or vice versa. Another facet noted frequently was that of fatigue, where subjects complained of the effort required to maneuver the car on the slalom and during the back-up.

Unusual examples of driving behavior on the street portion of the project included the following: missing traffic lights or stop signs, placebo condition (2 subjects), drug condition (3 subjects); engaging in passing maneuvers without sufficient caution, placebo condition (4 subjects), drug condition (6 subjects); poor anticipation or poor handling of vehicle with respect to traffic flow, placebo condition (2 subjects), drug condition (6 subjects); not aware or inappropriately aware of pedestrians or stationary vehicles, drug condition (3 subjects); and preoccupied at traffic signal and did not respond to green light, drug condition (1 subject). The driver observer intervened rarely while the vehicle was being driven on city streets, in fact on only three occasions, once during the placebo condition and twice during the drug condition.

D. Course and Street—Physiological Measures

1. ANALYSIS OF DATA

In the analysis of driving skills on the course and on the street, a dose-related model was necessitated because of significantly different patterns of response with the low- and high-dose groups. Because no such consistent dose-related trends were evident with the physiological measures used on both the course and the street, the analysis of physiological data dealt with combined low- and high-dose groups.

2. HEART RATE, GSR, AND RESPIRATION

Table VI summarizes the heart rate data relevant to driving the course. First and second order effects occurred, the tachycardia induced by driving being potentiated by the drug. Specifically, there was a significant increase in heart rate on the baseline trials compared with the laboratory baseline ($t = 7.26$, $p < 0.001$), the increase being on the average 21.8 beats per minute. There was a further significant increase in heart rate on the drug trials compared with the baseline trials; the increase was on the average an additional 23.2 beats per minute for the general score and comparable significant increases were present for all tasks including braking. During driving, the placebo condition, however, resulted in a slight rise in heart rate. Whereas significant differences in heart rate occurred with the drug compared with the placebo trials for the general score (on the average of 21.8 beats per minute) and in a comparable manner for all tasks including braking, there was no dose-related response regarding heart rate.

The findings for the two GSR parameters (i.e., fluctuations and amplitude) indicate high arousal during the baseline condition (Table VI). For the driving baseline, the mean value was 8.4 fluctuations per minute.

14. Effects of Marijuana on Driving

TABLE VI

Course: Means for Baseline, Placebo and Drug, as well as t Tests[a] between Placebo and Drug Conditions and between Low and High Drug for Heart Rate

Task	Heart rate						GSR fluctuations					GSR amplitude			
	Baseline mean $N = 42$	Placebo mean $N = 13$	t placebo vs. baseline	Drug mean $N = 29$	t drug vs. baseline	t low vs. high drug	Baseline mean $N = 34$	Placebo mean $N = 12$	Mean d scores	Drug mean $N = 22$	Mean d scores	Baseline mean $N = 34$	Placebo mean $N = 12$	Mean d scores	Drug mean $N = 22$	Mean d scores
Slalom	99.9	102.9	0.12	122.8	9.62[b]	−0.68	8.5	8.3	−0.9	8.0	−0.2	0.55	0.51	−0.03	0.54	−0.01
Tunnel I	97.3	99.8	0.22	122.5	9.93[b]	−0.77	8.3	8.0	−0.9	8.8	0.8	0.43	0.34	−0.09	0.40	−0.03
Tunnel II	95.2	96.3	0.80	119.2	8.77[b]	−0.65	7.2	6.1	−1.2	7.6	0.4	0.39	0.27	−0.11	0.35	−0.05
Funnel	95.9	97.1	0.23	120.1	9.18[b]	−0.92	7.6	6.3	−1.8	8.1	0.8	0.42	0.29	−0.12	0.40	−0.02
Back-up	100.9	101.0	1.63	122.5	9.57[b]	−0.86	8.2	7.0	−1.8	6.8	−1.0	0.47	0.42	−0.09	0.48	0.03
Corner	99.9	100.8	1.22	122.2	8.04[b]	−0.66	10.5	10.1	−1.5	10.4	0.5	0.53	0.50	−0.07	0.49	−0.02
Risk	97.0	97.9	0.29	119.2	8.94[b]	−0.97	8.3	6.6	−1.5	8.6	0.2	0.43	0.32	−0.08	0.41	−0.04
General	98.0	99.4	0.72	121.2	9.38[b]	−0.81	8.4	7.5	−1.4	8.3	0.2	0.46	0.38	−0.09	0.44	−0.02
Braking	99.9	105.3	0.03	121.9	8.38[b]	−1.04	8.0	9.0	−1.7	9.4	2.5	0.74	0.57	−0.18	0.69	0.05
Laboratory		76.2														

[a] d scores used in the computation.
[b] $p < 0.001$.

As acquisition of a random (or a laboratory) baseline was not obtained, no unequivocal quantitative comparison can be drawn between a resting and task condition. Whereas the fluctuation rate did seem consistently high for all conditions (8.4 for baseline, 7.5 for placebo, and 8.3 for drug), no significant differences were noted between placebo and baseline, drug and baseline, or dose. The placebo group, however, showed a definite trend toward habituation (an overall decrease of 1.4 fluctuations per minute, although no task reached significance), while the drug group remained virtually the same (an overall increase of 0.2 fluctuations per minute).

The amplitude means add further support to the fluctuation trends (Table VI). The mean average amplitude of response was 0.46 of the maximal response recorded for the baseline group, and this indicates a relatively high arousal. Second, in the placebo condition all tasks showed a decline in amplitude (with funnel and back-up being significantly different from baseline). The drug condition followed this trend also, but not to the extent of the placebo condition (an overall mean decline for the placebo condition of 0.09 and for the drug condition of 0.02). As with fluctuations there was no dose-related response.

As mentioned earlier, respiration was only considered as a general function and not task related. Hence only four measures were compared: laboratory baseline, general driving rate, placebo driving rate, and drug driving rate. Driving the course significantly increased ($t = 2.30$, $p < 0.02$) the mean value of respiration from 15.4 (laboratory baseline) to 18.4. During driving after smoking, both the placebo and drug conditions showed decline of rate but only the drug condition was significantly different (mean placebo $d = -1.0$, $t = -0.19$; mean drug $d = -2.17$, $t = -2.71$, $p < 0.02$). As both the placebo and the drug conditions' rates decreased from their respective baselines, the t value (using d scores) between the groups was not significant. There was also no dose-related response regarding respiration rate.

Table VII summarizes the heart rate data relevant to driving on the street. Driving with the placebo condition did not result in a significant rise in heart rate when compared with the laboratory baseline (on the average 4.6 beats per minute). The drug condition, however, resulted in tachycardia, the increase being on the average of 22.3 beats per minute compared with the laboratory baseline and 17.7 beats per minute compared with the placebo condition. As may be noted from Table VII, comparison of the two experimental conditions resulted in consistent significant differences for all types of traffic patterns and events. With the exclusion of parking (which can be explained on a work model), the range of scores is much more restricted for the placebo than the

TABLE VII

City Streets: Means for Experimental Conditions, t Tests[a] between Experimental Conditions and Low and High Drug for Heart Rate

Traffic patterns and events	Heart rate					GSR fluctuations				Respiration		
	n	Placebo mean	Drug mean	t drug vs. placebo	t low vs. high drug	n	Placebo mean	Drug mean		n	Placebo mean	Drug mean
Residential through streets	27	79.2	96.0	8.56[b]	−1.03	16	1.87	2.33		15	16.4	14.7
Residential side streets	16	80.8	93.9	6.02[b]	−2.54[c]	14	1.99	2.58		10	17.3	14.9
Local commercial area	26	80.5	98.9	8.39[b]	−2.14[c]	17	1.89	2.49		14	16.7	14.1
Downtown	26	81.3	99.5	8.91[b]	−1.27	15	1.90	2.00		14	15.6	14.6
Higher speed area	28	81.8	103.9	9.12[b]	0.20	17	2.57	3.18		15	16.9	16.7
General for types	—	80.3	98.8	10.16[b]	−1.11	—	2.04	2.54		—	16.6	15.1
Turns	27	84.4	101.5	8.54[b]	−1.90	17	1.73	2.00		15	20.2	18.8
Through major intersections	27	82.4	100.3	8.48[b]	−1.08	17	1.34	1.62		12	19.4	18.6
Parking	13	91.4	102.9	2.48[c]	−2.34[c]	—				—		
General for events	—	84.8	101.6	9.12[b]	−2.13[c]	—	1.52	1.86		—	19.9	18.9
General	—	82.3	100.0	9.92[b]	−1.60	—	1.84	2.30		—	17.9	16.5
Laboratory		77.7									15.9	

[a] d Scores used in the computation.
[b] $p < 0.001$.
[c] $p < 0.05$.

drug condition, suggesting that the rise due to drug is reinforced by arousal. Dose-related responses occurred with two types of traffic patterns, one event and the events' composite score.

Table VII also summarizes the GSR fluctuation data. There was a slightly higher but statistically nonsignificant level of arousal for all traffic patterns and events during the drug (general mean score was 2.30) compared with the placebo condition (general mean score was 1.84). A trend toward dose-related response was observed for the GSR as well as the heart rate. Specifically, fluctuation rates were significantly higher for the high- compared with the low-dose drug groups for two types of traffic patterns (residential side streets and downtown) and for the types' composite score.

From the physiological data one can identify those tasks that resulted in the highest levels of arousal, and there does seem to be a definite pattern here for the various experimental conditions across the three physiological measures. Specifically, ranking the tasks with the highest arousal by experimental condition reveals that slalom occurs in 8 of the 9 combinations as does cornering in 8 of 9 combinations. One of these tasks, slalom, also resulted in the highest mean score of cones hit on the course for the various experimental conditions.

Relationships between types of traffic patterns and events for the street data were also analyzed by rank-order correlations (Table VIII). Both

TABLE VIII

City Streets: Rank-Order Correlations of Types of Traffic Patterns and Events within Electrophysiological Measures and Types of Traffic Patterns between Electrophysiological Measures

Experimental condition	Placebo–drug	Placebo	Drug
Heart rate	0.79[a]	—	—
GSR fluctuations	0.86[b]	—	—
Respiration	0.86[b]	—	—
Heart rate–GSR fluctuations	—	0.90[a]	0.10
Heart rate–respiration	—	0.20	0.10
Respiration–GSR fluctuations	—	0.60	0.70

[a] $p < 0.05$.
[b] $p < 0.01$.

types and events were used to determine relationships between experimental conditions for heart rate, then GSR and finally respiration, and, as may be noted from Table VIII, all those correlations were significant.

In comparing physiological measures, only types of traffic patterns were used and, of the six comparisons, only the heart rate and GSR comparison for the placebo condition was significant.

A patterning regarding level of arousal is evident on the physiological data between experimental conditions and across physiological measures. In all six comparisons "higher speed areas" resulted in the highest level of arousal. The second highest level of arousal was shared between "residential side streets" and "downtown traffic."

3. GRAPHIC REPRESENTATION OF PHYSIOLOGICAL MEASURES

Figure 2 illustrates the graphic comparisons of physiological measures during driving on the course and the street. For heart rate and respiration, the observed changes are recorded through the laboratory baseline, course baseline, course with condition, and street with condition. For GSR fluctuations, the observed changes are recorded through course baseline, course with condition, and street with condition; and for GSR amplitude through course baseline and course with condition.

E. Postdriving Interview

This was carried out only with those subjects who received marijuana, but within the context of the double-blind design. The subject was asked about his general impressions of the driving experience and recorded his answer. The subject was then asked to record any outstanding feature of the driving experience. The spontaneous statements by 35 of the 38 subjects (no data were available for the remaining 3 subjects) were on the whole rather brief, on the average 2 minutes per subject with a range of 1 to 4 minutes of recording time. The 82 nonmutually exclusive subjective statements were categorized as follows: unpleasant, e.g., less attentive (16), perceptual changes (13), anxious (10), confused (9), strangeness (8), nausea (3); pleasant, e.g., relaxed (8), increased awareness (5), drive slower (5), more attentive (5). As may be noted from the nature and distribution of responses, negative or unpleasant (72%) rather than positive or pleasant (28%) responses characterized the driving experience with marijuana.

Last, the subject was asked "would you have driven on city streets being as stoned as you are if you had not been participating in the test situation." Responses of the 38 subjects were distributed as follows: yes, 16 subjects or 42%; yes, but with reservations, 14 subjects or 37%; and no, 8 subjects or 21%.

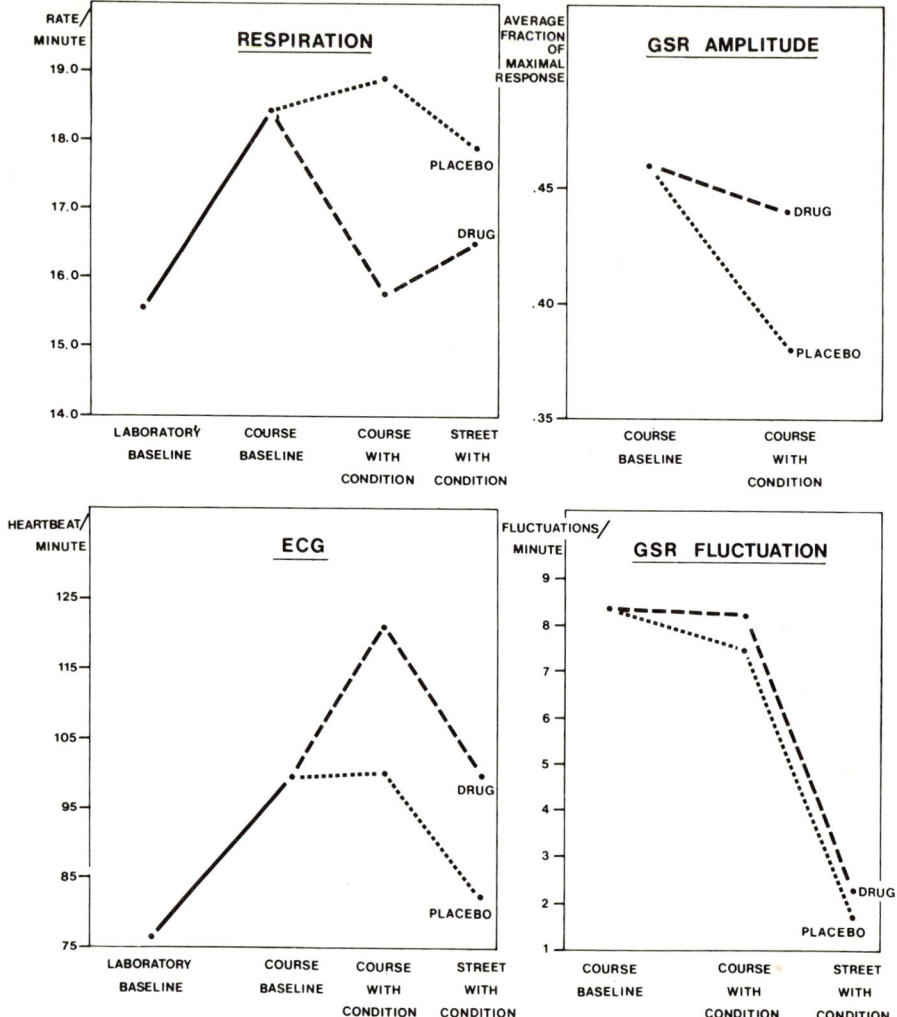

Fig. 2. Graph of observed ECG, respiration, GSR fluctuation, and GSR amplitude through laboratory baseline, course baseline, course with experimental condition, and street with experimental condition.

F. Driving Questionnaire

The first part of the questionnaire dealt with items regarding past driving history and attitudes regarding driving. Of the 64 subjects, five reported that their driver's licence had in the past been suspended (one because of impaired driving, one because of reckless driving, and three

14. Effects of Marijuana on Driving

for other reasons). Thirteen of the subjects had been involved in an accident that had resulted in a claim during the past two years, and two subjects were involved in more than one such claim. Rating of their own driving ability was distributed as follows: excellent, 19% (ratio of males to females 5:2); good, 72% (ratio of males to females 1:1); and fair, 9% (ratio of males to females 1:4). Responses to the question "do you think men are better drivers than women?" were distributed as follows: very strongly or strongly agree, 14% (ratio of males to females 4:1); agree, 44% (ratio of males to females 1:1); strongly or very strongly disagree, 34% (ratio of males to females 1:2); and refused to answer, 8% (ratio of males to females 2:1).

The second portion of the questionnaire sought information regarding an already established pattern of driving in the context of marijuana use; specifically, driving after having used marijuana and, second, smoking marijuana while driving. Driving after having smoked marijuana was reported by 80% of the sample (ratio of males to females 3:2) and driving while smoking marijuana by 55% of the sample (ratio of males to females 2:1). Regarding duration of this behavior, 38% of the group reported that they had been driving after using marijuana over a period of three years, and an additional 28% reported such behavior over a period of a year. Forty-two percent had driven while smoking marijuana during the past three years. The frequency during the past year of driving after smoking marijuana occurred on the average of once a month and the frequency of occurrence was less for driving while smoking marijuana. Driving after or while smoking marijuana was reported during daylight as well as at night.

The third portion of the questionnaire dealt with the amount of marijuana used in connection with driving and reported effects. The modal amount of marijuana smoked before driving was reported as more than one joint and somewhat lesser amounts were reported while driving. The 124 nonmutually exclusive subjective statements regarding effects after smoking (by 47 of the 51 subjects) or while smoking (by 32 of the 35 subjects) and driving were categorized as follows: unpleasant, e.g., anxious (23), less attentive (21), slower reflexes (10), poor judgment (8), bothered by light (6), lack of control (4); pleasant, e.g., drive slower (27), relaxed (13), enjoy driving more (9), drive more skillfully (3). The trend regarding the ratio of unpleasant (60%) to pleasant (40%) effects is accordingly consistent between the questionnaire data obtained before the driving experience and the postdriving interview (after a clinical trial). There was, however, a consensus regarding the global effects of marijuana on driving, namely, 61% of the group reported that marijuana slightly detracts from or impairs driving.

The last portion of the questionnaire dealt with restrictions regarding marijuana while driving as well as other drugs that are used before or while driving. Responses to the question "if marijuana is legalized should there be precautions regarding marijuana and driving?" were as follows: none, 12%; as with alcohol, 60%; other, 16%; and undecided, 12%. The use of other drugs in combination with marijuana before driving was reported by 28% of the sample, during driving by 13% of the sample. The use of alcohol in combination with marijuana before driving was reported by 64% of the sample, during driving by 20% of the sample.

IV. DISCUSSION

Driving ability as measured on the course was a composite of skill, judgment, and shifting set. The subjects, many of whom were students, presented as highly motivated and as high achievers and responded in a competitive manner to the challenge of driving in an experimental context. Whereas boredom and fatigue were also factors to contend with, these seemed to be of secondary import. The possibility was considered that unconscious if not conscious bias to demonstrate that marijuana did not affect driving would have led many of the volunteers to accumulate more cone hits during the experimental block. To offset this possible bias, none of the volunteers nor the research staff were aware which of the practice sets was designated as the baseline. Furthermore, this possible bias may not be as important as it seems at first glance in that 61% of the group reported on the questionnaire that marijuana slightly detracts from or impairs driving. Other corroborative evidence regarding ego involvement may be found in the comparison of subjective "high" and performance on the course. Specifically, 10 of the 21 subjects who correctly identified the placebo nonetheless remained involved and improved their performance significantly; of the remainder only 3 subjects showed a decline in performance and these were the 3 identified placebo reactors.

The nature of the driving tasks on the course was such that learning occurred with repeated trials, i.e., total scores improved of the order of 15% between successive practice blocks I to II to III (with the slope of the linear regression being significant). A comparable rate of improvement (17%) was predicted (from the linear regression) for the experimental block (IV). The advent of the drug, however, impeded learning: scores worsened to the extent of 29% from predicted for the low-dose group and 54% for the high-dose group. These rates of decline are reflected in the regression analysis where two of the tasks and total score of the low-dose group and five of the tasks and total score of the high-dose group were beyond the upper limits of the confidence interval. There was a substantially lesser rate of decline (8%) for the placebo group, and this decline could be explained by the performance of the 3 identified placebo reactors.

A learning model can also be used to explain the differential rate of change between the baseline block (III) and the experimental block (IV) for the three experimental conditions. The placebo group continued to improve significantly (mean improvement of score was 5.5), the low-dose group was somewhat impaired in learning (mean decline of score was 1.0), while the high-dose group was significantly impaired in learning (mean decline of score was 8.2). Also, both low- and high-dose groups showed significant mean declines in learning of 6.5 and 13.7 compared to the placebo group. Furthermore, there was a dose-related response, in terms of comparisons within and between experimental conditions. One would accordingly infer that marijuana interferes with driving skills, and that the effect on driving is dose related.

It would be misleading, however, to infer that marijuana had an invariate effect on the driving skills of this group of 64 volunteers, and this is borne out in further analysis of scores in terms of absolute change as well as change from a cutoff point. The use of a cutoff point leads to a more precise, albeit conservative inference, namely, 33% and 55% of the respective low- and high-dose groups showed significant decline in performance, 43% and 31% of the respective groups did not change significantly, and 24% and 14% improved to a significant extent. How does one explain these findings? First, there are individual differences regarding drug effect, notwithstanding dosage level. Second, change in sensorium is most apt to result in efforts at compensation, particularly in driving which does require a higher degree of alertness. But as with drug effect, there are individual differences in ability to compensate, as exemplified by those volunteers whose scores did not change significantly, or in fact to overcompensate, as reflected by those subjects who showed improvement in scores.

That differential effects on driving performance can be expected with a disinhibiting agent such as alcohol receives credence from the study by Coldwell *et al.* (1958) who found that only 56% (28 of 50) of their group were significantly impaired in driving performance in a restricted traffic-free area, after ingesting a defined dose of alcohol, venous blood concentration of 0.78 per mil (0.078%).

Driving ability as measured on the street was a composite of 11 behavioral components (general driving habits, cooperation, attitude, irritability, judgment, speed, care, confidence, tension, aggression, and concentration) in a context of varying traffic patterns (residential through streets, residential side streets, local commercial area, downtown, and higher speed area) and traffic events (turns, through major intersections, and parking).

In comparing course skills in a restricted, traffic-free area with driving and road performance on city streets, including downtown area, during peak hours of traffic flow, it should be borne in mind that the driving skills measured in these two experimental situations do not on the surface appear to be similar, and the scoring systems are certainly conceptually different. Nonetheless, there is a striking relationship between the percentages of decline, no change and improvement for the respective course and street groups. Again using a cutoff point, the significant rate of decline on the street was higher for both low (42%) and high (63%) dose groups when compared with the course (33% and 55% for respective dose groups) and the differences in percentages between the street and course portions of the study were constant regardless of dose; the rate of significant improvement on the street was also higher for both low (32%) and high (16%) dose groups when compared with the course (24% and 14% for respective dose groups); while the rate of no change was more or less equivalent on the street for both dose groups (26% for low and 21% for high) and below that noted for the course (43% and 31% for respective dose groups). On the street, as well as on the course, individualized responses to drug effect and varying degrees of compensation would account for the pattern of change in driving performance within dosage levels, with the more striking changes in impairment occurring with the high dose.

Those behavioral components most adversely affected by the drug while driving on the street were judgment and concentration, whereas those components that were affected to a lesser degree included general driving skills, irritability, speed, confidence, tension, and aggression. Furthermore, there was a significantly higher incidence of emergent events, but not degree of hazard for the drug compared with the placebo trials.

Factors that have been identified by other investigators as possible influences on driving performance, specifically sex, driving experience, and previous driving while under the influence of marijuana, did not turn out to be significant in either the course or street portions of the present study. Whereas unusual behavior on the course (including transient episodes of preoccupation and possible confusion) as well as on the street (including lack of awareness of pedestrians or stationary vehicles) were noted during the drug condition, intervention by the driver examiner occurred very rarely.

A second inference is accordingly warranted, namely, that marijuana interferes with driving performance in a real-life driving situation as well as in a restricted context. Furthermore, the high degree of consistency between independent measures of driving skills on the street as well as on the course lends credence to the findings regarding drug effects and dose-related effects.

That autonomic arousal is associated with emotion and stress is well accepted (Lacey and Lacey, 1970). Of vital functions affected during stress, the most dramatic and readily measurable changes occur in heart rate. The causal relationship between stress and tachycardia has been well documented, for example, with naval pilots during take-off and landing (Roman et al., 1967), during periods of stress in the daily lives of physicians (Ira et al., 1963), in ski jumpers (Imhog, 1969), and in fact as part of the orienting response to any new stimulus (Germana and Klein, 1968). More relevant to this study are the changes in heart rate during automobile driving (Taggart and Gibbons, 1967; Simonson et al., 1968).

The significant and consistent changes in heart rate recorded in this study could most readily be related to an interaction model of stress-habituation and drugs. The first order effect, namely driving, resulted in differential changes in heart rate on the course compared with the street. Specifically, heart rate increased by 29% (beats per minute) during baseline (practice driving) trials on the course compared with the laboratory measure. A directly comparable measure of heart rate was not available for driving on the street because of the nature of the experimental design. But an indirect measure was available, namely, difference in rate between the laboratory and the placebo condition, and this resulted in a 30% increment in heart rate on the course (to 99.4 bpm) compared with a 6% rise in rate on the street (to 82.3 bpm).

If one begins with the premise that driving on the street as well as the course is stressful and results in autonomic activation, and predriving baseline differences can be ruled out (laboratory baselines for the course and street groups were on the average 76.2 and 77.7 bpm), then the significant increase in heart rate noted on the course (30%) compared with the negligible increase on the street could be explained in terms of monitoring procedure and habituation. The physiological monitoring on the course was on a sampling basis, and in fact designed to document the stress induced by the course tasks which followed in very quick succession. The monitoring on the street was continuous and resulted in the confounding of increases in heart rate with return to normal rate that characterizes the more nonstressful periods of driving. Sampling of the driving experience studied, as well as their driving site (Trafalgar Square in London, England), might account for Taggart and Gibbons' (1967) findings of significant rise in heart rate. The same explanation may apply to Simonson *et al.* (1968) who noted distinct increases in heart rate with critical driving situations.

The second order effect, namely, the drug, potentiated the stress of driving, and the resultant tachycardia was more or less identical for those subjects who drove on the street compared with the course (of the order of 22%). The findings regarding tachycardia on the heels of marijuana are quite consistent with previous electrophysiological investigations in our laboratory which used an identical dose level of marijuana (Chapter 6). In contrast, the effect of placebo on heart rate was negligible, and this has also been demonstrated in our laboratory. The design of this study also permitted a measure of internal validation, namely, by comparing the heart rates for the discrete tasks on the course and then the types of traffic patterns and events on the street. Such an analysis revealed that heart rate measures were amazingly consistent between the tasks on the course and at a reduced rate between types of traffic and events on city streets. A dose-related response occurred only on the street and for two of the five types of traffic, one of the three types of events, and for events' composite score.

The second autonomic index of activation or arousal, GSR, is a less stable measure than heart rate because of the methodological problems associated with its determination (Edelberg, 1972), but is nonetheless widely used as a measure of stress. A number of driving studies have in fact used GSR as a measure of arousal or stress (Hulbert, 1957; Michaels, 1960; Taylor, 1964). The findings in this study with respect to GSR are less striking than the heart rate measure, but the stress-habituation-drug model still obtains. In comparing GSR fluctuation rates between the course and the street, the differences are equally striking and of the same order of magnitude for the placebo as drug conditions; ratio of fluctuations was 4:1 for the course compared with the street regardless of placebo or drug conditions. On the course, only the placebo group showed a trend toward habituation. On the street, there was a dose-related response.

Now to place the findings of this study into the context of other investigations that have dealt with GSR and driving. Michaels (1960) used a design in his driving study that is comparable to the present one—continuous monitoring of GSR, urban traffic including downtown area, relating measures to traffic events—and reported 1.71 to 2.42 GSR events per minute, with an average magnitude of 2.23 and 2.28. Inasmuch as one can compare GSR data between studies, there is a striking similarity between Michaels' findings and the GSR fluctuation rate noted in this study for the placebo (1.84) and drug (2.30) conditions. The markedly

14. Effects of Marijuana on Driving

higher GSR fluctuation rates on the course—practice (8.4), placebo (7.5), and drug (8.3)—indicate a much higher level of arousal compared with driving on the city streets, which is consistent with the experimental design. As will be recalled, the course was task-oriented and the appearance of the stimuli (cones) were predictable and constant, with sampled monitoring of discrete events in quick succession. On the city streets, stimuli were nonpredictable and variable, from an uneventful drive to one fraught with emergent situations, with the monitoring having been continuous.

An explanation for the differences in the GSR fluctuation data between the course and street might well be that on the course the subject was in a constant state of arousal and rearousal, more particularly the high-dose group who were hitting significantly more cones. On the street, on the other hand, subjects adopted their usual driving pattern and arousal occurred in relationship to encountered events. In terms of a realistic model of driving, the street portion of the study is probably a better indication of usual (normative) levels of arousal. The course, on the other hand, is more challenging, possibly in an artificial sense, and accordingly more anxiety inducing.

Taylor (1964) also measured GSR in subjects who drove their vehicles over a wide range of roads and during varying road conditions. His measure of GSR rates (combined frequency and response amplitude) is not comparable to Michaels' study or to the present one. Incidentally, Taylor related the pronounced variability between subjects, which is certainly not unusual in GSR data, to variables such as experience as a driver and the driver's age. One of his findings was that the variety of road and traffic conditions did not substantially affect GSR rate. The reliability of this finding would have to be questioned in light of the present study where "higher speed areas" resulted in substantially greater levels of GSR arousal compared with other traffic patterns or events.

Respiration as an index of stress has received much less attention in the literature than heart rate or GSR. In comparing the respiration data on the course with that obtained while driving on the street, and then relating the findings to similar comparisons for the heart rate data, the following emerged: For the laboratory-placebo conditions, respiration increased on both the course and the street, more so on the course, and these trends are consistent with the heart rate trends; for the laboratory-drug conditions, respiration increased slightly for both the course and the street, but more so on the street, and these trends are not consistent with the heart rate trends. The latter is the result of the fall in respiration rate during the drug compared with placebo conditions on both the course and the street. Whereas this finding is not consistent with previous investigations in our laboratory where the subjects were in a resting state, it does appear compatible with a study published by Domino (1972) in which he reports "a slight tendency for a minor decrease in respiration rate in certain subjects after smoking marijuana."

Within the context of homeostasis, one would theoretically expect an integration of physiological systems and a degree of concordance within and between indices of arousal. The findings in this study, in some measure at least, support this theoretical position. For the various tasks on the course, there was a high degree of internal consistency in arousal for heart rate and GSR across experimental conditions. Furthermore, the concordance remained high between heart rate and GSR during the baseline and placebo condition. That the drug resulted in differential effects in subjects is not surprising in view of performance scores on the course. On the street, the same pattern of high concordance was reflected for physiological measures across experimental conditions, but the relationships between physiological measures all but disappeared.

What is the relationship between retrospective reporting of the effects of marijuana on driving as derived from the questionnaire and subjective reporting directly after having smoked marijuana and driven on city streets, and, in turn, how do these relate to the objective findings regarding driving performance while under the influence of marijuana? Regarding the reported effects of marijuana on driving, the group under investigation evidenced a high degree of concordance between their retrospective and prospective reporting of effects, in terms of incidence of unpleasant effects and preponderance of unpleasant compared with pleasant effects. Regarding the relationship between effects and performance, here again there was a very high degree of concordance, specifically, 61% of the group reported on the questionnaire that marijuana slightly detracts from or impairs driving, and 42% and 63% of the respective low- and high-dose groups showed a significant decline in their driving performance on city streets.

V. CONCLUSION

Using group data leads to the conclusion that marijuana does have a detrimental effect on driving skills and performance in a restricted driving area, and even more so under normal conditions of driving on city streets. A closer scrutiny of individual differences in driving performance leads to a qualification of the conclusion, specifically, the effect of marijuana on driving is not uniform for all subjects but is in fact bidirectional; whether or not significant decline occurs in driving ability is dependent

14. Effects of Marijuana on Driving

on the subject's capacity to compensate and the dose of marijuana. For those subjects who improved their performance, the explanation may lie in overcompensation and possibly the sedative effect of the drug.

Whereas the street portion of this study approximated normal driving conditions, it should be stressed that the context of the driving experience even on city streets was experimental. The design of this study provided maximal safeguard in terms of a dual-control vehicle, a driver observer, and, in addition, the subjects were professionally screened and with rare exception emotionally stable. Given the experimental setting and set, safeguards, and the nature of the study sample, idiosyncratic behavior that might occur under normal driving conditions would be less likely to occur in a study such as the present one.

Other identified factors might lead to more stringent conclusions regarding the effects of marijuana on driving. The first is night driving, which may be more stressful. But an even more important unanswered question is the cumulative effect of alcohol and marijuana on driving (64% of the study sample reported using alcohol in combination with marijuana before driving). Third, the doses of marijuana used in this study were within the range of social marijuana usage (Le Dain, 1972); more heroic doses might be taken before driving. Fourth, the effect of marijuana on reactions and decisions during high speed is still another unknown.

What are the recommendations that emerge from this study? Driving under the influence of marijuana as well as alcohol should be avoided. More investigation is urgently required, with high priority given to studies that approximate normal conditions of driving and in which alcohol and marijuana are administered to the same subjects.

What are the implications of these findings in social and legislative planning? Here again, the attitudes and responses of the marijuana users included in this study may well be worthy of emphasis, specifically, only 12% of the group indicated that no precautions would be warranted regarding marijuana and driving if marijuana were legalized.

ACKNOWLEDGMENTS

Much of the credit for the initiation and the continuity of this study belongs to two individuals: the first, Ray Hadfield, Superintendent of Motor Vehicles, Department of Transport and Communications, British Columbia, who was instrumental in solving the myriad of administrative and legal details in order to get this study under way; the second, Campbell Clark, B.Sc., Research Technician who assisted in the integration of all facets of this study.

This research was supported by a grant from the British Columbia Alcohol and Drug Fund. The author wishes to express his appreciation to: Dr. A. M. Marcus, Associate Professor, Department of Psychiatry, University of British Columbia; Dr. H. Sanders, Associate Professor, Department of Pharmacology, University of British Columbia; Dr. M. Low, Associate Professor (Neurology), Department of Medicine, University of British Columbia, and Head, EEG Department, Vancouver General Hospital; Dr. P. Graystone, Assistant Professor, Department of Physiology, University of British Columbia; L. Gold and E. Roadburg, law students; A. Crancer, Office of Counter-alcoholic Measures, Washington, D.C.; and Dr. R. Miller, Le Dain Commission, Ottawa.

A special debt of gratitude is acknowledged to: The Hon. Alex Macdonald, Attorney-General of British Columbia; Alan Eyre, President, Dueck Motors; the residents of the Department of Psychiatry, Health Sciences Centre Hospital; the University of British Columbia and, in particular, the Department of Psychiatry, Health Sciences Centre Hospital.

REFERENCES

Bech, P., Rafaelsen, L., and Rafaelsen, O. J. (1973). *Psychopharmacologia* **32**, 373–381.
Binder, A. (1971). *Accid. Anal. & Prev.* **3**, 237–256.
Coldwell, B. B., Penner, D. W., Smith, H. W., Lucas, G. H. W., Rodgers, R. F., and Darroch, F. (1958). *Quart. J. Stud. Alc.* **19**, 590–616.
Crancer, A., Dille, J., Delay, J., and Haykin, M. (1969). *Science* **164**, 851–854.
Domino, E. F. (1972). *Psychopharmacol. Bull.* **8**, 17.
Dott, A. B. (1972). "Effect of Marijuana on Risk Acceptance in a Simulated Passing Task." DHEW Publ. No. (HSM) 72-10010. U.S. Dept. of Health, Education and Welfare, Washington, D.C.
Edelberg, R. (1972). In "Handbook of Psychophysiology" (N. S. Greenfield and R. A. Sternbach, eds.), pp. 367–418. Holt, New York.
Ellingstad, V. S., McFarling, L. H., and Struckman, D. L. (1973). "Alcohol, Marijuana and Risk Taking." Contract No. DOT-HS-191-2-301. Univ. of South Dakota, Vermillion.
Gale, E. N., and Guenther, G. (1971). *Brit. J. Addict.* **66**, 189–194.
Germana, J., and Klein, S. B. (1968). *Psychophysiology* **4**, 324–328.
Gostomzyk, J. G., Parade, P., and Gewecke, H. (1973). *Z. Rechtsmed.* **73**, 131–136.
Hulbert, S. F. (1957). *Percept. Mot. Skills* **7**, 305–315.
Imhog, P. R. (1969). *J. Appl. Physiol.* **27**, 366–369.
Ira, G. H., Whalen, R. E., and Boddonoff, M. D. (1963). *J. Psychosom. Res.* **7**, 147–150.
Kielholz, P., Goldberg, L., Hobi, V., Ladewig, D., Reggianni, G., and Richter, R. (1972). *Deut. Med. Wochenschr.* **20**, 789–794.
Klonoff, H. (1973). *Can. Med. Ass. J.* **108**, 145–150.
Lacey, J. I., and Lacey, B. C. (1970). In "Physiological Correlates of Emotion" (P. Black, ed.), p. 205. Academic Press, New York.
Le Dain Commission. (1972). "A Report of The Commission of Inquiry into the Non-Medical Use of Drugs." Information Canada, Ottawa.

Low, M., Klonoff, H., and Marcus, A. (1973). *Can. Med. Ass. J.* **108,** 157–165.
Michaels, R. M. (1960). *U.S. Pub. Roads* **31,** 53–71.
Moskowitz, H., McGlothlin, W., and Hulbert, S. (1973). "The Effects of Marjuana Dosage on Driver Performance." Contract No. DOT-HS-150-2-236. University of California, Los Angeles.
Nichols, J. L. (1971). "Drug Use and Highway Safety: A Review of the Literature." Report DOT-HS-012-1-019 (prepared for U.S. Department of Transportation).
Rafaelsen, O. J., Bech, P., Christiansen, J., Christrup, H., Nyboe, J., and Rafaelsen, L. (1973). *Science* **179,** 920–923.
Roman, J., Older, H., and Jones, W. (1967). *Aerosp. Med.* **38,** 133–139.
Simonson, E., Baker, C. A., Burns, N. M., Keiper, C., Schmitt, O. H., and Stackhouse, S. (1968). *Amer. Heart J.* **75,** 125–135.
Taggart, P., and Gibbons, D. (1967). *Brit. Med. J.* **1,** 411–412.
Tashkin, D. P., Shapiro, B. J., and Frank, I. M. (1973). *N. Engl. J. Med.* **289,** 336–341.
Taylor, D. H. (1964). *Ergonomics* **7,** 439–451.
Wilde, G. J. S., and Curry, G. A. (1970). "Psychological Aspects of Road Research: A Study of the Literature, 1959–1968." Queen's University, Kingston, Ontario.

SUBJECT INDEX

A

Achievement motivation, 95, 223, 243-250,
  see also Amotivational syndrome
Adrenocorticotropic hormone (ACTH),
  cannabinoid effects on activity of,
  177-180
Adverse reactions from marijuana, 32-33,
  see also Marijuana, adverse reactions,
  specific disorders
Affective disorder, 271
"Agnosia of succession," 161
Aggression
  comparison of marijuana with other drugs,
    352
  methodological problems in evaluating
    marijuana effects
    cumulative drug effects, 341-342
    drug-drug interaction, 341
    dose response characteristics, 340-341
    drug properties, 340
    environmental influences, 342
    individual variation, 342-343
    process factors, 343-344
    psychological influences, 342
    time action characteristics, 341
  methods of study
    field survey, 344-345, 347-354
    laboratory studies, 344-347
Alcohol
  aggression, 349-350, 352
  automobile driving, 360
  drl schedules, comparison with THC, 204,
    243-244
  goal directed serial alternation, effects on,
    31
  Korsakoff syndrome, development of, 160
  interaction with marijuana and THC, 54-69
    addiction research inventory, 64

conjunctival injection, 60
Cornell medical index, 64
delayed auditory feedback, 60-61
psychological effects, 68
physiological effects, 59-60
pursuit meter performance, 56-57
time production, comparison with THC,
  31
Amotivational syndrome, 34-35, 115-116,
  223, 226, 287-289
Anagrams test, 111
Anterograde amnesia, 161
Anticholinergic drugs, see Cholinergic
  functioning; Cannabinoids, comparison
  with anticholinergics and hippocampectomy
Anticholinergic-like effects, of marijuana,
  128-129, 150
Anticholinesterase, see Cholinergic functioning
Appraisal function, of central nervous
  system, 150
Army alpha test, 106
Ataxia, produced by marijuana, 59, 62
Atkinson-Shiffrin model of memory, 82,
  192, 193
Attention
  assessment of
    anagrams test, 111
    contingent negative variation (CNV),
      127, 129, 213
    field dependence, 104
    field independence, 104
    latent learning, 167, 213
    vigilance, 167, 213
  components of
    degree of selectivity, 104
    resistance to distraction, 104
    shifting, 104

399

and concentration, 167
effect of marijuana on
  attention focus, 109, 213-214
  CNV, 213-214
  degree of selectivity, 105
  hippocampal lesions and, 167
  latent learning, 214
  memory and, 89, 91, 213
  resistance to distraction, 105-111
  set shifting, 111-112, 214
  vigilance, 112, 213
  model of, 104
Atropine, see Cholinergic functioning; Cannabinoids, comparison with anticholinergics and hippocampectomy
Autokinetic effect, effects of marijuana on, 112

B

"Becoming a Marijuana user," 234
Bender Gestalt test, 107
Benton sentence repetition test, 131
Blood pressure, 256, 257
Brain syndrome
  acute, 281-285
  organic, 272
Brown-Petersen paradigm, 88-90, 167
Buss-Durkee self report, 346

C

Cancellation test, 107
Cannabinoids, see also Marijuana, Tetrahydrocannabinol
  comparison with ACTH and hippocampectomy, neuroendocrine effects
    behavioral, 178-179
    pharmacological, 179-180
  comparison with anticholinergics and hippocampectomy, animal and human behavior
    attention, 167
    active avoidance, 168
    conditioned fear, 167
    drl schedules, 170, see also Time perception
    extinction, 169
    habituation, 170-171
    maze behavior, 165

memory, 166
passive avoidance, 170, 176, 199-200
sequential behavior, 166
state dependent learning, 169-170, 206-212, see also State dependent learning
pharmacological effects
  antiepileptic actions, 171-172
  EEG, 171
  hippocampal theta rhythm, 171-172, 175
  hippocampal afterdischarge, 172
  hypothermia, 176
  limbic system, 171
Carbachol, 174-175
Cerebral atrophy, 34, 35
Cerebral dysfunction, 141
Cholinergic functioning, see also Cannabinoids, comparison with anticholinergics and hippocampectomy
  anticholinergic drugs and, 164
  anticholinesterase and, 164
  acetylcholine
    metabolism, 174
    release, 173
    uptake, 175
  cholinergic blockade, 173
  drinking center, hypothalmus, 174
  muscarinic receptors, 173
  gating, 164
  hippocampus, 164
  memory formation, 164
Cigarette smoking and marijuana use, 311
Closure speed test, 105
Cloze analysis, 109
Cognition, general, effects of marijuana on, 122-124, 158-160
Compensatory behavior and tolerance, 323
Concept formation, effects of marijuana on, 91, 146, 150
Conditioned fear, 167
Confabulation, 110, see also Memory
Conjunctival injection, 54, 256, 257
Consciousness, 75
Contingent negative variation (CNV), 31, 127, 133, 143, 144, 148, 149, see also Attention, assessment
Continuous performance test, 107, 237
Counterbalanced design, 11
Crime, see Aggression

Subject Index

D

Delayed auditory feedback, effects of marijuana on, 51-52, 59, 66
Depersonalization inventory, 29
Derealization, 29, 39
Dextroamphetamine, 31
Digit symbol substitution, 28, 106, 107
Dishabituation, 170-171
Dissociation, 92, *see also* State dependent learning
Double blind procedure, 28, 47
Drew, W. G., 114
Driving performance
  behavioral components of, 376-377, 389-390
  effect of marijuana
    comparison with alcohol, 359-360
    course driving, 372-373
    dose response relationship, 389
    driving experience under, 379
    driving questionaire, 386-387
    history of, 359-362
    methodological problems in evaluation, 21-22
    physiological changes, 380-386
    post-driving interview, 385
    predisposing factors, 2, 3
    sex differences, 379
    street driving, 70, 374-377
    subjective evaluation of, 377-378
    unusual behavior and, 379-380
  physiological changes correlated with, 361, 391-394
Drug(s), *see* specific substances
  nonspecific actions of, 94, 95
Drug-taking disposition, 311

E

EEG abnormality, 127, 128
  pharmacological effect, 125, 126, 141, 143, 148, 222
Escalation
  to dangerous drugs and marijuana use, 41, 257, 304-335
  extrinsic factors related to, 327-332
  intrinsic factors related to, 320-325
    biochemical, 322-325
    pharmacological, 320

pseudopharmacological, 320-321
  longitudinal data, 319
  problems of evaluation
    logical issues
      causal mechanisms, 320-327
      descriptive studies, 305-313
    methodological issues
      causal mechanisms, 327-335
      descriptive studies, 313-319
  theories of
    disturbed personality, 325
    Nahas theory of, 323-325
    sophisticated stepping stone, 325-326
    subcultural, 327-332
    tolerance-disillusionment model, 324
"Escape from violence," 354
Euphoria, from marijuana, 33, 37, 58
Evoked potential, 126, 127, 143, 148

F

Fixed rehearsal procedure, 86
Free recall task, *see also* Memory
  advantages for drug research, 83
  theoretical analysis of, 81
Flashback, 29, 36, 152
Functional relationship, 190

G

Gas chromatography, 47-48
Gating function, *see also* Hippocampus, inhibition
  nonspecific, 163-164
  specific, 164
Glare recovery time and marijuana, 112
Goal directed serial alternation (GDSA), 29, 91, 106, 159
Grip strength, 46
GSR, 143, 148, 362
Guilford number facility test, 114

H

Habituation, effects of marijuana on, 214-215
Hallucinations, 39
  dose response relationship, 26, 27
Hallucinogens, and marijuana use, 317
Halstead category test, 131

Halstead-Reitan battery, effects of marijuana on, 107, 136-141
Halstead tactual performance test, 131
Hand steadiness, 46
Heart rate
  dose response relationships, 25, 26, 126
  pharmacological effects, 63, 126, 128, 143, 148, 222
Hemicholinium, comparison with cannabinoids, 173, 175
"Hemp drug insanity," 286
Hippocampus, *see also* Cannabinoids, comparison with anticholinergics and hippocampectomy
  cholinergic system and memory, 164
  inhibition, 163-165
  memory, 160-166
    alternative explanation, 163
    cholinergic synapse, 164
    interference, 162
    intrusion errors, 159, 161
    Korsakoff-like deficit, 161-162
    narrative material, 161
    psychic blindness, 161
    short-term memory, 162
    temporal lobe deficit, 160
Homeostasis, and cannabis use, 394
Hyperalgesia, effects of THC on, 199
Hypothermia, 176

I

Idiosyncratic reactions, 348
Inhibition, *see* Hippocampus, inhibition
Interference and hippocampal lesions, 162
Internal clock, *see also* Memory, Time perception
  marijuana effects on, 159, 196, 202
Interresponse time (IRT), 203-204
Intrusion errors, 95-96, 159, 161

J

Jackson personality research form, 95

K

Kluver-Bucy syndrome, 161
Koh's block design test, 107
Korsakoff syndrome, 160

L

Latent learning, 167, 213
Leary, T., 42
Legalization of marijuana, issues,
  aesthetic, 25
  biological, 25, 26-39
  social, 25
LeDain commission, 2-3, 14, 18, 19, 121, 123, 125, 145, 224, 359-361
Limbic system, effects of cannabinoids on, 150-151, 160
Limited hold (LH), 203
Lysergic acid (LSD)
  cross-tolerance with marijuana, 27
  effects on nonspatial single alternation, 195-197

M

MacQuarrie test of mechanical ability, 33
Marijuana, *see also* Cannabinoids, Tetrahydrocannabinol
  adverse reactions to, *see* specific conditions
    determinants of, 278
    general, 32-33, 278-279
    psychopathology, 34, 293-294
    unusual experiences, 17-18
  alcohol and, *see* Alcohol
  analysis of, 47
  areas of investigation, 3
  clinical research model, 6-8
  demographic variables describing use, 2
  dose response relationships, *see also* specific conditions
    comparison with LSD, 26-27, 195-197
    conjunctival injection, 60
    Cornell medical index, 53, 64
    drug correlation scale, 64
    goal directed serial alternation, 29
    mood, 26
    neuropsychological test battery, 140-141
    pursuit meter, 56-58
    scaling of drug effects, 26
    subjective reactions, 64
  drugs and
    correlation scale, 53
    use of with, 274-295, 305-316, *see also* Escalation
  half life, 13, 37

Subject Index

intoxication with
  environmental influences, 250-254
  expectancy, 16
  history of use, 235
  potency, 234
  set and setting, 240-242, 250-252
inventory, self-reporting, 9
neurophysiological actions, 129
peak effect, 54
physiological changes, 26-27, see also specific conditions
puff inspiration, determination of, 48
reinforcement for use, 17
social dose, 260, 262
socially relevant dose, 145
Marijuana research programs
  driving, planning of
    course, 364-366
    tasks, course, 365
  liability insurance, 19-20
  physiological measures, 364, 368, 371-372, 380-386
    procedures, course and city streets, 367-371
    screening procedures, 362
    standardizing dosage, 363
    volunteer criteria, 362
  initiation
    acknowledgment and certificate form, 5-6
    consent form, 5
    human experimentation committee, 5
    release form, 5
    university endorsement, 4-5
  logistics
    rating scale, intoxication, 14
    screening procedures, 10
    smoking procedure, 13
    standardizing dosage, 12
    subjective evaluation of effects, 16-19
    volunteer criteria, 10
  methodological problems in, see also Aggression
    dependent variables, choice of, 8
    driving, 20-22
    motivational variables, 66-67, 69, 71
    pharmacology, 7
    set and setting, 7
    smoking procedure, 48-49, 54, 245

    standardizing dosage, 12, 47, 363
    purpose of memory research, 74-75
Marijuana users
  "Becoming a Marijuana User," 234
  chronic, effect on
    academic achievement, 116
    approaches to study, 222-230
    attention, components of, 113-114
    intellectual functioning, 223
    organicity, 34
    psychic dependence, 38
    physical dependence, 38, 223
    psychopathology, 34
    psychomotor performance, 124, 223
    sleep, 236
  chronic versus naive
    clinical studies of, 115-116
    general differences, 28, 46, 104-108
    pharmacological differences in reaction to marijuana, 236
    psychomotor performance in, 236-237
    subjective responses to marijuana and placebo, 237-240
    tolerance, 28
  personality characteristics of, 293-294
Maze behavior, effects of marijuana on, 197-198
Memory
  assessment
    Atkinson-Shiffrin model of, 191-192
    Benton sentence repetition, 131
    category clustering, 97
    delayed matching, 193-194
    digit span, 78
    distractor paradigm, 89, 132
    free recall, 78-83
    memory monitoring, 99
    memory scanning, 78-79
    narrative recall, 28-29, 91, 109
    nonspatial single alternation, 195
    oddity problem, 194
    passive avoidance, 194
    picture recognition, 131
    reaction time, 79
    retrieval paradigm, 97
    serial position curve, 82
    spontaneous alternation, 198
    availability versus assessibility, 97
  components of

conceptual store, 76-77
event knowledge store, 76-77
long term storage, 76-77, 191-192
sensory register, 76-77, 147, 191-192
short term store, 76-77, 191-192
consciousness and, 79
control processes, 77
directions for research on marijuana, 97
dual trace notion of, 78
effect of marijuana on
  Atkinson-Shiffrin model of, 82, 192-193
  Brown-Peterson task, 89, 167
  chronological memory, 159
  compensation, 160
  confabulation, 160
  decay, 193
  delayed matching, 194-195
  delayed recall, 84-85, 92-93
  delayed recognition, 84, 92-93, 109
  digit recall, 110
  distractor paradigm, 89, 167
  goal directed serial alternation, 29
  immediate memory, 27-28, 32, 95
  interference, 147-148, 193
  Korsakoff-like deficit, 160
  memory scanning, 79-81
  and motivation, 248
  narrative material, 28-29, 91, 109
  nonspatial single alternation, 195
  nonverbal memory, 98
  oddity performance, 194
  primacy effect, 84-85, 88, 193
  recall, 81, 83-85, 257
  recency effects, 84-85, 193
  recognition, 257
  retrieval, 96
  serial position curve, 87-88, 93, 192-193
  short term memory, 81
  spontaneous alternation, 198
  storage versus retrieval, 83-85, 108-109, 147
  temporal distintegration, 29
encoding, 77
event knowledge partition, 77
memory set, 78-79
short term memory, 76-79
short term versus long term memory, 191-192
rehersal buffer, 77
serial position curve, 81-83, 193, *see also* Marijuana memory
unitary versus dualistic conceptions, 190
Miller, L. L., 32
"Mind expansion," 40
Motivation, 95, 233, 243-250, *see also* Amotivational syndrome
Mystical terminology, 39

N

Narcotic addiction, and marijuana use, 305-310
National Commission on Marijuana and Drug Abuse, 2, 224
Neural model, for marijuana and behavior, 151-152
Neuroendocrine effects of marijuana on,
  ACTH, 177
  corticosterone uptake, 177
Neurological impairment from marijuana, 232
Neuropsychological test battery, description of, 131-132, 135-140
Nonrehearsal buffer, 89

P

Panic anxiety reaction, 279-281
Paranoia, 67
Paresthesia, from marijuana, 158
Persistance, and drug use, 311-312
Placebo reaction, 65-66, 378
Polygenetic theory, *see* Escalation
Potency, variability of in cannabis, 318
Problem solving, as affected by marijuana, 91
Propranolol, 28-29
Psychic dependence, 38
Psychiatric illness, 266-299
  correlation with, 289-292, 295, 296
    versus causation, 277
  data interpretation, 276
  definitions, problems with, 267-269
  diagnostics, problems with, 269-272
  experimental methods, 274-275
  intercurrent, 285-287
  psychodynamic theory, 267
  research limitations, 272-274
Psychiatric questions, descriptive terms, 267, 268

Subject Index

Psychomotor performance, *see also* specific tasks
assessment
foot tapping, 132
grooved pegboard, 32
Halstead finger tapping test, 132
Halstead tactual performance test, 131
Klove grooved steadiness test, 132
Klove maze coordination, 132
Klove static steadiness, 132
pursuit meter, 49-50
factors influencing effects of marijuana,
inability to concentrate, 67
lack of coordination, 67-68
loss of motivation, 66-67
Pulse rate, 26
Pursuit meter, 28, 49, 56-59, 112
description of, 49-50, 66
Pursuit rotor, 112, 257

R

Randomized block design, 54
Reaction time, 46, 107, 108
"Recreational drug," 40
"Reefer madness," 228
Rehearsal, 77, 82, 86-90, 192-193
Respiration, 143
Retrograde amnesia, 161
Rhinopharyngitis, 35

S

Safety, effects of marijuana on, 70-71
Salivary flow, 129
Schizophrenia, 36, 272
Scientific terminology, 39
Scopolamine, *see also* Cannabinoids, comparison with anticholinergics and hippocampectomy
effects on nonspatial single alternation, 195-197
Seashort tonal memory test, 131
Sedative-hypnotics, and marijuana use, 309
Sensory modality differences, 145
Setting, 53, 234, *see also* Marijuana, intoxication, Marijuana research, methodological problems
Serial position curve, *see* Memory, assessment
Sex differences, 135, 145

Simulated driving, 108, *see also* Driving performance
effects of marijuana and alcohol, 32
Sleep, 128
Sociogenic drugs, 328
Sociopathy, 271
Species generality, 190
Speech, effects of marijuana on, 28, 158
Spontaneous alternation, 198
State dependent learning, 92, 94, 96-98, 110-111, 169-170, 206-212
asymmetrical, 92, 98, 169-170, 208-209, 211-212
definition, 92
drug discrimination paradigm, 169-170, 206, 207, 209-211
task parameters, 208-209
transfer paradigms, 169-170, 206-209
symmetrical, 98, 169-170, 208-209, 211-212
Static equilibrium, 46, 52, 53
Sternberg memory scan paradigm, 78
Stress and autonomic arousal, 391
Stroop test, description of, 52
Styles of drug use, 314
Subcortical mediation, and marijuana, 150
Subculture, and drug use, 306
Subjective drug effects questionnaire, 238

T

Tachycardia
marijuana induced, 26-27, 148
stress and, 391
Tapping speed, 46
Tart, C. T., 73
Telemetry, 364
Temporal disintegration, *see* Time perception
Temporal integration inventory, 29
Temporal lobe patients, 161, *see also* Hippocampus
Tetrahydrocannabinol (THC), *see also* Cannabinoids, Marijuana
amount available in marijuana cigarette, 55
behavioral effects in animals
active avoidance, 199-200
exploration, 198
fear, 200-201
freezing, 201

maze behavior, 98
nonspatial single alternation, 151
passive avoidance, 199-200
state dependent learning, 169-170, 206-212
distribution in monkey brain, 151, 172
interation with propranolol, 24, 28
metabolites of, 150
pharmacology of
 blood pressure, 26
 body temperature, 26
 chemosis, 27
 conjunctival injection, 60
 corticosterone uptake, 172
 EEG, 34
 muscular weakness, 27
 tachycardia, 27, 148
time perception, effects on,
 drl schedules, 31
 goal directed serial alternation, 159
 temporal disintegration, 159
 time production, 31
Time perception
 correlation with physiological factors, 206
 effect of marijuana on
  attention and, 111
  drl schedules, 31, 170, 203-205, 243-244
  goal directed serial alternation, 91, 106
  internal clock, 196, 202
  motivation and, 246-247
  nonspatial single alternation, 195-196
  overestimation, 30
  time discrimination, 204-205
  time estimation, 203
  time production, 30, 203
  time reproduction, 203
  time tags, 202
  underestimation, 30
 methods of measurement, 203
 relationship to memory, 202-203, 205-206
Thought processes, effects of marijuana on, 158-159
Titration, of marijuana intake, 254-261
Tolerance
 behavioral versus physical, 323
 compensatory behavior, 249
 effects of marijuana on
  in animals, 36, 227
  to behavioral effects, 223-225
  to euphoric effects, 37
  in man, 36, 224, 291
  metabolic tolerance, 37
  to pharmacological effects, 223-225
  "reverse" tolerance, 36
  to subjective effects, 225
 "reverse" tolerance, 37
 species differences, 323
 tolerance-disillusionment model of, 324
Trail making test, 112, 115, 131

W

Witkin embedded figures test, 105
Wobble board, 52, 62